CONTENTS

W9-ATL-277

PREFACE

Computer technology and the speed with which it accomplishes work has revolutionized practice management in medical offices. Tasks such as billing and practice reporting that took days to perform in the past can now be completed in a few hours. Important, cost-saving benefits occur when a medical office begins to use a computer for routine office tasks.

For example, as a medical office assistant, you can dedicate your attention to patients instead of laboring over procedure codes and mathematical calculations; mistakes in patient accounts will diminish when the human element is reduced; and the practice's financial status will be instantly determinable at all times.

The purpose of **The Medical Manager**® Student Edition is to familiarize you with computerized account management and to help you develop the confidence and skills necessary to become a successful user of medical account management software. In this interest, specially designed practice exercises, located throughout the text, provide you with opportunities to apply what you have learned in each unit, and build your skills as you progress through the course.

After completion of this course, you should be able to go into any medical office and perform computerized account management duties within a short period of time, even when the software is different from the version you will use in this course. Understanding the capabilities of **The Medical Manager** and the relationship of the software to record keeping in a medical office empowers you to develop creative solutions to financial (as well as organizational) dilemmas. This not only helps you to increase profitability for your medical office or organization but also to gain respect from your colleagues and other medical office professionals.

ORGANIZATION OF THE UNITS

This edition of **The Medical Manager** follows patients from their first visit through insurance billing for services rendered. Unit 1, *Using The Medical Manager*, begins with the basics of the flow of information in the medical office and how to start using **The Medical Manager**. Unit 2, *Building Your Patient File*, teaches you how to enter new patient data including guarantor and insurance information. Based on the patients entered data in Unit 2, Unit 3, *Posting Your Entries*, instructs how to post entries for services provided. Unit 4, *Editing Prior Entries*, teaches the important skill of editing entries, and Unit 5, *Office Management/Appointment Scheduling*, introduces appointment scheduling and information on hospital rounds and procedure codes. Unit 6, *Practice Management*, introduces insurance billing, and Unit 7, *Report Generation*, explains the various reports available through **The Medical Manager**. Unit 8, *Advanced Functions*, provides you with the basics of the advanced functions of **The Medical Manager**, including unique payment, aging reports, and the display patient data feature. Unit 9, *Today's Medical Office*, includes information on the Health Insurance Portability and Accountability Act (HIPAA), including electronic data interchange, electronic medical records, and protecting patient privacy.

LEARNING MADE EASY

Whether you are taking your first medical office course or are continuing your training, **The Medical Manager** Student Edition is designed to make learning simple and straightforward. Each unit is meant to build, step-by-step on the knowledge gained in the previous one while, at the same time, introduce concepts that will be covered in the next unit. The following features contribute to making the time you spend in this course enjoyable, as well as productive:

◆ *Learning Outcomes*, which tell you what you can expect to know by the time you finish the unit, are listed at the beginning of every unit. You should review these sections when you have finished each unit to check your comprehension of the topics covered.

◆ *Unit Summaries* have been added to the end of each unit. These summaries provide you with information on the important concepts of the chapter. You can use these as review tools.

◆ Knowledge about medical offices and medical office procedures is combined with information about computers, so you will learn the *why* of an operation as well as the *how*.

◆ Examples of *actual medical forms* are provided to simulate actual office procedures using the type of source documents typically used in the medical office.

◆ *Notes in the margins* emphasize important points in the text.

◆ Carefully developed exercises help you evaluate what you have learned:
  (1) *Applying Your Knowledge* asks you to perform computer operations.
  (2) *Testing Your Knowledge* asks you to answer questions about the material in the units.
  (3) *Concepts Evaluations*, offered after Units 4 and 9, test your understanding of the concepts underlying the data entry principles.
  (4) At the end of Unit 2, a *Comprehensive Entry Exercise* is provided to ensure you grasp the basics of **The Medical Manager** before moving on to more complex tasks.
  (5) The end of Unit 8 provides a *Comprehensive Evaluation*. This evaluation offers an opportunity to complete a data entry exercise that encompasses all of the content covered within the first 8 units.

◆ *Step-by-step instructions* guide you through each computer application, so you never have to worry about having advanced computer knowledge.

◆ *Sample computer screens* in the text match the screens you see on your computer, so you can be sure that your work is correct.

◆ A detailed *Glossary* is included at the back of this book to provide you with easy access to any work meanings that are new to you.

◆ The principles and procedures taught via **The Medical Manager** courseware are similar to other account management software, so you should be able to transfer your knowledge to any account management system with ease.

◆ Comb-binding allows this book to lie flat for ease of data entry.

◆ Includes a unit that discusses changes occurring in the health care industry and the future of medical office computerization.

◆ A special file included on the Student Disk allows you to print health insurance claim information on actual CMS-1500 forms.

◆ Directions clearly separate step-by-step instructions from conceptual material.

◆ A troubleshooting section is included in the Instructor's Manual to help your instructor quickly resolve problems that may arise while using the software.

CHANGES IN THIS EDITION

◆ *Version 10 for Windows®* This edition uses Version 10 of **The Medical Manager** software. This version is current with the version that you will likely encounter when you take a job at an office that uses **The Medical Manager.** Accordingly new text and art have been added to reflect this new version.

◆ NEW! A *Quick Reference Guide* keyboard template has been included in this edition. This easily removed guide fits neatly on your keyboard. It should be used to easily locate and navigate your way through **The Medical Manager**.

◆ Unit 1, *Using **The Medical Manager***, represents the combination of Version 9.20 Unit 1 *Today's **Medical Manager***, and Unit 2, *Using the **Medical Manager***. This allows the "basics" to appear all in one chapter.

◆ Version 9.20 Unit 4, *Posting Your Entries*, has been broken down into two separate units, Unit 3, *Posting Your Entries* and Unit 4, *Editing Your Entries*. This organizational change emphasizes the importance of the editing functions of **The Medical Manager**.

◆ *Patient Information Form* has been revamped so that the patient information appears before the guarantor's name to simulate more closely what the student may see in the medical office.

◆ Exercises have been rearranged so they are introduced from "simple entry to more complex."

◆ Additional exercises have been added to this edition.

◆ A *workbook* is available with its own data disk, offering additional exercises for reinforcement of skills covered in the book.

◆ Procedure and diagnoses codes have been updated to reflect the current standards in use in the health care industry.

SUPPLEMENTARY ITEMS

The Medical Manager *Student Edition Version 10 for Windows Educational Software Site License*
ISBN # 1-4018-4996-2
This is the software that must be installed on every student's computer in order for the student data disks to run.

*Workbook to Accompany **The Medical Manager** Student Edition Version 10 for Windows.*
ISBN # 1-4018-2575-3

◆ Includes its own data disk in the back of the book.

◆ Offers students additional exercises to reinforce skills taught in the
   The Medical Manager *Student Edition Version 10 for Windows.*

*Instructor's Manual to Accompany **The Medical Manager** Student Edition Version 10 for Windows.*
ISBN # 1-4018-2576-1
FREE to the instructor, this manual includes

◆ learning outcomes, key concepts, teaching recommendations, and suggestions on enhancing the class discussion.

◆ explanations of the concepts and data entry key strokes tested in the *Applying Your Knowledge, Comprehensive Exercise,* and *Comprehensive Evaluation* exercises.

- answers to the *Testing Your Knowledge* and *Concept Evaluations*.
- two comprehensive tests and a comprehensive set of exercises that enable instructors to evaluate student progress in learning to use **The Medical Manager** software.
- appendices covering installation instructions, error reporting and recovery, data structures, file backup and restoration, printing solutions and configurations, additional instructor resources, including transparency masters of medical forms, screens, and terminology, and frequently asked questions.
- troubleshooting guide and Delmar Learning's Technical Support FAQs.
- an *Instructor CD-ROM* packaged with the Instructor's Manual, that includes all of the content of the paper Instructor Manual, a link to **The Medical Manager** Resource Center, correctly completed exercises, and a tutorial that walks you through the features of **The Medical Manager** Student Edition.

The Medical Manager Student Edition Version 10 for Windows Lab Pack
ISBN # 1-4018-2577-X

Workbook to Accompany **The Medical Manager** *Student Edition Version 10 for Windows Lab Pack*
ISBN # 1-4018-2579-6
These packs include replacement data disks if a student disk is lost or damaged.

INSTALLATION REQUIREMENTS

The Medical Manager® software programs will reside on and run from the hard drive of the computer. The specific installation requirements are, as follows:
- A computer with an Intel®-compatible processor (486 or higher)
    - A 486 processor MUST have a DX designation (including a math coprocessor; not an SX designation), or
    - A 586 (Pentium) processor
- 300M of hard drive space
- At least 16MB of RAM
- 1.4-MB floppy disk drive
- Windows® 98 or newer

A FEW WORDS OF ADVICE

As is the case with paper files and records, the electronic patient record used in a computerized medical practice management system, such as **The Medical Manager**, is only as reliable as the data entered into it by its users. Therefore, it is very important that proper measures be taken to ensure not only that the data entered is accurate but that this data is backed-up with sufficient frequency as to guarantee its continued availability to the practice. In **The Medical Manager** Student Edition, a deliberate effort has been made to assist students in developing patterns of accurate and responsible procedures for using **The Medical Manager** software. Of course, the objective of this effort is to ensure that students take this conscientious behavior with them into the environment in which they will interact with real patients.

Remember that any time you begin learning a new computer program, it is normal that you experience a certain amount of frustration. Take your time and, if at all possible, read through the material before the actual class session. It is also helpful to remember that computers perform correctly only when they are given the correct instructions. When you give an instruction the computer does not understand, it will give you something you do not want or nothing at all. When you make a mistake entering information (such as a patient's name or number, procedure or diagnosis code, or any of the other items in the application problems), the computer will not know you made a mistake and will give you an answer based on your input, regardless of whether it is correct or not. Although you may not recognize an error when you make it, incorrect information will, in all probability, show up as future problems. The computer waits for you, the user, to provide an exact instruction that it understands, and then performs that operation accordingly. Therefore, when an error occurs, there is a very large possibility that it is simply due to user error. The best way to avoid this frustration is not only to read instructions carefully but also stop and ask for assistance if you feel you have entered the correct information but are not getting a correct response.

CONCLUSION

The health care financing industry is undergoing a great change, and the United States Congress can be expected to legislate many important new guidelines over the next several years. As physicians attempt to stay abreast of these guidelines and other financial issues that affect their profitability, medical financial management software will become an even more important tool for use in managing their medical offices. As this change becomes evident, personnel skilled at using **The Medical Manager** and programs like it will be in even greater demand. After completing this course, you will feel confident in your knowledge of medical billing, as well as in the fact that, with this much respected skill, your services will be highly marketable in the medical community.

ABOUT THE AUTHOR

Richard Gartee is Director of Design Strategy at Medical Manager Research & Development, Inc., the company that authors **The Medical Manager** software. He serves as part of **The Medical Manager** program design team. He also developed the original dealer and end-user training programs under which more than 200 dealerships and 24,000 medical offices have been trained.

Richard Gartee is one of the original coauthors, and editor of **The Medical Manager** documentation, as well as numerous specialized training guides. He designs new modules of **The Medical Manager** software. He serves as Medical Manager Research & Development, Inc.'s liaison to IBM, Blue Cross/Blue Shield, and other companies in the computer industry as well as the U.S. Department of Commerce International Trade Administration and various universities. He is listed in Who's Who in America and Who's Who in the Computer Industry.

A FEW WORDS OF ACKNOWLEDGMENT

The author would like to extend special thanks to Ruby Moore who worked diligently to develop and test this new version of **The Medical Manager** Student Edition. Additionally, reviewers are solicited to ready the author's first efforts and make suggestions based on the content and their experience with students; the author then incorporated their suggestions into the final book. The insights and recommendations of all involved have helped make this a better product. Special thanks to all whom offered feedback throughout the revision planning for the book.

Reviewers for version 10 of The Medical Manager Student Edition

Aimee Burnham
BS
Director of Education
Branford Hall Career Institute
Springfield, MA

Cindi Brassington
MS, CMA
Assistant Professor of Allied Health
Quinebaug Valley Community College
Danielson, CT

Pamela DeNobile
CMA, CCS-P, CPC
Compliance Coordinator
Pinnacle Medical Group
Bradenton, FL

Pamela Fleming
RN, MPA, CMA, CPC
Associate Professor/Program Coordinator
Quinsigamond CC
Worcester, MA

Virginia Hannan
Adjunct Faculty
Bryant & Stratton Institute
Williamsville, NY

Kris Hardy
CMA, CDF
Medical Assistant, Medical Coder/Biller Program Director
Brevard Community College
Melbourne, FL

Arlene Miller
AS
Instructor
Sarasota County Technical Institute
Sarasota, FL

U N I T 1

Using The Medical Manager

LEARNING OUTCOMES

After completing this unit, you should be able to:

◆ Describe the flow of information in a medical office.

◆ Explain why the appointment schedule is important.

◆ Explain patient eligibility.

◆ Discuss the function of an encounter form.

◆ Describe three methods for collecting insurance payments.

◆ Discuss several types of health insurance coverage.

◆ Name and describe three types of health insurance plans.

◆ Discuss managed care insurance coverage.

◆ Discuss the role of computers in today's medical office.

◆ Describe the purpose of **The Medical Manager** software.

◆ Start **The Medical Manager** system.

◆ Input and process data.

◆ Print reports from support files.

◆ Back up the daily data files.

◆ Navigate effectively through **The Medical Manager** software.

Medical offices may be privately owned and operated by one or more physicians or by a for-profit company that employs physicians. Local, state, or federal governments may also establish them. Usually, the government-controlled medical offices are larger than private practices and employ many more physicians. Often, they serve "uncompensated care" patients who are unable to pay and are located in a metropolitan areas or in a wing of a city- or state-owned hospital.

In any case, it is important to note that most medical offices operate in a similar manner: All daily activities are built around the treatment of patients. Supplemental activities such as appointment scheduling, account billing, and financial management are based on patient treatments.

Note: The term "medical assistant" is used frequently throughout the Student Edition. The author realizes that, in some cases, it would be more appropriate to use a different title such as certified medical assistant, clinician, or nurse. However, "medical assistant" is used as a general term to indicate any member of a medical office's personnel.

FLOW OF INFORMATION IN A MEDICAL OFFICE

Information flows in a circle in a medical office. Communication usually starts with an appointment scheduled between the medical assistant and the patient, and it ends with the patient making arrangements with the medical assistant for payment or for another appointment. The following discussion illustrates the flow of information and highlights several points of communication that are typical to most medical offices. As you read, refer to the Flow of Information chart shown in Figure 1-1.

Figure 1-1 Flow of Information in a Medical Office

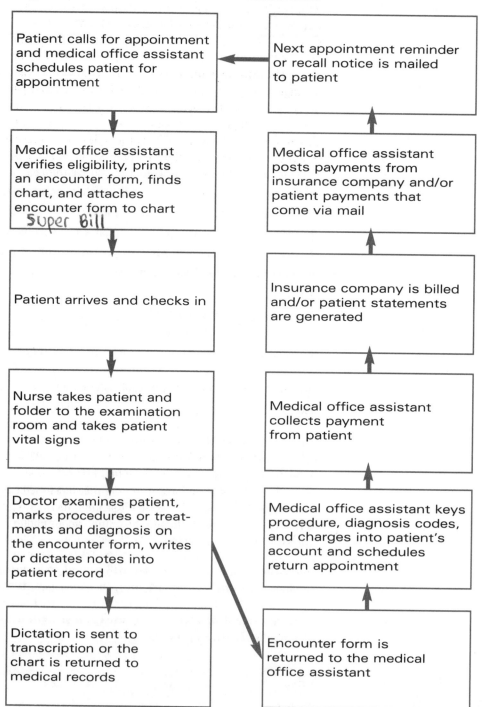

Patient calls for appointment and medical office assistant schedules patient for appointment

Medical office assistant verifies eligibility, prints an encounter form, finds chart, and attaches encounter form to chart
Super Bill

Patient arrives and checks in

Nurse takes patient and folder to the examination room and takes patient vital signs

Doctor examines patient, marks procedures or treatments and diagnosis on the encounter form, writes or dictates notes into patient record

Dictation is sent to transcription or the chart is returned to medical records

Next appointment reminder or recall notice is mailed to patient

Medical office assistant posts payments from insurance company and/or patient payments that come via mail

Insurance company is billed and/or patient statements are generated

Medical office assistant collects payment from patient

Medical office assistant keys procedure, diagnosis codes, and charges into patient's account and schedules return appointment

Encounter form is returned to the medical office assistant

Appointment Scheduling

Efficient operation of the medical office depends on correct scheduling of appointments, an activity requiring clear thinking and good judgment. Whether appointments are scheduled manually in a daily appointment book or by computer using **The Medical Manager** software, the entire staff depends on the smooth flow of patient traffic in order to maintain a workable schedule. Appointments must be made so they allow sufficient time for each patient's medical condition to be treated thoroughly, yet without wasteful time gaps.

Scheduling of appointments is based on the severity of each patient's medical condition and the available time slots. This responsibility requires that you ask questions about each patient's complaint to determine whether the symptoms are severe enough for an immediate appointment. If the patient's call is urgent, you must make time during the day for the patient to see the physician. For less urgent conditions, you will suggest available times and work with the patient to schedule a convenient appointment.

Appointments for patients and other visitors are recorded in an appointment book or in **The Medical Manager** system. Compare Figures 1-2 and 1-3. With either arrangement, the appointment schedule serves as the daily planning guide by showing (1) the names of all patients to be seen each day, (2) the time of each patient's appointment, (3) each patient's telephone number, and (4) a brief reason for the visit. From this information, the doctors and other office personnel determine approximately how much time is needed for their portion of the patient's treatment and which medical instruments and supplies will be required for the examination. One advantage of a computerized appointment scheduling system is that time slots can be designated for desired types of appointments, as shown in Figure 1-3.

Appointments are scheduled for varying amounts of time based on the patient's symptoms and on the particular medical specialty, but most practices develop a formula for scheduling that will help you determine the amount of time needed for each patient. The table below shows a typical scheduling formula for an internal medicine practice.

Scheduling Formula for Internal Medicine Practice

New patients	30 minutes
Patients for consultation	45 minutes
Patients requiring complete physical examination	45 minutes
All other patients (minor illnesses, routine checkups)	15 minutes

Appointments are scheduled manually in a daily appointment book or electronically in **The Medical Manager** system's Appointment Scheduler. With an appointment book, you will search for empty slots, or "holes" in the schedule by flipping through each page until you find an appropriate opening. With a computerized system such as **The Medical Manager** software, you can key in information about the appointment, and the computer will search for an appointment opening.

Medical office appointment books are divided by days of the week, usually with each day separated into 15-minute segments. As many segments as necessary are blocked out in order to provide for each examination. For example, a new patient visit would use two 15-minute segments, as shown in Figure 1-3. Look for 'Deborah Evans' as an example.

When a patient requests an appointment, ask for a specific description of the symptoms. If, in your judgment, the complaint is serious enough to justify an immediate examination, look through the day's schedule for the first vacant time period. If no openings exist, find a time when the patient can be "worked in."

Offer patients one or two alternative times and schedule the appointment according to their wishes. To increase efficiency, it is a good idea to ask new patients to arrive

Figure 1-2 Sample Appointment Book Page from a Group Practice

	Dr. Monroe / June 6	Dr. Simpson / June 6	Dr. Carrington / June 6
8 00/15/30/45	Hospital / Rounds	Hospital / Rounds	Hospital / Rounds
9 00/15/30/45	Mary Radno / New Pat / 296-4110 — Seldon Larson / New Pat / 741-6021	Susan Miles / New Pat / 296-8140 — James Lewis / New Pat / 763-6011	Allison Rogers
10 00/15/30/45	Sandy Dearing / Flu / 741-4181 — Ray Buck / Kidney Problem — Nancy Dripdale / Sinuses / 741-6222 — Rose Hillel / Chest Pain / 763-2499	Manley Johnson / New Pat / 296-4192 — Randy Agnew / Athlete's Foot / 466-3249 — Denise Lawler / Hernia Recheck / 296-7102	Celina Sellers / New Pat / 296-3109 — Betsy Brunfeld / New Pat / 763-2069
11 00/15/30/45	John Thomas / Warts / 763-2026 — Mike Ward / Ear Draining / 763-7104	Nelson Brunner / Diarrhea / 296-8329 — Ralph Bater / Sore Throat / 466-1000 — Sammy Dale / Headaches / 763-2190 — Denny Samuelson / Reme Stitch / 924-1904	Kimberly Russell / New Pat / 466-0102
12 00/15/30/45	Lunch	Lunch	Lunch
1 00/15/30/45	James Snowden / Bruised Back / 296-5290 — Salvador Lee / Stomach Pain / 466-6201 — Tina Maybrey / Menstrual Pain / 296-4996	Deborah Helion / Pain in Leg / 763-2943	Sam Gaines / Preg. Recheck / 466-9843 — Linda Long / Malig. Recheck / 296-2314 — Danielle Lacy / Preg. Recheck / 296-7142 — Claine Laudeback / Preg. Recheck / 296-1012
2 00/15/30/45	Joseph Feldon / Diabetes Check / 466-2964	Wallace Langley / Boil on Neck / 466-1904 — Anne Darrell / CPQ / 296-1972	Wanda Darrell / Preg. Recheck / 763-2411 — Gilley Lucy / Malig. Recheck / 741-0210 — Helen Lloyd / Preg. Recheck / 296-7102
3 00/15/30/45	Martha Reynolds / Blood Pressure / 296-8104	Mandy Hall / CPQ / 466-3579	Mr. & Mrs. Colin Womach / Preg. Consult / 466-1063
4 00/15/30/45	Eva Rouse / Back Pain / 466-3101 — Andrew Chen / CPQ / 466-3101	Robert Prentice / CPQ / 296-7234	Mr. & Mrs. Mel Brownley / Preg. Consult / 462-1115 — Nadine Wells / Preg. Consult / 296-3102
5 00/15/30/45	Matthew Hayes / Consult / 763-2104	Lorie Pierce / Pierce & Weinstein Accountants (Her Office)	Anita Ziegler, President American Heart Association
6 00/15/30/45	Partner's Meeting — Dr. Monroe, Simpson, Carrington	Partner's Meeting — Dr. Monroe, Simpson, Carrington	Partner's Meeting — Dr. Monroe, Simpson, Carrington
7 00/15/30/45			
8 00/15/30/45			

Overbooking refers to double scheduling.

at the office at least 15 minutes ahead of their scheduled appointment time so they can complete forms needed to open a financial account and set up clinical records.

Medical offices sometimes *overbook* their patients. This means they schedule more patients than the physician can see during a reasonable amount of time. Overbooking

Figure 1-3 Sample Appointment Screen from **The Medical Manager** (Multi-Doctor view)

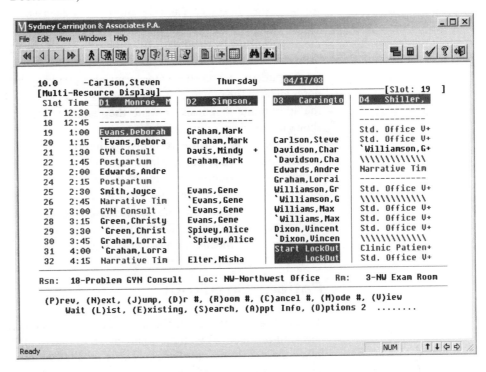

is not recommended because it often delays the schedule and frustrates the patients, physician, and staff. Avoid overbooking unless an emergency patient or a very sick patient must see the doctor immediately. Many physicians like to schedule a 30-minute break once or twice a day to compensate for delays. These time slots may be blocked so that no appointments may be scheduled during these time periods.

Emergency patients receive top priority.

An emergency patient should receive top priority and should be allowed to see the physician immediately, even though the emergency may delay other patients. When emergencies occur, you should call all patients who may be affected by the delay and offer to reschedule their appointments for another time. Advise patients already in the office of the emergency and give them the option of waiting for the physician or rescheduling their appointments.

Patient Eligibility

To ensure that the patient's insurance is in effect or that the patient will be covered for particular services that are scheduled to be performed, the practice often needs to verify the patient's insurance eligibility with the insurance company. This can be done either by phone or by using a computerized system such as **The Medical Manager**. Eligibility is particularly important to managed care practices. The ability for a primary care physician to ensure that a patient is on his/her patient roster is very valuable in the day-to-day operation of the practice. Using software such as **The Medical Manager's** automated insurance eligibility verification (AEV) system allows the practice to submit electronically a list of patients who are scheduled for the following day and receive verification of the eligibility overnight as opposed to doing it on a patient-by-patient basis on the day of the appointment. Alternatively, some practices verify the patient's eligibility at the time the appointment is scheduled. This is typically done in specialty practices to ensure that the insurance company will cover procedures before appointment time is booked.

Encounter Forms

An encounter form serves as a communication device between the doctor and the front office. An encounter form is a printed list of the most common procedures and treatments performed by the doctor. By making a checkmark following each examination, the doctor uses the encounter form to indicate the procedure or treatment performed for the patient. Some encounter forms also provide a list of the most common diagnoses given in the practice. If this is the case, the doctor will also place a checkmark by the appropriate diagnosis or write the diagnosis in the space provided. Figure 1-4 shows a typical encounter form.

The encounter form is returned to the front desk after each examination so the medical assistant can transfer information from it to the patient's account. As a bookkeeping tool, encounter forms monitor the accounting of patients seen during the day. At the end of the day, the number of encounter forms should match the number of patients seen that day; and the number of charge entries posted should equal the total of all procedures marked. Encounter forms are printed in numerical order, and any missing number means charges were not posted or an encounter form was voided.

Patient Checkout

A medical assistant posts charges and payments to each patient's account during the checkout process. When patients are asked to return for additional treatment or for a follow-up visit, the doctor indicates a return interval on the encounter form, and the front desk assistant makes the appointment, usually before the patient leaves the office. When appointments are made far in advance, the patients' names are placed in a recall file so that they may be reminded as the appointment date approaches.

Methods for Collecting Payment

Three methods for collecting payments in a medical office follow:

1. *Patient pays in full and files an insurance claim.* Some medical offices require patients to pay the full amount of their bill at the time of the visit. These offices provide the patient with an encounter form that includes the information required in order to file a claim with an insurance plan. The patient then staples the encounter form to a claim form (the plan normally provides the practice with the necessary forms to give to the patient) and mails it to the insurance claim center. The patient is then reimbursed by the insurance plan at a later date.

2. *Patient pays, but the medical office files the claim form.* Some medical offices file claims for patients. In this case, the patient may be required to pay at the time of the visit, and the insurance plan reimburses the patient. This idea is gaining in popularity because errors in billings are reduced, and physicians may be paid sooner for their services.

3. *Insurance plan pays medical office; the patient pays remainder.* Most medical offices file the insurance claims, accepting "assignment of benefits" for at least some of the insurance plans (Assignment of benefits is addressed in Unit 2). Payment is then sent directly to the doctor. When the insurance check arrives, the patient is responsible for any portion not covered by the insurance plan. In many cases, the patient due portion is calculated and collected at the time of the visit. For some plans, this portion is called the patient copay.

Figure 1-4 Sample Encounter Form

Sydney Carrington & Associates P.A.
34 Sycamore Street   Suite 300
Madison, CA 95653

Date: 01/10/2003

Voucher No.: 1059

Time: 10:00

Patient: Thomas Williams
Guarantor: Terry L. Williams

Patient No: 120.3
Doctor: 1 – J. Monroe

☐ CPT	DESCRIPTION	FEE
OFFICE/HOSPITAL CONSULTS		
☐ 99201	Office New:Focused Hx-Exam	_____
☐ 99202	Office New:Expanded Hx-Exam	_____
☐ 99211	Office Estb:Min/None Hx-Exa	_____
☒ 99212	Office Estb:Focused Hx-Exam	$30.00
☐ 99213	Office Estb:Expanded Hx-Exa	_____
☐ 99214	Office Estb:Detailed Hx-Exa	_____
☐ 99215	Office Estb:Comprhn Hx-Exam	_____
☐ 99221	Hosp. Initial:Comprh Hx-	_____
☐ 99223	Hosp.Ini:Comprh Hx-Exam/Hi	_____
☐ 99231	Hosp. Subsequent: S-Fwd	_____
☐ 99232	Hosp. Subsequent: Comprhn Hx	_____
☐ 99233	Hosp. Subsequent: Ex/Hi	_____
☐ 99238	Hospital Visit Discharge Ex	_____
☐ 99371	Telephone Consult - Simple	_____
☐ 99372	Telephone Consult - Intermed	_____
☐ 99373	Telephone Consult - Complex	_____
☐ 90843	Counseling - 25 minutes	_____
☐ 90844	Counseling - 50 minutes	_____
☐ 90865	Counseling - Special Interview	_____
IMMUNIZATIONS/INJECTIONS		
☐ 90585	BCG Vaccine	_____
☐ 90659	Influenza Virus Vaccine	_____
☐ 90701	Immunization-DTP	_____
☐ 90702	DT Vaccine	_____
☐ 90703	Tetanus Toxoids	_____
☐ 90732	Pneumococcal Vaccine	_____
☐ 90746	Hepatitis B Vaccine	_____
☐ 90749	Immunization; Unlisted	_____

☐ CPT	DESCRIPTION	FEE
LABORATORY/RADIOLOGY		
☐ 81000	Urinalysis	_____
☐ 81002	Urinalysis; Pregnancy Test	_____
☐ 82951	Glucose Tolerance Test	_____
☐ 84478	Triglycerides	_____
☐ 84550	Uric Acid: Blood Chemistry	_____
☐ 84830	Ovulation Test	_____
☐ 85014	Hematocrit	_____
☐ 85031	Hemogram, Complete Blood Wk	_____
☐ 86403	Particle Agglutination Test	_____
☐ 86485	Skin Test; Candida	_____
☐ 86580	TB Intradermal Test	_____
☐ 86585	TB Tine Test	_____
☐ 87070	Culture	_____
☐ 70190	X-Ray; Optic Foramina	_____
☐ 70210	X-Ray Sinuses Complete	_____
☐ 71010	Radiological Exam Ent Spine	_____
☐ 71020	X-Ray Chest Pa & Lat	_____
☐ 72050	X-Ray Spine, Cerv (4 views)	_____
☐ 72090	X-Ray Spine; Scoliosis Ex	_____
☐ 72110	Spine, lumbosacral; a/p & Lat	_____
☐ 73030	Shoulder-Comp, min w/ 2vws	_____
☐ 73070	Elbow, anteropost & later vws	_____
☐ 73120	X-Ray; Hand, 2 views	_____
☐ 73560	X-Ray, Knee, 1 or 2 views	_____
☐ 74022	X-Ray; Abdomen, Complete	_____
☐ 75552	Cardiac Magnetic Res Img	_____
☐ 76020	X-Ray; Bone Age Studies	_____
☐ 76088	Mammary Ductogram Complete	_____
☐ 78465	Myocardial Perfusion Img	_____

☐ CPT	DESCRIPTION	FEE
PROCEDURES/TESTS		
☐ 00452	Anesthesia for Rad Surgery	_____
☐ 11100	Skin Biopsy	_____
☐ 15852	Dressing Change	_____
☐ 29075	Cast Appl. - Lower Arm	_____
☐ 29530	Strapping of Knee	_____
☐ 29705	Removal/Revis of Cast w/Exa	_____
☐ 53670	Catheterization Incl. Suppl	_____
☐ 57452	Colposcopy	_____
☐ 57505	ECC	_____
☐ 69420	Myringotomy	_____
☐ 92081	Visual Field Examination	_____
☐ 92100	Serial Tonometry Exam	_____
☐ 92120	Tonography	_____
☐ 92552	Pure Tone Audiometry	_____
☐ 92567	Tympanometry	_____
☐ 93000	Electrocardiogram	_____
☐ 93015	Exercise Stress Test (ETT)	_____
☐ 93017	ETT Tracing Only	_____
☐ 93040	Electrocardiogram - Rhythm	_____
☐ 96100	Psychological Testing	_____
☐ 99000	Specimen Handling	_____
☐ 99058	Office Emergency Care	_____
☐ 99070	Surgical Tray - Misc.	_____
☐ 99080	Special Reports of Med Rec	_____
☐ 99195	Phlebotomy	_____
☐	_____	_____
☐	_____	_____
☐	_____	_____
☐	_____	_____

ICD-9 CODE DIAGNOSIS	
☐ 009.0	Ill-defined Intestinal Infect
☐ 133.2	Establish Baseline
☐ 174.9	Breast Cancer
☐ 185.0	Prostate Cancer
☐ 250	Diabetes Mellitus
☐ 272.4	Hyperlipidemia
☐ 282.5	Anemia - Sickle Trait
☐ 282.60	Anemia - Sickle Cell
☐ 285.9	Anemia, Unspecified
☐ 300.4	Neurotic Depression
☐ 340	Multiple Sclerosis
☐ 342.9	Hemiplegia - Unspecified
☐ 346.9	Migraine Headache
☐ 352.9	Cranial Neuralgia
☐ 354.0	Carpal Tunnel Syndrome
☐ 355.0	Sciatic Nerve Root Lesion
☐ 366.9	Cataract
☐ 386.0	Vertigo
☐ 401.1	Essential Hypertension
☐ 414.9	Ischemic Hearth Disease
☐ 428.0	Congestive Heart Failure

ICD-9 CODE DIAGNOSIS	
☐ 435.0	Basilar Artery Syndrome
☐ 440.0	Atherosclerosis
☐ 442.81	Carotid Artery
☐ 460.0	Common Cold
☐ 461.9	Acute Sinusitis
☐ 474.0	Tonsillitis
☐ 477.9	Hay Fever
☒ 487.0	Flu
☐ 496	Chronic Airway Obstruction
☐ 522	Low Red Blood Count
☐ 524.6	Temporo-Mandibular Jnt Synd
☐ 538.8	Stomach Pain
☐ 553.3	Hiatal Hernia
☐ 564.1	Spastic Colon
☐ 571.4	Chronic Hepatitis
☐ 571.5	Cirrhosis of Liver
☐ 573.3	Hepatitis
☐ 575.2	Obstruction of Gallbladder
☐ 648.2	Anemia - Compl. Pregnancy
☐ 715.90	Osteoarthritis - Unspec
☐ 721.3	Lumbar Osteo/Spondylarthrit

ICD-9 CODE DIAGNOSIS	
☐ 724.2	Pain: Lower Back
☐ 727.6	Rupture of Achilles Tendon
☐ 780.1	Hallucinations
☐ 780.3	Convulsions
☐ 780.5	Sleep Disturbances
☐ 783.0	Anorexia
☐ 783.1	Abnormal Weight Gain
☐ 783.2	Abnormal Weight Loss
☐ 830.6	Dislocated Hip
☐ 830.9	Dislocated Shoulder
☐ 841.2	Sprained Wrist
☐ 842.5	Sprained Ankle
☐ 891.2	Fractured Tibia
☐ 892.0	Fractured Fibula
☐ 919.5	Insect Bite, Nonvenomous
☐ 921.1	Contus Eyelid/Perioc Area
☐ v16.3	Fam. Hist of Breast Cancer
☐ v17.4	Fam. Hist of Cardiovasc Dis
☐ v20.2	Well Child
☐ v22.0	Pregnancy - First Normal
☐ v22.1	Pregnancy - Normal

Previous Balance	Today's Charges	Total Due	Amount Paid	New Balance

Follow Up

PRN _____ Weeks _____ Months _____ Units _____

Next Appointment Date: _____   Time: _____

I hereby authorize release of any information acquired in the course of examination or treatment and allow a photocopy of my signature to be used.

_____

INSURANCE PAYMENTS

Health care costs in the United States have skyrocketed so rapidly in the last ten years that some families generally cannot afford the services of physicians and hospitals. Since someone has to pay for health care, most Americans purchase insurance protection individually or through an organization, such as an employer.

By purchasing health insurance, people are able to be more financially prepared for the high cost of an unexpected illness or injury. Over the last two decades, escalating health care costs have generated several alternative financing plans besides the traditional private office, fee-for-service arrangement. A variety of health care insurance options are available to patients today, including individual and group insurance, health maintenance organizations (HMOs), preferred provider organizations (PPOs), independent practitioner associations (IPAs), Medicare, and Medicaid. These are more fully explained in the following section, *Health Care Financing Plans.*

Although patients are ultimately responsible for paying their medical account, with insurance they usually have to pay only a small portion of the costs of an illness or accident themselves, and some form of insurance pays for the remainder. Because the livelihood of the physician and staff of a medical facility depends on income from insurance sources, managing insurance payments is a fundamental responsibility of the medical office.

Types of Health Insurance Coverage

Health insurance can be separated into three categories: basic coverage, major medical coverage, and comprehensive coverage. The amount of premium a subscriber or purchaser pays determines the degree of protection a policy offers.

Basic insurance covers general physician, hospital, and surgical fees.

Although insurance policies vary widely, certain general benefits are available in most basic policies. The physician's fee, hospital expenses up to a maximum amount, and surgical fees, as determined in the contract, are generally covered by basic insurance. Payment may be based on a "usual and customary fee," or the contract may specify a stated amount. Many policies require a deductible or copayment from the patient, which requires that the patient typically pay the first $100, $200, or more of annual medical costs in addition to 20 percent of the remaining charges. For example, the patient whose medical expenses amount to $500 during one year might be required to pay a $200 deductible and an additional $60 ($500 - $200 x 20 percent), and the insurance plan would pay the remaining $240.

Hospital benefits for basic insurance may pay a certain dollar amount for a specified number of days, or they may pay full charges for a specific type of room, usually semiprivate, for a specified number of days. Inpatient services such as laboratory tests, radiographs, operating room, anesthesia, surgical dressings, and some outpatient services, although not all, are usually included. Some plans cover extended care at a skilled nursing facility after a patient is released from a hospital. A basic policy usually covers all or a large portion of maternity care.

Major medical insurance takes up where basic insurance leaves off.

Major medical insurance is sometimes called catastrophe insurance because it is designed to help offset huge medical expenses that result from a lengthy illness or serious accident. Most major medical policies include a deductible amount as well as a coinsurance provision that calls for an additional percentage (usually 20 percent) to be paid by the patient. Benefits, which range from $10,000 to unlimited coverage, are determined by the amount of the premium. They cover health services and supplies beyond those available in basic policies, including special nurses, rental of medical equipment, prosthetic devices, and related items.

Comprehensive insurance combines basic and major medical.

The benefits of basic insurance and major medical insurance are combined for comprehensive major medical coverage. A small deductible usually covers broad medical treatment under one policy.

Health Care Financing Plans

Blue Cross and Blue Shield are nonprofit insurers.

Commercial carriers are for-profit insurers.

HMOs offer pay-in-advance membership for health care.

PPOs offer medical services at preset fees.

Medicare protects Americans 65 years of age and older and disabled people.

Medicaid provides health coverage for the poor.

TRICARE and CHAMPVA are other government programs.

Worker's Compensation insurance is provided by the employer

No Fault - car related or accident

Americans have a choice of several major types of health care financing plans. They are Blue Cross and Blue Shield, commercial insurance companies, HMOs, PPOs, Medicare and Medicaid, and other government programs.

Blue Cross and Blue Shield plans are organized under the laws of the individual states and are regulated by boards of directors made up of public representatives, physicians, and other health care providers. "The Blues," as they are called, are nonprofit organizations. In most states, Blue Shield plans pay for the services of physicians and other providers, and Blue Cross plans pay for hospital services. A patient may subscribe to either or both plans.

Aetna Life and Casualty, Prudential Insurance, Equitable Life Assurance Society, The Travelers Company, and other similar companies are for-profit organizations that offer individual or group basic health and major medical insurance for an annual fee or *premium*.

HMOs are groups that offer pay-in-advance memberships instead of traditional insurance. For a monthly or annual prepayment, each insured person is guaranteed physician and hospital services for little or no additional charge. Patients are attracted to HMOs because they guarantee the patient will have no unexpected medical costs. In return, patients are required to use physicians named by the HMO, with some exceptions for emergencies and out-of-town care. HMOs emphasize "wellness," and "wellness checks" as a method of reducing expenses.

PPOs provide medical services to the insurers at preset, usually lower, fees in return for a large number of referrals. In a preferred provider organization, a large buyer of group insurance (such as a major corporation or a union) agrees to send all members of the group (usually employees of a company) to physicians or hospitals affiliated with the PPO in return for volume discounts of approved, allowable services by physicians.

Medicare was developed in 1965 by the federal government to protect the elderly and the disabled population. Medicare medical insurance pays 80 percent of allowable physician's fees and related medical charges, minus a deductible. Medicare hospital insurance pays for most but not all of a patient's hospital treatment and related expenses.

Medicaid, also developed in 1965, is a financial assistance program sponsored jointly by the federal government and the states to provide health care for the poor. Benefits offered are similar to other insurance programs, although the plans differ from state to state. Medicaid generally pays the deductible amount charged under Medicare and the 20 percent not covered by Medicare medical insurance for eligible patients. (In general, Medicaids patient do not have to pay for health care services.)

TRICARE is the Department of Defense's health care program. It was formerly called CHAMPUS [the Civilian Health and Medical Program of the Uniformed Services (Army, Navy, Air Force, Marines, and Coast Guard)]. This program covers medical care for uniformed service personnel and their families that is not directly related to the military. Although it is similar, TRICARE is completely separate with a totally different beneficiary population than CHAMPVA, described below.

CHAMPVA refers to the Civilian Health and Medical Program of the Veterans' Administration and covers (1) dependents of totally disabled veterans whose disabilities are service-related, and (2) surviving dependents of veterans who have died from service-related disabilities.

Although the benefits are similar, these government programs (Medicare, Medicaid, TRICARE, and CHAMPVA) are administered separately with significant differences in claim filing procedures and preauthorization requirements.

Worker's Compensation insurance laws in each state require employers to purchase insurance that provides health care and income to employees and their dependents when the employee suffers a work-related injury, illness, or death. The employer pays all insurance premiums for Worker's Compensation insurance in return for protection from financial liability. The primary purpose of Worker's Compensation insurance is to return the employee to work. This includes providing medical treatment, hospital care, surgery, and therapy from the time of injury or diagnosis of an illness until recovery.

Changes in health care laws will cause insurance companies to offer additional alternatives during the next several years. It is always a good idea to use the media to stay abreast of these changes.

MANAGED CARE

Health insurance coverage that is termed *managed care* is becoming increasingly prevalent. The main goal of managed care plans is to keep medical costs down and, at the same time, to ensure the patient receives the quality medical care he or she needs. Managed care plans try to keep medical costs under control by providing incentives for the physician to keep the patient healthy. This helps prevent unnecessary or costly medical procedures and avoids the need to hospitalize the patient. Costs are also controlled by predefining a price, called a *contractual rate*, for services the physician performs and negotiating with the managed care plan to determine which medical services will or will not be covered, called the *service limitations*, under the plan. This means that the physician knows how he or she will be reimbursed for each service provided to the patient as well as for which services he or she will be reimbursed.

The growth of managed care is changing the way physicians do business and care for their patients, and both physicians and patients are benefiting from this change. In the managed care relationship, the patient is enticed to see a contracted physician because the portion of the charge the patient must pay is usually much less than the charge for seeing a noncontracted physician. The physician is motivated to participate in this relationship in order to have access to all the members of the insurance plan (this can increase his or her patient base).

How Managed Care Is Different

The difference between managed care plans and traditional health insurance is that managed care plans involve a contract between the physician or group of physicians and the insurance carrier. The insurance carrier requires that physicians accept a certain amount of money, a *contractual rate*, for the services they provide and also specifies what portion the patient will pay. This portion is called the *copayment*, or *copay*. In traditional health insurance plans, patients are free to choose whichever physician or health care provider they wish, the providers are free to charge their usual and customary charge, and the patients pay the difference between what the physician has charged and what their insurance company is to cover.

How Managed Care Works

There are many variations in managed care plans, but many of them involve a payment method called capitation. In a capitated plan, patients select a primary care physician (PCP). The patients choose their PCP from a list (of approved physicians or directly) provided by the plan. The PCP is often paid a fixed amount monthly, called a *capitation payment*, per patient, regardless of whether or not the PCP sees each patient during that time period.

Except in an emergency, whenever patients need medical services, they must always contact their PCP first. The PCP evaluates their condition and decides either to treat the patient himself or herself or refer them to a specialist for more in-depth care. For this reason, the PCP may be referred to as the managed care *gatekeeper*.

The PCP cannot always treat the patient for every condition. Therefore, the PCP may refer the patient to a specialist or another facility. A specialist is a physician or other health care provider who has specialized training in a particular area of medicine. The patient must get a referral from their PCP before receiving care from a specialist. Usually, these referrals must be preauthorized by the managed care plan.

The referrals from a PCP may vary greatly. The referrals may limit the number of visits a patient can make to a particular specialist, the total dollar amount of the specialist's services, the valid date range within which the referral must be used, or the specific procedures that can be performed by the specialist. The PCP can often send the patient only to other providers who have also contracted with the plan for special rates, again to help keep costs down.

As a medical practice begins to enter into managed contracts with insurance plans, the use of a computerized managed care system is necessary for the practice to keep track of all the capitated payments, special rate schedules, and referral limits of their contract with the plan.

Managed Care in Action

During a typical visit to the PCP's office, the patient's eligibility is verified against a list, the *eligibility roster* (Figure 1-5), of all plan members who selected the participating physician as their PCP. The patient is then seen by the PCP and treated or referred to a specialist or facility for further care.

The patient typically pays a visit copay plus any amount designated by the plan such as additional copayments for certain procedures, payment for noncovered services, or the patient due amount of discounted fee-for-service procedures. The PCP bills the plan for any services not included in the capitation coverage.

If the patient is referred to a specialist, the referral must be authorized and sent to the specialist or facility. The PCP must not only adhere to the plan contract but also ensure that the patient sees the specialist or goes to the facility. Because the PCP is responsible for the patient's care, the authorized services must be monitored and results from the referral obtained and recorded.

Specialty Care Needs

Unlike the PCP who must operate within the limits of the plan contract, the specialist or facility must operate within the limits set by each individual referral. It is the spe-

Figure 1-5 Eligibility Roster

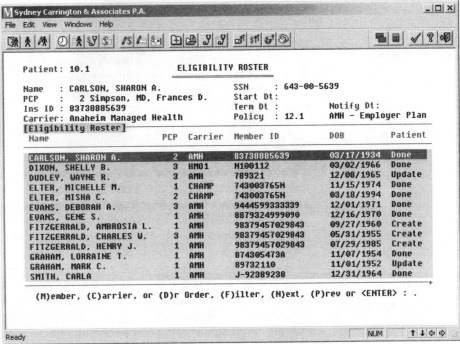

cialist's responsibility to stay within the referral limits or risk not receiving full payment for the services rendered to the patient.

As patients are scheduled, the medical office assistant must verify the patient has valid insurance coverage and that the visit is authorized by a referral from the patient's PCP. Services must be performed within the limits set by the referral, such as a time period, a set number of visits, a dollar amount, specific procedure codes, or general referral reasons. The services performed by the specialist are reported back to the PCP in the form of *Referral Results*.

APPLYING YOUR KNOWLEDGE

EXERCISE 1: Flow of Patient Information

STEP 1

You are asked to explain the flow of patient information in a medical office to a newly hired medical assistant. Make an outline of the points you will cover.

EXERCISE 2: Appointment Scheduling Process

STEP 2

Medical practices use similar methods for scheduling appointments. Prepare a brief description of a typical appointment scheduling process. Discuss overbooking.

EXERCISE 3: Types of Insurance

STEP 3

A friend of yours asks you to describe three different types of insurance that are available to medical patients. Write the answer you will give.

EXERCISE 4: Managed Care

STEP 4

Describe how managed care works in a physician's office.

ROLE OF COMPUTERS IN TODAY'S MEDICAL OFFICE

Clinical and Management Uses

Computers tell a physician whether a surgical patient's vital signs are normal, and they track the course of the patient's health after surgery. Computers record and calculate the costs of the patient's treatment and prepare insurance forms for billing purposes, and as in the case of **The Medical Manager** system, computers are used for managing medical practices.

Computers are widely used in private practices for record keeping, patient accounting, billing, insurance form preparation, appointment scheduling, payroll, word processing, and database management. Although laboratory testing by computer is not as prevalent in private practice as in hospitals, physicians may use computers to determine proper dosage, judge the effect of one drug when taken with another, and determine the influence a previously ingested drug has on laboratory tests.

The use of computers in medical practices has grown dramatically as physicians recognize that their income can be increased through proper auditing of patient accounts, follow-up of claims submitted to insurance companies and government agencies, and inventory control. Word processing and database management have revolutionized patient record keeping and reduced the risk of medical malpractice because of the efficiency with which medical reports can be processed. The bottom line of the influence of computers in the health care industry is that, overall, computers save physicians time and money and make the day-to-day management of their practices easier.

The Medical Manager Software

The advantage of using computers for practice management is the subject for the remainder of this book. **The Medical Manager** is the name of the software program that will be used to teach you about practice management. **The Medical Manager** system is a sophisticated computer program that helps you manage the essential daily activities of a medical office. Several of the practice management advantages of **The Medical Manager** software are discussed below.

Increased Income. An important benefit of computerized practice management is an increase in revenue. Professional, computerized statements result in faster payment from both patients and insurance carriers. Patients tend not to question the validity of a computerized statement, and insurers usually process computerized forms more quickly and more accurately. The time normally required to complete practice management tasks is reduced to a fraction of what it would normally take; time saved is money earned.

Greater Accuracy. Once procedure codes have been entered into **The Medical Manager** system from the encounter form, it is simple for the computer to formulate an accurate charge for the patient's visit. Correct fees are consistently charged to patients in a computerized system because the fees are stored in the computer's memory.

Reduced Mundane Paperwork. Everything is automated in **The Medical Manager** software; therefore, staff time spent on posting, billing, insurance, recalls, and management information is drastically reduced. The time saved may be reallocated to more productive tasks such as patient and insurance collection follow-up, recall follow-up, and patient communication.

Minimization of Duplication. Recording financial and clinical information is repetitive work, and the duplication of effort wastes time and increases errors. With **The Medical Manager** system, all services and financial transactions need to be entered only once. The computer then uses this information, as needed, to process data. The information entered is available to the medical office in a variety of ways to accommodate medical office needs.

Faster Insurance Processing. Time-consuming tasks, such as typing insurance forms, are eliminated in **The Medical Manager** software because forms are created automatically by the computer system and can be mailed on a daily or weekly basis. Government and private insurance claims are processed more quickly and fewer rejections are received that are due to missing information or typographical errors.

Electronic Media Claims. A growing number of insurance carriers can receive insurance claims through a telephone modem. This eliminates paperwork for both the insurance carrier and the doctor's office. For many carriers, especially Medicare, this means much faster payment to the doctor. The waiting period for receiving payment for claims, normally taking up to six weeks, can be shortened dramatically with electronic claims processing.

Professional Image. Forms generated by **The Medical Manager** system are neatly printed without typographical errors and contain accurate, complete information. This method helps provide an image of professionalism for the practice.

USING THE MEDICAL MANAGER

The Medical Manager system is a comprehensive practice management software program for medical offices that allows many activities to be completed using a computer.

This means work is done more quickly and efficiently with fewer errors. Some tasks that can be completed using **The Medical Manager** software are listed below.

◆ Schedule patient appointments.

◆ Create encounter forms.

◆ Post patient charges and payments.

◆ Produce a patient receipt.

◆ Complete insurance claim forms.

◆ Prepare the daily deposit slip.

◆ Age accounts receivable.

◆ Compile a variety of reports.

As you use **The Medical Manager** software, you will also learn more about routine medical office functions, such as working with patient accounts; filing insurance claims with public and private carriers; maintaining up-to-date records; and communicating effectively with patients, insurance companies, and businesses.

STARTING UP THE MEDICAL MANAGER

The Medical Manager is installed on the computer.

The Medical Manager software should have been stored on the hard drive of your computer previously. You should check with your instructor to confirm that this is the case; then follow the steps below to begin working with the software.

STEP 1

Turn on the computer and wait for the operating system prompt or desktop to appear on the screen. Locate the icon shown in Figure 1-6 and proceed to the next step.

Figure 1-6 **The Medical Manager** Icon

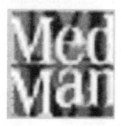

STEP 2

Insert the Student Disk that came in the back of the text-workbook into the floppy disk drive.

STEP 3

Place the mouse pointer on **The Medical Manager** icon shown in Figure 1-6 and double-click the mouse button. This will load the information stored on the Student Disk into the computer's memory. The log-on screen for **The Medical Manager** system, shown in Figure 1-7, will appear.

STEP 4

Type user number '**1**', and press **ENTER**.

STEP 5

Type the student password '**ICAN**' and press **ENTER**. You may use either upper- or lower-case letters.

Password is a safety device.

STEP 6

Key the date, '**01102003**,' and press **ENTER**. (This is the system date for this text-book and is not meant to be today's actual date.) Note that this field is self-formatting

Figure 1-7 Log-On Screen for **The Medical Manager** system.

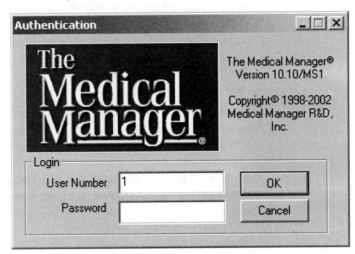

and the computer automatically adds slashes to separate the month from the day and year as soon as ENTER is pressed.

Dates may be entered in either the form 'MMDDYY' (6 digits) or 'MMDDYYYY' (8 digits). When the cursor leaves a date field, the date will appear as 'MM/DD/YY', and when the cursor returns to a field already containing a date the full eight characters will be shown unformatted. For example, if the user enters '041403', the date will display as '04/14/03' when the cursor leaves the field, and as '04142003' when the cursor returns to the field.

Note that when entering a two-digit year ('MMDDYY' format) the following rules apply:

1. If the last two digits of the year entered are '29' or less, the system will automatically assume that the year begins with '20.' For example, '01/01/01' will be formatted as '01/01/2001.'

2. If the last two digits of the year entered are '30' or greater, the system will automatically assume that the year begins with '19.' For example, '01/01/99' will be formatted as '01/01/1999.'

Note: The date you enter when you log into The Medical Manager *system is important. You should not change it unless you are specifically told to do so. When you are instructed to change the date, change it very carefully, making sure to enter the correct information. If the date is entered incorrectly, you will not be able to use your files without technical assistance. Never advance further than desired because the date can never be backdated.*

STEP 7

The Main Menu (Menu 1) as shown in Figure 1-15 on page 21, of **The Medical Manager** software appears after the date is entered and its appearance confirms that you have successfully logged into **The Medical Manager** software. This completes the process for starting up **The Medical Manager** system.

THE MEDICAL MANAGER WINDOW

Now that you are at the Main Menu (Menu 1), it is important that you understand the basic features of **The Medical Manager** window, the screen that displays **The Medical Manager** software. **The Medical Manager** window has a title bar, a menu bar, a toolbar, and a status bar. In addition, a special toolbar is associated with the

Figure 1-8 **The Medical Manager** System Main Toolbar

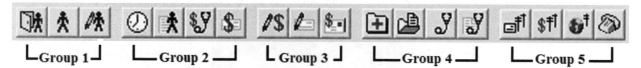

Appointments screen. This section will devote special attention to **The Medical Manager** system toolbar (Figure 1-8), as it can be used as a primary resource for many functions of operating **The Medical Manager** software.

Note: Not all toolbar features and functions of The Medical Manager *software will be covered in the Student Edition, however, an overview of these items follows.*

The main toolbar (also referred to as the *top toolbar*), located across the top of **The Medical Manager** window, allows the user to "direct chain" to primary modules within the current window, open an additional window, and perform frequently used tasks. When the mouse pointer is resting over a toolbar button the system automatically displays the name of the button on the status bar and a screen tip is displayed just below the button. An expanded view of the main toolbar buttons is as follows:

Reading from left to right, the buttons on the left side of the toolbar allow the user to access the following modules:

Group 1	New Patient Entry, Display Patient Data, and Edit Patient Records
Group 2	Appointment Entry, Encounter Forms, Procedure Entry, and Payment Entry
Group 3	Edit Activity Records, Edit Payment Records, and Collections System
Group 4	Electronic Chart Menu, View Patient Chart System, Clinical History, and Managed Care System
Group 5	Electronic Media Claims, Electronic Remittance, Network Services, and Phone System

The remaining control buttons on the main toolbar (Figure 1-9) allow the user to do the following:

New Window Button	Opens an additional window that displays the Main Menu (Menu 1) without having to log in again and keeps the current patient.

Figure 1-9 Control Buttons on **The Medical Manager** Toolbar

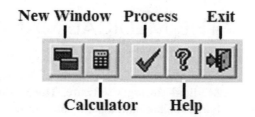

Calculator Button	Opens a calculator window. Once the calculation is performed, the value automatically displays in the input field.
Process Button	Saves information entered when a screen is completed, or starts printing a report.
Help Button	Opens a help window for the current field.
Exit Button	Exits from a screen (or part of a split screen) without storing the information entered, exits a menu or module to the next higher level menu, or stops the printout of a report; this is the Escape key (Esc) in **The Medical Manager** Student Edition.

A Quick Reference Guide for **The Medical Manager** has been included in the Student Edition. Locate the Quick Reference Guide at the back of this book and detach it, carefully tearing along the perforated edge. Follow the instructions on the Quick Reference Guide, folding the perforated keyboard template and detaching it from the reference guide. The keyboard template can be laid on your keyboard above the function keys. The Quick Reference Guide should be saved and may be used to quickly locate and navigate your way through **The Medical Manager** for the duration of this course.

NAVIGATING THE MEDICAL MANAGER SOFTWARE

Several different methods are available for navigating throughout **The Medical Manager** software:

Keyboard. The normal keyboard commands of **The Medical Manager** system, some of which have already been explained in this unit, may be used to navigate the system. Using the keyboard, you may also use a feature called *direct chaining*. Direct chaining allows the user to quickly change to another program within **The Medical Manager** software. For example, keying '/pro' at any menu prompt or Patient Retrieval screen and pressing ENTER will automatically take the user to the Procedure Entry Patient Retrieval Screen. Similarly, keying '/pay' and pressing ENTER will take the user to the Payment Entry Patient Retrieval Screen. A list of frequently-used direct chaining options are listed on the removable Quick Reference Guide.

Direct Chaining. Direct chaining may also be used to move quickly between menus. For example, keying '/m2' and pressing ENTER will take the user directly to Menu 2 (the File Maintenance Menu). In any case in which a menu number is listed, you may use direct chaining by entering '/m' together with the actual menu number shown and pressing ENTER. A list of frequently used menu numbers that may be used in direct chaining are listed on the Quick Reference Guide.

EXIT Button. The EXIT button, located at the right edge of the top toolbar controls (Figure 1-9), is of particular importance in the Student Edition, because it allows you to leave a screen at any time and return to the previous screen without saving the data you have been working on in that screen. Besides clicking on the EXIT button, you may also press ESCAPE (this key is usually labeled "Esc") located on the upper left corner of your keyboard. Note, however, that in an office, another key may be defined as the EXIT key. Each time the ESCAPE key or EXIT button is pressed, the next higher level menu is displayed until you reach the Main Menu (Menu 1).

Status Bar. The status bar is located at the bottom of **The Medical Manager** system screen (shown in Figure 1-15) and contains buttons for moving the cursor up and down to the previous and next item, and for paging to the previous and next page. An expanded view of the status bar is shown in Figure 1-10.

Figure 1-10 Navigation Buttons in **The Medical Manager** Software

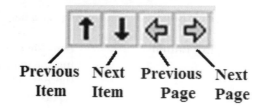

Previous Item Next Item Previous Page Next Page

Reading from left to right, the navigation buttons on the status bar allow the user to perform the following functions.

Buttons	Functions
Previous Item	Moves the cursor to the previous selectable item or field
Next Item	Moves the cursor to the next selectable item or field
Previous Page	Displays the previous page of information
Next Page	Displays the next page of information

Mouse. The mouse may also be used for navigating. The table shown in Figure 1-11 provides an explanation of each function.

Figure 1-11 Using the Mouse for Navigation

Mouse Button	Action	Function
Left Button	Single click	Selects an item
Left Button	Double click	Selects and activates the following items:
		Menu Items
		Help Windows
		Help Windows Items
		Input Fields
		Command Lines and Prompts
		Options and Valid Entries
Middle Button	Single click	Opens a help window for the current field
Right Button	Single click	Displays a shortcut menu listing the most frequently used modules
Wheel	Roll the wheel forward and back	Moves the cursor up and down the page

SPECIAL FEATURES

Displaying a Calendar Window. A calendar window (Figure 1-12) is available for all date fields by pressing the Help button ('?') on the top toolbar or by typing a question mark ('?') and pressing ENTER.

Note: Once a date is selected, it automatically closes the calendar window and displays the date in the field.

Figure 1-12 Sample Calendar Window

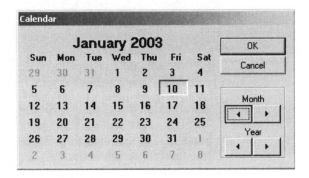

Sizing a Window. **The Medical Manager** software window may be dropped down, or minimized, by using the minimize button (Figure 1-13) on the upper right corner of the window. The window may be resized to the full screen using the maximize button (also shown in Figure 1-13).

Figure 1-13 The Minimize, Maximize, and Close Buttons

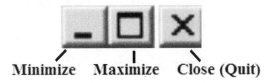

Minimize   Maximize   Close (Quit)

The windows close button in the upper right corner of the window will properly exit **The Medical Manager** if the student is at a menu or at a patient retrieval screen (patient retrieval discussed in Unit 2). Note that it does not perform the same function as pressing **The Medical Manager's** Exit key or using the Exit button in **The Medical Manager's** toolbar shown in Figure 1-9.

In addition, users may resize the window by placing the mouse on any side or corner of the window and dragging the mouse to either increase or decrease the size of the active window.

Online Documentation and Online Content Help. For physician offices using **The Medical Manager** software, online documentation and content help may be invoked from the Help menu at the top of the screen. However, these options are not available in the Student Edition of **The Medical Manager** software.

SPECIAL KEYS FOR ENTERING OR EDITING DATA

If you are already logged into **The Medical Manager** system, press **ESCAPE** several times until you return to the Main Menu (Menu 1). If you are starting a new class session, log into **The Medical Manager** system by following the instructions provided at the beginning of this unit.

There are a variety of keys and buttons that are used for entering or editing data in **The Medical Manager** software. Before proceeding with the next section, take a few moments to familiarize yourself with their functions, shown in Figure 1-14. Note that directions for completing these tasks using Windows buttons are also provided.

Figure 1-14 Data Entry Keys

Edit Keys	Function
← →	Use left and right arrow keys to move the cursor within a field OR position the mouse pointer at the desired location on the screen and click to relocate the cursor.
↑ ↓	Use up and down arrow keys to move the cursor between fields OR position the mouse pointer at the desired location on the screen and click.
Backspace	Use the Backspace key to erase from right to left within a field.
Delete	Use the Delete key to erase from left to right within a field; may also use CTRL-G.
Insert	Use during the edit of an existing field to toggle between Insert (add new characters at current position) mode and Overwrite (write over existing characters with new text) mode; may also use CTRL-I.
End	Use to move cursor to first blank space to the right of data already entered in a field; may also use CTRL-E.
F10	Use to erase any characters in the field being edited; also called the Clear field key; may also use CTRL-X.
ENTER or RETURN	Use to enter data in a field after keying is complete.
HOME or ? Key	Use to invoke a Help window listing of data (available only when prompted by the instruction "or ? for Help"); clicking on the Help button ('?') on the upper right side of the top toolbar will also invoke a help window.
Page Up	Use within Help windows to display the previous page of help information; operates whenever the (P)revious option is available OR click on the up arrow button (↑) at the right edge of the bottom toolbar to revert to the previous page.
Page Down	Use within Help windows to display the next page of help information; operates whenever the (N)ext option is available OR click on the down arrow button (↓) at the right edge of the bottom toolbar to advance to the next page.
F1	Use to process data, save your work, or initiate the printout of a report; also called the PROCESS key; may also use CTRL-P OR click on the PROCESS button ('√') on the right side of the top toolbar to process.
ESCAPE	Use to escape from a screen without storing the information entered; also called the Exit key; may also use ESC (escape to previous screen) or ESC-1 [escape to Main Menu (Menu 1)] OR click once on the EXIT button on the right side of the top toolbar to Escape to the previous screen.
Top of Form	Use to advance the attached printer to the top of the form; use CTRL-T.

Note: In a Windows environment, you can often substitute using the mouse pointer and one click (instead of manual keystrokes) to highlight an item on the screen; double-clicking will highlight and choose an item on the screen.

THE MAIN MENU

In this section, we will practice using some of the special keys, explained above, using the Main Menu (Menu 1) in **The Medical Manager** system. You will start each exercise in the text, and all future office procedures and operations, from the Main Menu (Menu 1). Therefore, it is a good idea to completely familiarize yourself with how the Main Menu (Menu 1) works.

The Main Menu (Menu 1) of **The Medical Manager** software appears after the date is entered. If you are already logged onto **The Medical Manager** system and not at the Main Menu (Menu 1), return to the Main Menu (Menu 1) by pressing ESCAPE. If you are not currently logged into the system, follow the instructions shown at the beginning of this unit to reenter the software. The Main Menu (Menu 1) screen is shown in Figure 1-15.

Figure 1-15 The Main Menu (Menu 1) Screen

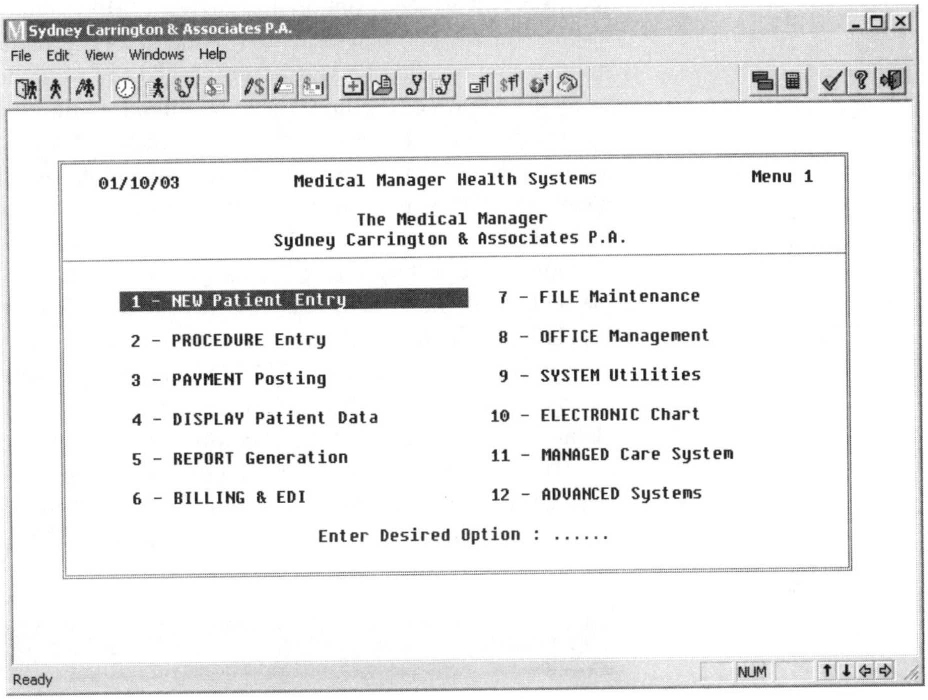

Computer menus are like restaurant menus.

When you go to a foreign restaurant for dinner, you may be given a menu of food choices from which you may order items by number. You will probably order a salad, an entrée, vegetables, drink, and dessert, although you may not know their exact pronunciation. Using computer menus, as explained below, is very similar.

The Medical Manager system works in much the same way in that you may select programs by number without knowing the program name. Some items on menus invoke programs, some lead to other menus. The first menu you see is the Main Menu (Menu 1), from which you may choose the task you wish to perform first. The Main Menu (Menu 1) is identified by the "Menu 1" message in the upper right corner of the screen. As you work through the units in this text-workbook, you will learn the meaning of all the numbered choices in the Main Menu (Menu 1).

Main Menu (Menu 1) is identified by "Menu 1" in the upper right corner of the computer screen.

All functions in **The Medical Manager** software begin by starting with the Main Menu (Menu 1). Users select the program they wish to work with by choosing an item (accomplished by entering an item number) and then pressing ENTER to select it. The system will then go to the menu of another program option within **The Medical Manager** software. Note, however, that all program menus in the software are ordered in a hierarchy with the Main Menu (Menu 1) being the highest. Any time you wish to return to a previous menu, all you have to do is press EXIT. In fact, **The Medical Manager** software is so advanced that not only will this return you to the previous menu, but also the option that you originally selected (i.e., the numbered menu item that you chose to go to the subsequent menu) will be highlighted.

Working with the Menu System

Begin working with the Main Menu (Menu 1) by using the arrow keys to move the highlight bar to option **12**, ADVANCED Systems, and press **ENTER** to select it. The Advanced Systems Menu (Menu 24) will appear. To demonstrate how menus function in a hierarchy, simply press **ESCAPE** and notice that you will be returned to the Main Menu (Menu 1). Notice also that option 12, ADVANCED Systems, will be highlighted because this is the last option you chose.

Make sure you are at the Main Menu (Menu 1) before proceeding. Type '**12**' and press **ENTER** to select option 12, ADVANCED Systems. Notice that the system goes again to the Advanced Systems Menu (Menu 24). Note that manually keying the option number and pressing ENTER accomplished the same task you initially completed by using the arrow keys to move the highlight bar to the option and then pressing ENTER.

Another way of selecting items on a menu is to use the mouse. At the Advanced Systems Menu (Menu 24), move the mouse pointer to option **1**, CUSTOM Menus, and double-click. The option will be simultaneously highlighted and selected. The Custom Menu (CMenu 1) will appear. EXIT twice to return to the main menu (Menu 1).

Finally, you will use direct chaining to go quickly between menus. At the prompt at the bottom of the screen, key '**/c2**' (this means "go to Custom Menu 2") and press **ENTER**. Notice that you have accomplished similar tasks in several different ways.

Now, instead of pressing ESCAPE until you reach the Main Menu 1, key '**/m1**' (this means, of course, go to Menu 1) and press **ENTER** and you will be returned to the Main Menu (Menu 1). Note that direct chaining will be addressed more in-depth later in the text. However, whenever you see a menu option number in parentheses, you can quickly go to the numbered option by typing a forward slash ('/'), followed by an 'm' for menu or 'c' for custom menu, the menu number, and then pressing the ENTER key.

APPLYING YOUR KNOWLEDGE

EXERCISE 5: Registering Your Name

In this exercise, you will learn to use additional editing keys while registering your name using the Student Registration process.

STEP 1 You should already be logged into **The Medical Manager** system and at the Main Menu (Menu 1). Type '**/c2**' and press **ENTER** to begin this exercise.

STEP 2 From the Operating System Utilities Menu (CMenu 2), choose option **11**, Student Name Registration. Remember that there are several ways to choose this option and a combination of methods may be used to accomplish any given task within **The Medical Manager** software. The Student Registration screen shown in Figure 1-16 will appear.

STEP 3 Key in your first name as you want it to appear and press **ENTER**. Key your last name as you want it to appear and press **ENTER**.

Note: Do not enter the student name, Paul Wilson. This is the student name used, for demonstration purposes, throughout the Student Edition.

Figure 1-16 Student Entry Screen

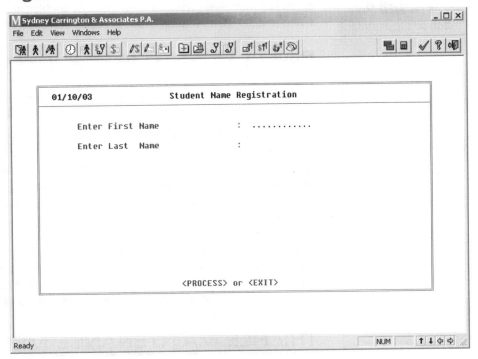

STEP 4

When you have keyed both your first and last names and checked them for accuracy, press the **F1** key or click on the PROCESS button ('√') on the top toolbar to process the screen and save your name to the disk. After processing, the screen will flash briefly while information is being updated. When the registration process is completed, your screen will return to the Operating System Utilities Menu (Custom Menu 2). You will not see your name change take effect until you exit and reenter **The Medical Manager**.

EXITING AND REENTERING THE MEDICAL MANAGER SOFTWARE

Now is a good time to pause to learn how to exit **The Medical Manager** software and reenter at a later time. Although it is important for you to know how to start up the software, you must also know how to stop at the end of your current class session and start during the next class session without destroying any information you have stored. This is also important because you may wish to go back to a previous screen from time to time, or you may have reason to return to the Main Menu (Menu 1).

You may exit a screen at any time.

Practice exiting **The Medical Manager** system. Press **ESCAPE** or click on the EXIT button on the top toolbar until the following prompt appears: "Do You Wish to Exit **The Medical Manager**? (Y/N)." Key 'Y'; press **ENTER**, and you will be exited out of **The Medical Manager** software. You must do this at the end of each session or you may lose data you entered during class. Any other response will return you to **The Medical Manager** system's Main Menu (Menu 1).

You may also exit **The Medical Manager** system from any menu, custom menu, or patient retrieval screen by going to the File menu at the top of the window. Using the mouse, click on File and a drop-down list of options will appear. Click on EXIT and you will be exited out of **The Medical Manager** software. Finally, as with almost any other Windows software, you may click on the X shown on the right side of the title bar (shown in the upper right corner of your screen), but only when your screen is at a Menu prompt or a Patient Retrieval Screen. Refer to Figure 1-17 for a list of options for exiting the software.

UNIT 1 Using The Medical Manager

23

To reenter, double-click on the MED MAN icon on the desktop.

This break to learn how to exit and reenter is important, because you may be near the end of your class period. If time remains, double-click on the icon shown in Figure 1-6 to re-enter **The Medical Manager** software and continue.

Figure 1-17 Ways to Exit **The Medical Manager** Software

Key	Action
ESCAPE	Used to return user to previous screen without saving; used continuously, this key will eventually invoke the prompt: 'Do You Wish to Exit The Medical Manager? (Y/N).'
X	Used in Windows programs to exit the current application.
Exit Button	Used to return user to previous screen without saving; used continuously, this key will eventually invoke the prompt: 'Do You Wish to Exit The Medical Manager? (Y/N)'.
File-Exit	Drop-down menu options selected, in order, to exit **The Medical Manager** software session.
/quit	Direct chaining command keyed at any menu or patient retrieval screen used to exit **The Medical Manager** software session.

THE FILE MAINTENANCE MENU

Besides learning to work from the Main Menu (Menu 1), the starting point for all program functions within **The Medical Manager** software, it is also important that you learn about the File Maintenance Menu (Menu 2). If this is a new class session, log onto **The Medical Manager** system by following the instructions provided at the beginning of this unit. If you are already logged onto **The Medical Manager** system, press **ESCAPE** or click on the EXIT button until you return to the Main Menu. From the Main Menu (Menu 1), choose option **7**, FILE Maintenance, and press **ENTER**. The File Maintenance Menu (Menu 2), shown in Figure 1-18 will appear.

Figure 1-18 File Maintenance Menu (Menu 2) Screen

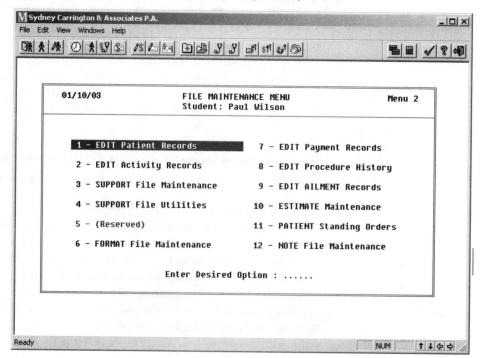

```
01/10/03              FILE MAINTENANCE MENU              Menu 2
                        Student: Paul Wilson


        1 - EDIT Patient Records        7 - EDIT Payment Records

        2 - EDIT Activity Records       8 - EDIT Procedure History

        3 - SUPPORT File Maintenance    9 - EDIT AILMENT Records

        4 - SUPPORT File Utilities     10 - ESTIMATE Maintenance

        5 - (Reserved)                 11 - PATIENT Standing Orders

        6 - FORMAT File Maintenance    12 - NOTE File Maintenance


                    Enter Desired Option : ......
```

When information is stored in **The Medical Manager** software, it is stored in files. The File Maintenance Menu (Menu 2) provides an easy method for making additions or modifications to the files. Existing information can be expanded; new information can be added; and old information may be deleted. By selecting an option from the File Maintenance Menu (Menu 2), you are able to work with specific types of information available from within the system.

The first option you will choose from the File Maintenance Menu (Menu 2) is option 3, SUPPORT Files Maintenance (Menu 13). To do so, key '**3**' at the prompt and press **ENTER**. You may also double-click on option 3 using the mouse. This will replace both entering the option number manually and pressing ENTER to select it. The screen in Figure 1-19 will appear.

Note: After this point, you will not necessarily be reminded to press ENTER after keying an instruction.

Figure 1-19 Support Files Maintenance Menu (Menu 13) Screen

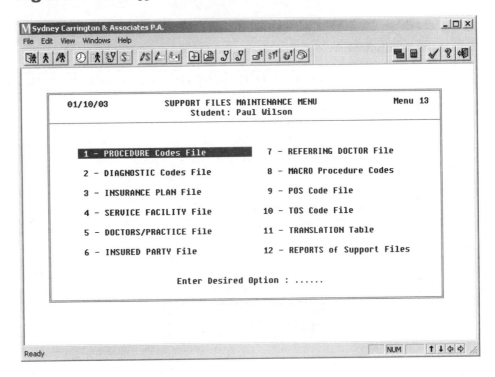

APPLYING YOUR KNOWLEDGE

EXERCISE 6: Using Help Windows

Using what you have learned regarding menus and navigating **The Medical Manager** software, complete the following exercise using the Support Files Maintenance Menu (Menu 13). If you are unsure about how to proceed, refer to the text at the beginning of this unit regarding data entry keys and working with the Main Menu (Menu 1).

The Support Files Maintenance Menu (Menu 13) allows you to input procedure codes, diagnosis codes, names and addresses of insurance plans, names of referring physicians, and related information that will be used frequently. The first activity you will complete is the addition of a referring doctor to the support file.

STEP 1

If this is a new class session, log onto **The Medical Manager** system by following the instructions provided at the beginning of this unit. If you are already logged onto **The Medical Manager** system, press **ESCAPE** or click on the EXIT button until you return to the Main Menu. From the Main Menu (Menu 1), press the right arrow key to highlight option **7**, FILE Maintenance. Press **ENTER** to select it. You may also double-click on this option using the mouse. This will replace both entering the option number manually *and* pressing ENTER to select it. Refer back to Figure 1-18 for an illustration of the File Maintenance Menu (Menu 2) screen. From here, press the down arrow key twice and press ENTER or double-click the mouse to select option **3**, SUPPORT File Maintenance. Finally, press the right arrow key and press ENTER or double-click the mouse to select option **7**, REFERRING DOCTOR File, from the Support File Maintenance Menu (Menu 13). The Referring Doctor Maintenance screen shown in Figure 1-20 will appear.

Figure 1-20 Referring Doctor Maintenance Screen

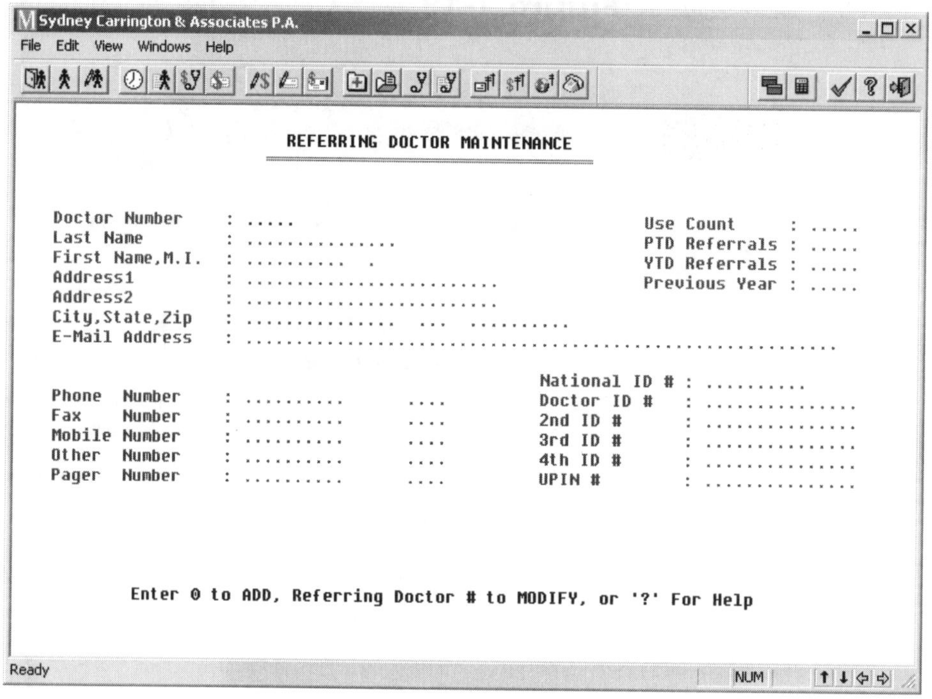

THE POINT AND SELECT FEATURE

Making Menu Selections

As you learned in Exercise 1, all menus come up with either the first menu selection or the last used selection highlighted. The highlight bar is symbolized in Figures 1-15, 1-18, and 1-19 by the shaded box positioned over the menu item. To make a menu selection, the user may key the number of the desired item and press ENTER, use the arrow keys to highlight the desired item and press ENTER, or use the mouse to place the pointer over the desired item and then double-click. The point and select feature is also used in various of **The Medical Manager** software's help windows, which we will be learning more about in this section.

Using Help Windows

Use the keyboard or mouse to Point and Select.

The point and select feature provides an alternative method of making selections on menus, selecting information to be edited, and making choices when using help windows. This feature allows the user to reduce keystrokes, and thereby increases accuracy when making selections on menus, editing information, and when using Help windows.

With Point and Select, the user points by pressing the arrow keys to move a highlighted bar to the desired selection, and then makes the selection by pressing ENTER. This feature may be used instead of directly typing a reference number and pressing ENTER. As with other Windows applications, the user may also use the mouse pointer to point to the desired selection, and then double-click to select the item.

Editing Information

Pressing the Home key is the same as keying a ? and pressing ENTER or clicking on the Help (?) button on the desktop.

STEP 2

Screens that list items available for editing appear with a highlighted bar automatically positioned over the first selection or with a prompt at the bottom of the screen that contains "Enter '?' for Help." The Referring Doctor Maintenance screen is of the latter type.

To display a list of referring doctors that may be edited, in the doctor number field press the Home key or enter a '?' and press **ENTER**. Using the mouse, you may choose to click on the Help button ('?') on the top toolbar instead. A screen similar to Figure 1-21 should be displayed.

Figure 1-21 Referring Doctor List

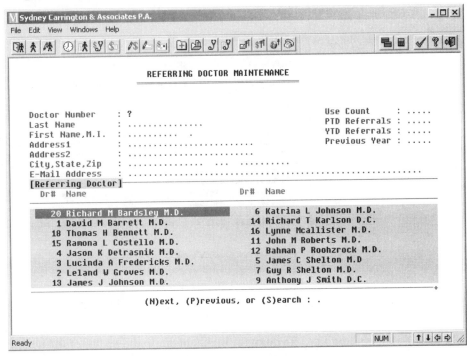

To (M)odify, key 'M' and press ENTER.

To select the first referring doctor for edit, press **ENTER**. The doctor's information will be displayed. To modify information in **The Medical Manager** system, key the letter '**M**' when prompted to "(M)odify or (D)elete", and press **ENTER** to see how this works. Do this now, and the cursor will position itself on the doctor's last name.

Using Help Windows

All Help windows come up with the first selection highlighted. The Help window provides access to lists of things that the user might otherwise have to look up on paper, then key manually into a field. An example of this is a list of cities and their corresponding zip codes. Help windows often have choices in the order in which items are displayed, such as name or code order.

STEP 3

Move the highlight bar using the arrow keys, the Tab key, or the mouse.

Press the down arrow key until the cursor is positioned in the city field OR move the mouse pointer to this field and click once. Press the Home key OR click on the Help button ('?') on the top toolbar. The Zip Code Help window for Referring Doctor Maintenance shown in Figure 1-22 will appear.

The highlight bar may be moved within the window by use of the up and down arrow keys. Moving the mouse pointer to an item and clicking on the item will also move the highlight bar to the desired location. Sometimes the Help window has sufficient space to display the list in two or more columns like the Zip Code Help window shown in Figure 1-22. In these cases, the left and right arrow keys may also be used to move the highlight bar between columns, or the user may simply position the mouse pointer at the desired screen location and click to relocate the cursor. (Figure 1-23).

Figure 1-22 Same Zip Code Help Window

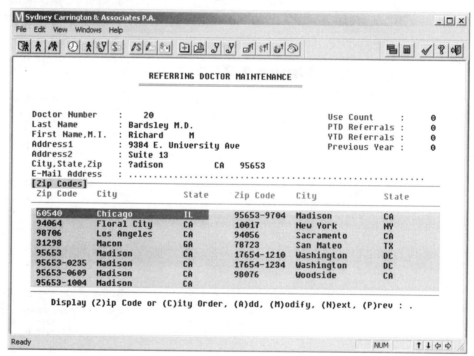

To move the highlight bar to the middle of the window, press the Tab key. To move it to the bottom of the window, press the Tab key again. To return the highlight bar to the top of the window, press the Tab key once again. Remember that the mouse can be used, at any point, to replace these keystrokes.

Plus sign (+) in the right corner of a window means more information is available.

If there are too many items to fit on one screen, **The Medical Manager** system will display a plus sign (+) in the lower and/or upper right corners of the window. The next portion of the list, called a page, can be seen by pressing the Page Down key or by typing (N)ext and pressing ENTER. To see a previous portion of the list press the Page Up key or type (P)revious and press ENTER. You may also use the mouse pointer to

Figure 1-23 Summary of Help Window Features

Help Window Keys	Function
← →	Left and right arrow keys; use in multicolumn windows to move the highlight bar between columns.
↑ ↓	Up and down arrow keys; use to move the highlight bar to the desired selection OR use the mouse to click on the up or down arrow button on the status bar at the bottom of the screen to go to the previous (using the ↑ arrow button) or the next (using the ↓ arrow button) line on **The Medical Manager** screen.
Tab key	Use the Tab key to jump quickly through a window. When pressed several times in sequence, the Tab key moves the light bar first to the middle of screen, then to the bottom, then back to the top again.
Page Down key or (N)ext	Use to display the next page of items OR use the mouse to click on the right arrow button (→) on the bottom toolbar to view data on a subsequent page.
Page Up key or (P)revious	Use to display the previous page of items OR use the mouse to click on the left arrow button (←) on the bottom toolbar to view data on a previous page.
ENTER or RETURN	Use to select the item that is currently highlighted OR use the mouse pointer to point to an item, then double-click to select it.
HOME or ? Key	Use to invoke a Help window listing of data (available only when prompted by the instruction "or ? for Help"); clicking on the Help button (?) on the upper right side of the top toolbar will also invoke a Help window.
+	Plus sign; when a plus sign occurs at the lower right corner of a window it indicates more help information is available on the next page. When a plus sign appears at the upper right corner of a window, it indicates more help information is available on a previous page. Use the mouse to click on the left arrow button (←) to view data on a previous page or to click on the right arrow button (→) to view data on a subsequent page.
Lightbar	Marks the cursor location in the Help window. In some windows, movement of lightbar controls display of data on main part of the screen. You may also move the lightbar by positioning the mouse pointer on a desired item and clicking once.
Select	Use to select a help item; move the lightbar to the desired item and press ENTER; you may also use the mouse to select an item by double-clicking on the item.
ESCAPE	Use ESCAPE to leave the Help window and return to the current screen without making a selection OR click on the EXIT button on the right side of the top toolbar.

click on the left arrow (←) and right arrow (›) buttons located on the bottom toolbar to go to the previous or next portions of the list.

Pressing the down arrow key on the last item of the page, when there is a plus sign in the lower corner of the window, will also cause the next page to be displayed. Pressing the up arrow key on the first item of a page with a plus sign in the upper right corner of the window will cause the previous page to be displayed. Again, you can use the left arrow (←) and right arrow (›) buttons located on the bottom toolbar to move through multiple pages of information.

Practice using the down arrow key, the left arrow key, the up arrow key, the right arrow key, the Tab key, the arrow buttons on the bottom toolbar, and the mouse pointer to practice moving in the Help windows. When you have tried the various options, press **ESCAPE** or click on the EXIT button on the top toolbar.

You may use the ESCAPE key to exit a Help window when you do not wish to select an item from the list, yet you wish to remain in the Edit screen. Using the mouse pointer, you may also click on the EXIT button on the right corner of the top toolbar. In this example, press **ESCAPE** again. Do not make any changes to the referring doctors' data in this exercise.

> *EXIT when you want to leave a help window without making a selection.*

Note: In a Windows environment, you can often substitute using the mouse pointer and one click (instead of manual keystrokes) to highlight an item on the screen; two clicks will automatically select a specific item on the screen.

ENTERING REFERRING DOCTOR INFORMATION

> *A referring doctor may refer a patient to a specialist. **The Medical Manager** system automatically assigns the next available doctor number.*

Physicians often refer their patients to other doctors who specialize in the treatment of certain conditions or diseases. For example, a family physician would probably refer an individual with a broken arm to an orthopedic specialist. A patient with heart problems would be referred to a cardiologist.

The Referring Doctor File adds, modifies, or deletes the names of referring doctors. It informs the practice of how many current patients were referred by each referring doctor.

APPLYING YOUR KNOWLEDGE

EXERCISE 7: Adding a Referring Doctor

You will now enter a new referring doctor. If you are not currently in the Referring Doctor Maintenance screen, press **ESCAPE** or use the mouse pointer to click on the EXIT button at the right edge of the top toolbar until you return to the Main Menu (Menu 1).

Using the keyboard or the mouse, select option **7**, FILE Maintenance, then option **3**, SUPPORT File Maintenance. When the menu appears, select option **7** for the REFERRING DOCTOR File. The Referring Doctor Maintenance screen shown previously in Figure 1-20 appears.

STEP 1

Information about several referring doctors is already entered in your system. Key '**0**' to add a new referring doctor and press **ENTER**. The question, "Do You Wish to Open New Referring Doctor? (Y/N)" will appear. Answer '**Y**'. **Do not enter a number here yourself because The Medical Manager system will automatically assign the next available doctor number.**

STEP 2   Enter the last name of the doctor, '**Summerfield MD**.' To include degrees such as M.D. or D.O., you should put them in the Last Name field as shown above (i.e., "Summerfield MD"). Note that the last name field is not long enough to enter 'M.D.' so you must enter only 'MD.' Now key the first name, '**Justine**,' and press **ENTER** before entering the middle initial, '**A**.'

STEP 3   Press **ENTER** to advance to the next field and enter the street address '**3434 Alafaya Trail Blvd**' **and** press **ENTER**. At the secondary address field prompt, enter '**Suite 2000**' then press **ENTER**. At the city, or zip code field, press the Home key or click on the Help button ('?') on the top toolbar to invoke a Help window for this field. Press the down arrow key and then **ENTER** or use the mouse pointer to double-click and select the first listing for '**Madison, CA**.' The city, state, and zip will automatically be completed for you.

STEP 4   Press **ENTER** twice to skip to the e-mail field and advance to the next field. Key the telephone number '**9167655347**.' Remember that because this field is self-formatting, this will appear as 916-765-5347 when ENTER is pressed. Press **ENTER** to skip the Phone Extension field.

STEP 5   Key the telephone number '**9167655346**' into the fax telephone number field. Press **ENTER** through the remaining telephone numbers and extensions until your cursor is in the Doctor ID field.

STEP 6   Enter the doctor ID '**872-02-0283**' and press **ENTER**. At the 2nd ID prompt, enter '**MD-7293-0293-0**' and press **ENTER**. Remember to key hyphens in ID numbers when you need to use them.

STEP 7   Skip each of the remaining fields by pressing **ENTER** at each one. Your completed screen should be similar to Figure 1-24. You may use the arrow keys or the mouse to return to any previous field, and you may use the editing keys shown in Figure 1-14 to make any corrections. When all of the data matches, process the screen by pressing the **F1** key or by clicking on the PROCESS button ('√') on the top toolbar.

Figure 1-24 Completed Referring Doctor Maintenance Screen

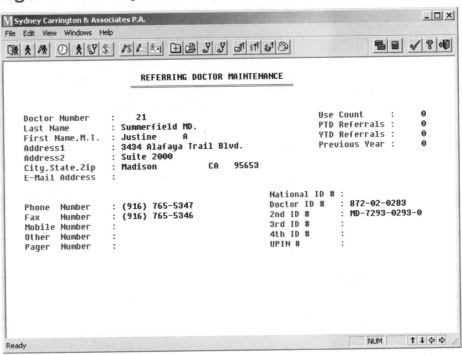

SUPPORT FILES

Support files provide a convenient way of standardizing data about events within the practice, as well as across the health care industry. They provide a way to enter a short code instead of typing a long description. This reduces errors and speeds up entry of routine data.

In addition to the Referring Doctors file that was previously discussed, **The Medical Manager** system maintains several other important support files. In most practices these files will already be set up for you by the administrators who originally set up **The Medical Manager** system. Although you will not usually be called on to create these files, a good understanding of their contents and purposes will help you because you will use the information from the support files in nearly every exercise in this text-workbook.

Procedure Codes

Procedure codes identify each service or treatment performed.

Physicians' Current Procedural Terminology, Fourth Edition (CPT-4), established in 1966 by the American Medical Association, is a standard medical coding system used by insurance carriers and medical offices to provide a uniform code to accurately describe and identify the services, procedures, and treatments performed for patients by the medical staff. These codes, the name of the procedure or service, the fee for each service, and other related information can be stored in **The Medical Manager** system for repetitive use.

Procedure codes are entered at the Support Files Maintenance Menu.

For example, almost every patient who visits the medical office will be charged for a patient visit. The procedure code for this will range from 99201 through 99215, depending on the complexity of the examination and the amount of time spent with the patient. By entering the procedure code, for example, 99213, the fee for the service, and the description "Office Visit" into the computer in advance, you can quickly record this information for every patient who is treated. This eliminates the need for rekeying the entire description. Insurance claim departments review procedure codes carefully to determine that the charge for each procedure identified by the code is fair and standard.

Diagnosis Codes

Diagnosis codes identify the medical condition.

Diagnosis codes are used to identify illnesses and diseases. The most common diagnosis codes are the ICD-9-CM codes contained in the books *International Classification of Diseases, 9th Edition, Clinical Modification*, which are available from the American Medical Association. The codes themselves are developed and maintained by the World Health Association, an agency of the United Nations.

Medicare, Medicaid, Blue Cross/Blue Shield, and most private insurance plans require diagnosis codes on their claim forms. Use diagnosis codes on all claim forms for faster processing and quicker payment. The first three digits of an ICD-9 code identify the primary diagnosis, and any additional digits define the diagnosis area further.

A diagnosis code on a claim form is important because the insurance carrier needs to validate the reason for treatment before the doctor will be reimbursed. In addition, procedure codes and diagnosis codes must be matched correctly, or a claim may be delayed or returned unpaid.

Insurance Plan Information

Insurance plans reference the insurance company's billing location and rules.

Health insurance companies pay the major portion of many physicians' fees; therefore, medical offices should have complete information about a patient's health insurance carrier, including the name, the location of the insurance plan, the telephone number, and related information.

Because some insurance carriers offer several different plans, **The Medical Manager** system permits multiple plans to be set up for each carrier. These can be different address locations, or different fee, profile, or billing arrangements. Plans can be managed care plans or fee-for-service plans.

Service Facility Information

Service facilities refer to the place where treatment was performed.

Information about all medical facilities where the physician treats or consults patients should be stored in **The Medical Manager** software. Service Facility Information can be viewed or changed by accessing the Service Facility File, which is option 4 on the Support Files Maintenance Menu (Menu 13).

APPLYING YOUR KNOWLEDGE

EXERCISE 8: Printing Support File Reports

A report of each of the support files can be generated automatically by **The Medical Manager** software and printed for easy office reference. In this section, you will print reports for each of the files that have been discussed. The Support File Report Menu (Menu 14) includes the eleven types of reports listed below.

1. Procedure Code Report
2. Diagnostic Code Report
3. Insurance Plan Report
4. Service Facility Report
5. Doctor/Practice Report
6. Insured Party Report
7. Referring Doctor Report
8. Ailment Report
9. Profile/Fee Set-Up Reports
10. Translation Table Report
11. Standing Orders Report

Follow the steps below to print Support Files Reports.

STEP 1   Return to the Support Files Maintenance Menu (Menu 13). If you are at some other menu, press **ESCAPE** or click the EXIT button on the top toolbar until you reach the Main Menu (Menu 1). Using the keyboard or mouse, select option **7**, FILE Maintenance, then option **3**, SUPPORT File Maintenance. Then, select option **12**, REPORTS of Support Files. The screen shown in Figure 1-25 will appear.

STEP 2   Enter '**2**' for the DIAGNOSTIC Code Report. The screen shown in Figure 1-26 will appear.

STEP 3   The defaults for the choices shown in this screen are (C)onsole, (C)ode, and (A)ll. Select the default options by pressing **ENTER** at each of these three fields, then press **F1** or click the PROCESS button ('√') on the top toolbar to process. Compare the Diagnosis Code Report shown in Figure 1-27 with your screen, which should be similar.

Figure 1-25 Support File Report Menu Screen

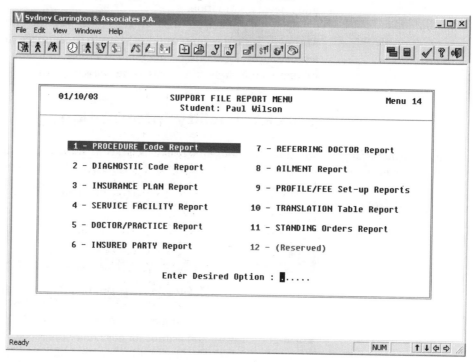

Figure 1-26 Diagnosis Code Report Selection Screen

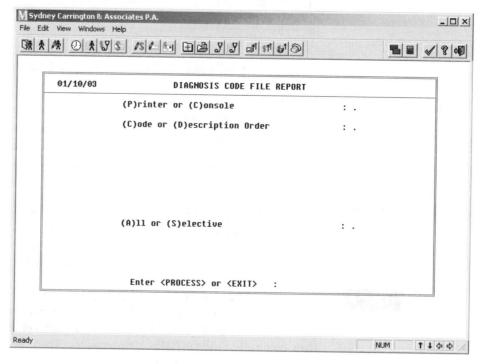

STEP 4

Make sure your printer is on, has paper in it, and is online. Press **ESCAPE** twice OR using the mouse, click the EXIT button on the toolbar two times. You will run the Diagnosis Code Report again. However, this time key '**P**' for (P)rinter and press **ENTER** for each of the other defaults. When **F1** is pressed or the PROCESS button ('√') is

Figure 1-27 Diagnosis Report by Code on the Console

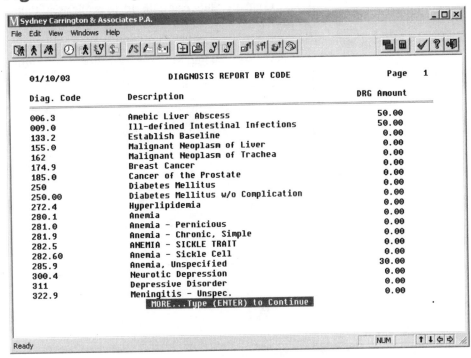

clicked on the top toolbar, the report will be sent to the printer instead of your screen. Check your work carefully as a comparison screen is not provided.

Note: This procedure will be used often in the following units.

EXERCISE 9: Printing Additional Support File Reports

To apply further the knowledge you have gained so far in this unit, you will print reports that will be handed in to your instructor. Follow the instructions carefully and check your work against the figures provided. Remember that reports of Support Files can be requested from the Support Files Report Menu (Menu 14) as many times as you like; so if you make a mistake you have the option of starting over. Note that the following steps are used repeatedly to generate each of the reports you would like to print.

STEP 1   Return to the Support Files Maintenance Menu (Menu 13). If you are at some other menu, you may press ESCAPE or click the EXIT button on the top toolbar until you reach the Main Menu (Menu 1). Then, using the keyboard or mouse, select option **7**, FILE Maintenance, then option **3**, SUPPORT File Maintenance.

STEP 2   Select option **12**, REPORTS of Support Files. From the Support File Report Menu (Menu 14), select one of the following report options and choose the options indicated in bold. Don't forget to press **F1** or click the PROCESS button ('√') on the top toolbar to process and your selected report will be generated.

Note: Pressing ENTER after each of your reports is generated should return you to the Support File Report Menu (Menu 14) so you can complete the remainder of the exercise.

Print one copy of the Insurance Plan Report, the Service Facility Report, the Doctor/Practice Report, and the Referring Doctor Report using the options shown in the following list. Your printouts should be similar to those shown in Figures 1-28 to 1-31. Compare your printouts to these figures, then hand the reports in to your instructor.

INSURANCE PLAN Report	(**P**)rinter	(**S**)ummary	(**A**)lphabetic	(**A**)ll
SERVICE FACILITY Report	(**P**)rinter	(**A**)ll	(**A**)lphabetic	(**A**)ll
DOCTOR/PRACTICE Report	(**P**)rinter	(**N**)umeric	(**A**)ll	
REFERRING DOCTOR Report	(**P**)rinter	(**N**)umeric	(**A**)ll	

Figure 1-28 Insurance Plan Report

```
01/10/03                        INSURANCE PLAN REPORT BY NAME                    Page    1
                                   Student: Paul Wilson
                                       All Entries
     Plan Info                   Address                 Phone Numbers
     =========================================================================================================
CHAMP  Champus                   Active Duty & Dependents   Voice: (800) 552-6612   Managed : N   Use Count : 0
   3   Champus                   1210 HARBOR DRIVE          Fax  :                  Program : 7   Assignment: Y
       Class: UB    Plan :       Washington, DC 17654-1210  Elig.:                  Form # : 1    Format # : 1

CHAMP  Champus                   Veterans Administration    Voice: (800) 552-6612   Managed : N   Use Count : 0
   4   Champus-VA                1210 HARBOR DRIVE          Fax  :                  Program : 7   Assignment: Y
       Class: UB    Plan :       Washington, DC 17654-1210  Elig.:                  Form # : 1    Format # : 1

CASA   Cross and Shield Plans                               Voice: (800) 345-7689   Managed : N   Use Count : 0
   6   Cross and Shield Ins Plan 435 Embarcadero            Fax  : (916) 345-1508   Program : 6   Assignment: Y
       Class: EMC   Plan :       Madison, CA 95653          Elig.:                  Form # : 1    Format # : 1

EMPTRU Employees Trust Insurance Workmans Comp Claim Dept.  Voice: (312) 456-7865   Managed : N   Use Count : 0
   8   Employees Trust Insurance 3 Carnation Drive          Fax  :                  Program : 7   Assignment: Y
       Class: WC    Plan :       Chicago, IL 60540          Elig.:                  Form # : 1    Format # : 1

EPSLON Epsilon Life & Casualty                              Voice: (800) 908-7654   Managed : N   Use Count : 0
   5   Epsilon Life & Casualty   P.O. Box 189               Fax  :                  Program : 7   Assignment: Y
       Class: EMC   Plan :       Macon, GA 31298            Elig.:                  Form # : 1    Format # : 1

FRGBEN Fringe Benefit Center                                Voice: (800) 999-1234   Managed : N   Use Count : 0
  12   Fringe Benefit Center     123 Mission Corners        Fax  :                  Program : 7   Assignment: Y
       Class:       Plan :       San Mateo, TX 78723        Elig.:                  Form # : 1    Format # : 1

HMO1   Health Maint. Org.        Provider Benefit Plan      Voice: (800) 999-1234   Managed : P   Use Count : 0
  11   Health Maint. Org.        6632 3rd Avenue            Fax  :                  Program : 7   Assignment: Y
       Class: HMO   Plan :       New York, NY 10017         Elig.:                  Form # : 1    Format # : 1

MEDCAL Medi-Cal Insurance                                   Voice: (415) 987-0987   Managed : N   Use Count : 0
   1   Medicaid Insurance        123 Capitol Street         Fax  :                  Program : 1   Assignment: Y
       Class: EMC   Plan :       Sacramento, CA 94056       Elig.:                  Form # : 1    Format # : 1

MEDI   Medicare                  Claims Dept - Box 443A     Voice: (800) 879-6789   Managed : N   Use Count : 0
   2   Medicare                  760 University Street      Fax  : (315) 222-1001   Program : 2   Assignment: Y
       Class: EMC   Plan :       Washington, DC 17654-1234  Elig.: (800) 879-4000   Form # : 1    Format # : 1

MEDIP  Medicare Plus                                        Voice: (800) 675-4354   Managed : N   Use Count : 0
  10   Medicare Plus             34567 Arvor Ave.           Fax  :                  Program : 7   Assignment: Y
       Class: HMO   Plan :       Madison, CA 95653          Elig.:                  Form # : 1    Format # : 1

PANAMC Pan American Health Ins.                             Voice: (213) 456-7654   Managed : N   Use Count : 0
   7   Pan American Health Ins.  4567 Newberry Rd.          Fax  :                  Program : 7   Assignment: Y
       Class:       Plan :       Los Angeles, CA 98706      Elig.:                  Form # : 1    Format # : 1

BENIND Beneficial Industrial Co. Attn. J. Jones            Voice: (800) 654-2323   Managed : N   Use Count : 0
   9   Worker's Compensation     4567 Main Street           Fax  :                  Program : 7   Assignment: Y
       Class: WC    Plan :       Floral City, CA 94064      Elig.:                  Form # : 1    Format # : 1


                        ****  Number Printed : 12  ****
                        ****  Number Active  : 12  ****
```

Figure 1-29a Service Facility Report, Page 1 of 2

```
01/10/03              SERVICE FACILITY REPORT BY NAME          Page    1
                          Student: Paul Wilson

No.      Service Facility                    Identification Numbers
=============================================================================
   6     Blood & Plasma Center               ID 1: 23-4493982
         47554 N.W. 34th Street              ID 2:
         Madison, CA 95653                   ID 3:
         Type  : L [Lab]                     ID 4:
                                             ID 5:
                                             NatID:


   7     Childrens Hospital                  ID 1: CA2832-23890283
         900 Sand Hill Road                  ID 2: .
         Madison, CA 95653                   ID 3:
         Type  : H [Hospital]                ID 4:
                                             ID 5:
                                             NatID:


  11     Doctors Laboratory                  ID 1:
         11445 W. Tennison                   ID 2:
         Madison, CA 95653                   ID 3:
         Type  : L [Lab]                     ID 4:
                                             ID 5:
                                             NatID:


  10     Jefferson Memorial Hosp.            ID 1:
         11556 NW Easter Ave.                ID 2:
         Madison, CA 95653                   ID 3:
         Type  : H [Hospital]                ID 4:
                                             ID 5:
                                             NatID:


  15     Lakeland Services                   ID 1: 74843422
         762 Alamedia Way                    ID 2:
         Lake Land, Ca 95693                 ID 3:
         Phone : (916) 555-6666              ID 4:
         Fax   : (916) 555-7788              ID 5:
         Modem : (916) 555-7789              NatID:
         Type  : L [Lab]


   9     Madison Central Surgery             ID 1:
         11556 W. University Ave.            ID 2:
         Madison, CA 95653                   ID 3:
         Type  : H [Hospital]                ID 4:
                                             ID 5:
                                             NatID:


   1     Madison Convalescent Home           ID 1: 3459865
         34 Sycamore  Suite 100              ID 2:
         Madison, CA 95653                   ID 3:
         Type  : S [Not Found]               ID 4:
                                             ID 5:
                                             NatID:
```

Figure 1-29b Service Facility Report, Page 2 of 2

```
01/10/03              SERVICE FACILITY REPORT BY NAME              Page    2
                          Student: Paul Wilson

No.        Service Facility                      Identification Numbers
================================================================================
  2        Madison General Hospital             ID 1: CA24556-69029
           3456 Grant Road                      ID 2: HSP1112328
           Madison, CA 95653                    ID 3:
           Type  : H [Hospital]                 ID 4:
                                                ID 5:
                                                NatID:


  8        Madison Surgery Center               ID 1:
           25334 SW 1st Ave.                    ID 2:
           Madison, CA 95653-0235               ID 3:
           Type  : H [Hospital]                 ID 4:
                                                ID 5:
                                                NatID:


 12        MetLab Services                      ID 1:
           5850 W. Cypress St.                  ID 2:
           Madison, CA 95653                    ID 3:
           Phone : (800) 282-6695               ID 4:
           Type  : L [Lab]                      ID 5: Lab Demo
                                                NatID:


  5        Miramonte Nursing & Rest             ID 1: R23-475759399
           76543 EL Monte Ave                   ID 2:
           Madison, CA 95653                    ID 3:
           Type  : S [Not Found]                ID 4:
                                                ID 5:
                                                NatID:


  4        Regional Hosp. of Madison            ID 1: CA02934E2E32
           675 Sand Hill Road                   ID 2:
           Madison, CA 95653                    ID 3:
           Type  : H [Hospital]                 ID 4:
                                                ID 5:
                                                NatID:


  3        Resource Laboratory                  ID 1: 44-0202
           4567 Anderson                        ID 2: 9876893AA
           Madison, CA 95653                    ID 3:
           Type  : L [Lab]                      ID 4:
                                                ID 5: Lab Damon
                                                NatID:


 13        Vista Trauma Institute               ID 1: E63892
           581 S. W. 80rd Avenue                ID 2: MNAX-338100-A
           Madison, CA 95653-0609               ID 3:
           Phone : (916) 555-7231               ID 4:
           Fax   : (916) 555-2190               ID 5:
           Modem : (916) 555-2191               NatID:
           Type  : H [Hospital]


 14        Westside Convalescence               ID 1: WC1577554
           West Oak Boulevard                   ID 2: WstConv
           Woodside, CA 98076                   ID 3:
           Phone : (916) 555-8129               ID 4:
           Fax   : (916) 555-8128               ID 5:
           Modem : (916) 555-8127               NatID:
           Type  : S [Not Found]



                   ****  Number Printed : 15  ****
                   ****  Number Active  : 15  ****
```

Figure 1-30a Doctor/Practice Report, Page 1 of 2

```
01/10/03                           DOCTOR/PRACTICE REPORT BY NUMBER                        Page    1
                                          Student: Paul Wilson
                                              All Entries
Dr. No.   Name/Address                 Identification Numbers
===================================================================================================
                                                                      UPIN #           :
   0      Student: Paul Wilson
          34 Sycamore St. Suite 300    Social Sec. No.  : 345-67-9865  Other ID No. 1  :
          Madison, Ca. 95653           National ID No.  :              Other ID No. 2  :
                                       Employer ID No.  : 988765R      Other ID No. 3  :
          (916) 398-7654               State ID No.     : 12345678952-13 Other ID No. 4 :
                                       Medicaid ID No.  : 45643         Other ID No. 5  :
          Class      : A               Wrk. Comp. ID No.: 8765987
          Department : 0               Blue Cross ID No.: 4356987
          Fin. Group : 0               Medicare ID No.  : 4356987
          Secur. Grp.: 0
          Location   :
          User ID    : 0
          Ref. Dr. # : 0



                                                                      UPIN #           : 4432094A
   1      Monroe MD, James T
          11554 Woodside Lane          Social Sec. No.  : 456-78-9065  Other ID No. 1  :
          Madison, CA 95653            National ID No.  :              Other ID No. 2  :
                                       Employer ID No.  : 908768900    Other ID No. 3  :
          (916) 987-6543               State ID No.     : 34565        Other ID No. 4  :
                                       Medicaid ID No.  : 2327656778   Other ID No. 5  : 4000000423
          Class      : A               Wrk. Comp. ID No.: 434565-23
          Department : 0               Blue Cross ID No.: 466778       Fee Schedule #        : 1    [Standard Fee]
          Fin. Group : 1               Medicare ID No.  : 466778       Medicare Override Fee# : 0
          Secur. Grp.: 1                                               Medi Override Profile # : 0
          Location   :                                                 Supervisor: N
          User ID    : 0
          Ref. Dr. # : 0               E-Mail Address   :
                                       Default Specialty:



                                                                      UPIN #           :
   2      Simpson M.D., Frances D
          675 Hidden Hill Court        Social Sec. No.  : 234-56-7643  Other ID No. 1  :
          Madison, CA 95653            National ID No.  :              Other ID No. 2  :
                                       Employer ID No.  : 12143454657  Other ID No. 3  :
          (916) 867-7799               State ID No.     : 34355        Other ID No. 4  :
                                       Medicaid ID No.  : 1334455-67   Other ID No. 5  :
          Class      : A               Wrk. Comp. ID No.: 235466
          Department : 0               Blue Cross ID No.: 235685       Fee Schedule #        : 1    [Standard Fee]
          Fin. Group : 1               Medicare ID No.  : 235685       Medicare Override Fee# : 0
          Secur. Grp.: 1                                               Medi Override Profile # : 0
          Location   :                                                 Supervisor: N
          User ID    : 0
          Ref. Dr. # : 0               E-Mail Address   :
                                       Default Specialty:
```

Figure 1-30b Doctor/Practice Report, Page 2 of 2

```
Dr. No.   Name/Address              Identification Numbers
=====================================================================================================================
   3      Carrington M.D., Sydney J                                            UPIN #           : 55724033A
          890 Elise River Rd.       Social Sec. No.  : 345-67-9865             Other ID No. 1   :
          Madison, CA 95653         National ID No.  :                         Other ID No. 2   :
                                    Employer ID No.  : 9088765R                Other ID No. 3   :
          (916) 948-7654            State ID No.     : 123678952-13            Other ID No. 4   :
                                    Medicaid ID No.  : 45643                   Other ID No. 5   : 5647382910
          Class     : A             Wrk. Comp. ID No.: 8765987
          Department : 0            Blue Cross ID No.: 435678                   Fee Schedule #         : 1     [Standard Fee]
          Fin. Group : 2            Medicare ID No.  : 435678                   Medicare Override Fee# : 0
          Secur. Grp.: 2                                                       Medi Override Profile # : 0
          Location  :                                                          Supervisor: N
          User ID    : 0            E-Mail Address   :
          Ref. Dr. # : 0            Default Specialty:


   4      Shiller, RPT, Sandra A                                               UPIN #           :
          405 Thayer St. #4         Social Sec. No.  : 908-67-5432             Other ID No. 1   :
          Madison, CA 95653         National ID No.  :                         Other ID No. 2   :
                                    Employer ID No.  :                         Other ID No. 3   :
          (916) 696-5607            State ID No.     :                         Other ID No. 4   :
                                    Medicaid ID No.  :                         Other ID No. 5   :
          Class     : B             Wrk. Comp. ID No.:
          Department : 0            Blue Cross ID No.:                         Fee Schedule #         : 1     [Standard Fee]
          Fin. Group : 1            Medicare ID No.  :                         Medicare Override Fee# : 0
          Secur. Grp.: 1                                                       Medi Override Profile # : 0
          Location  :                                                          Supervisor: N
          User ID    : 0            E-Mail Address   :
          Ref. Dr. # : 0            Default Specialty:




                              ****   Number Printed : 5  ****
                              ****   Number Active  : 5  ****
```

Figure 1-31a Referring Doctor Report—All entries, Page 1 of 3

```
                              Student: Paul Wilson
                                 All Entries
Dr#   Name/Address             Phone Numbers              ID Numbers             Referrals
============================================================================================

  1  Barrett M.D.,David M      Phone : (916) 678-3324     ID1: 567-42-2200       PTD:     0
     2345 Emerson Street       Fax   :                   ID2: 1393216MS         YTD:     1
     Suite M                   Mobile:                    ID3:                   Prev Yr: 0
     Madison, CA 95653         Other :                    ID4:
                               Pager :                    UPIN:
                                                          Nat ID:


  2  Groves M.D.,Leland W      Phone : (916) 678-9012     ID1: M10033-44556-A    PTD:     0
     Madison Medical Group     Fax   :                   ID2:                   YTD:     0
     Suite 710                 Mobile:                    ID3:                   Prev Yr: 0
     Madison, CA 95653         Other :                    ID4:
                               Pager :                    UPIN:
                                                          Nat ID:


  3  Fredericks M.D.,Lucinda A Phone : (916) 908-3321     ID1: 367-44-5832       PTD:     0
     90 W Camelia Way          Fax   :                   ID2: 8946M8:659        YTD:     0
     Suite 101                 Mobile:                    ID3:                   Prev Yr: 0
     Madison, CA 95653         Other :                    ID4:
                               Pager :                    UPIN:
                                                          Nat ID:


  4  Detrasnik M.D.,Jason K    Phone : (916) 765-7898     ID1: 642-73-6576       PTD:     0
     78 Bayshore Dr.           Fax   :                   ID2: 752774678         YTD:     4
     Suite B                   Mobile:                    ID3:                   Prev Yr: 0
     Madisonville, CA 95653    Other :                    ID4:
                               Pager :                    UPIN:
                                                          Nat ID:


  5  Shelton M.D,James C       Phone : (916) 294-1010     ID1: 1089203           PTD:     0
     130 S. Prairie Dr         Fax   :                   ID2:                   YTD:     0
                               Mobile:                    ID3:                   Prev Yr: 0
     Woodside, CA 95653        Other :                    ID4:
                               Pager :                    UPIN: 102983745000
                                                          Nat ID:


  6  Johnson M.D.,Katrina L    Phone : (916) 230-7392     ID1: 234-62-9010       PTD:     0
     1983 Lane Dr              Fax   :                   ID2: SL45000           YTD:     0
                               Mobile:                    ID3:                   Prev Yr: 0
     Floral City, CA 95653     Other :                    ID4:
                               Pager :                    UPIN:
                                                          Nat ID:


  7  Shelton M.D.,Guy R        Phone : (916) 290-2987     ID1: 232-98-1919       PTD:     0
     P.O.Box 1209              Fax   :                   ID2:                   YTD:     0
                               Mobile:                    ID3:                   Prev Yr: 0
     Woodside, CA 95653        Other :                    ID4:
                               Pager :                    UPIN:
                                                          Nat ID:


  8  Wilson M.D.,Linda T       Phone : (916) 230-7392     ID1: 237-81-4321       PTD:     0
     1983 Lane Dr              Fax   :                   ID2: SL54000           YTD:     0
                               Mobile:                    ID3:                   Prev Yr: 0
     Floral City, CA 95653     Other :                    ID4:
                               Pager :                    UPIN:
                                                          Nat ID:
```

Figure .1-31b Referring Doctor Report—All entries, Page 2 of 3

Dr#	Name/Address	Phone Numbers	ID Numbers	Referrals	
9	Smith D.C.,Anthony J 1071 North Gate Blvd Suite 5000 Los Angeles, CA 98706	Phone : (917) 765-5678 Fax : Mobile: Other : Pager :	ID1: 1209735 ID2: MD-344-9378-0 ID3: ID4: UPIN: Nat ID:	PTD: YTD: Prev Yr:	0 0 0
10	Stevenson M.D.,Roger K 904 Dew Drop Cove Suite 300 Sacramento, CA 94056	Phone : (845) 763-5823 Fax : Mobile: Other : Pager :	ID1: 303860378 ID2: MD-234-7364-1 ID3: ID4: UPIN: 92019 Nat ID:	PTD: YTD: Prev Yr:	0 0 0
11	Roberts M.D.,John M 527 Playa Linda Ave Suite A Woodside, CA 98076	Phone : (834) 739-2831 Fax : Mobile: Other : Pager :	ID1: 65358462 ID2: MD-736-0380-1 ID3: ID4: UPIN: Nat ID:	PTD: YTD: Prev Yr:	0 0 0
12	Roohzrock M.D.,Bahman P 8260 Palmetto Dr. Suite A Floral City, CA 94064	Phone : (409) 639-8838 Fax : Mobile: Other : Pager :	ID1: 124589-01 ID2: MD-123-3456-1 ID3: ID4: UPIN: Nat ID:	PTD: YTD: Prev Yr:	0 0 0
13	Johnson M.D.,James J 1290 Paloma Place Suite C Madison, CA 95653-0235	Phone : (917) 128-6393 Fax : Mobile: Other : Pager :	ID1: 8269873 ID2: MD-798-9128-9 ID3: ID4: UPIN: Nat ID:	PTD: YTD: Prev Yr:	0 0 0
14	Karlson D.C.,Richard T 717 S.W. 17th Terrace Chicago, IL 60540	Phone : (536) 787-3682 Fax : Mobile: Other : Pager :	ID1: 6538710-1 ID2: MD-2830-8367 ID3: ID4: UPIN: Nat ID:	PTD: YTD: Prev Yr:	0 0 0
15	Costello M.D.,Ramona L 8973 Belle Isle Dr Suite 1 Madison, CA 95653-0609	Phone : (407) 653-4022 Fax : Mobile: Other : Pager :	ID1: 73689-01 ID2: MS-8364-001 ID3: ID4: UPIN: Nat ID:	PTD: YTD: Prev Yr:	0 0 0
16	Mcallister M.D.,Lynne 901 N. Main Street Suite 2 San Mateo, TX 78723	Phone : (536) 702-3932 Fax : Mobile: Other : Pager :	ID1: MD-A0192-102 ID2: ID3: ID4: UPIN: Nat ID:	PTD: YTD: Prev Yr:	0 0 0

Figure 1-31c Referring Doctor Report—All entries, Page 3 of 3

```
01/10/03                         REFERRING DOCTOR REPORT BY NUMBER                        Page    3
                                      Student: Paul Wilson
                                          All Entries
     Dr#   Name/Address                Phone Numbers              ID Numbers              Referrals
     ================================================================================================
     17   Vizcarrondo M.D,Rosalyn M    Phone : (524) 820-2778     ID1: 123-76-9836        PTD:      0
          1053 Galleria Blvd           Fax   :                    ID2: MD-023-8265-0      YTD:      0
          Suite 15                     Mobile:                    ID3:                    Prev Yr:  0
          Sacramento, CA 94056         Other :                    ID4:
                                       Pager :                    UPIN:
                                                                  Nat ID:

     18   Bennett M.D.,Thomas H        Phone : (901) 876-2891     ID1: 920-09-0921        PTD:      0
          708 Floral Street            Fax   :                    ID2: MD-828-9102-02     YTD:      0
          Suite F                      Mobile:                    ID3:                    Prev Yr:  0
          Floral City, CA 94064        Other :                    ID4:
                                       Pager :                    UPIN:
                                                                  Nat ID:

     19   Summerfield M.D,Horrace J    Phone : (916) 765-5347     ID1: 999-32-0881        PTD:      0
          3434 Alafaya Trail Blvd      Fax   :                    ID2: MD-6743-1225-0     YTD:      0
          Suite 2000                   Mobile:                    ID3:                    Prev Yr:  0
          Madison, CA 95653            Other :                    ID4:
                                       Pager :                    UPIN:
                                                                  Nat ID:

     20   Bardsley M.D.,Richard M      Phone : (916) 635-8483     ID1: 873-98-0932        PTD:      0
          9384 E. University Ave       Fax   :                    ID2: MS-0238-923        YTD:      0
          Suite 13                     Mobile:                    ID3:                    Prev Yr:  0
          Madison, CA 95653            Other :                    ID4:
                                       Pager :                    UPIN:
                                                                  Nat ID:

     21   Summerfield MD,Justine A     Phone : (916) 765-5347     ID1: 872-02-0283        PTD:      0
          3434 Alafaya Trail Blvd.     Fax   : (916) 765-5346     ID2: MD-7293-0293-0     YTD:      0
          Suite 2000                   Mobile:                    ID3:                    Prev Yr:  0
          Madison, CA 95653            Other :                    ID4:
                                       Pager :                    UPIN:
                                                                  Nat ID:




                            ****  Number Printed : 21  ****
                            ****  Number Active  : 21  ****
```

EXERCISE 10: Printing the Procedure Code Report

All of **The Medical Manager** system reports run basically the same as those printed here. Variations may occur, but the experience gained in this exercise is applicable to other reports of all types in **The Medical Manager** software.

In this exercise, you will print the Procedure Code File Report, which provides several additional report options not shown in the previous reports you printed.

STEP 1   Press **ESCAPE** to return to the Support File Report Menu (Menu 14), key '**1**' and press **ENTER** to select option 1, PROCEDURE Code Report OR use double-click on option 1 to highlight and select it. The screen shown in Figure 1-32 will appear.

STEP 2   Print the Procedure Code Report using the following options:

(**P**)rinter

(**C**)ode Order

Figure 1-32 Procedure Code File Report Selection Screen

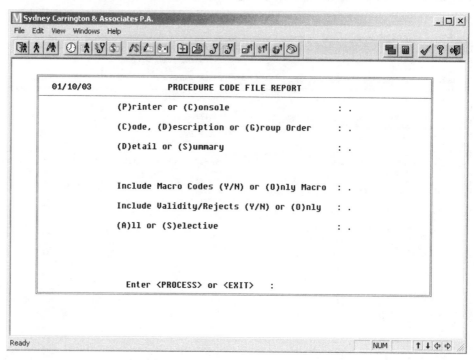

(**S**)ummary

(**Y**) to include macro codes

ENTER to accept default to include Validity/Rejects

(**A**)ll to include all procedure codes

1 to select Profile Fee Schedule

STEP 3

Press **ENTER** three times to accept default responses of 0 for the remaining Profile/Fee Schedule options, then press **F1** to process or click on the PROCESS button ('√') on the top toolbar. Compare your report with Figure 1-33. Hand in your Procedure Code Report By Code to your instructor.

DAILY FILES BACKUP

Backup is performed daily to protect the practice files.

Technical difficulties, power failures, improper key combinations, and a variety of other factors could cause you to lose information stored on your Student Disk. Therefore, you should make a backup copy of your files daily in order to protect your work. Similarly, in a medical office, the office manager makes a backup daily to protect all the practice's files.

Figure 1-33 Procedure Code Report

```
01/10/03                          PROCEDURE REPORT BY CODE                      Page   1
                                     Student: Paul Wilson
                                         All Entries

Srv. Code   Group   Description                                              Standard Fee
==========================================================================================
00452       10      Anesthesia for Radical Surgery                                  37.50
29075       6       Cast Appl.-Lower Arm                                            48.00
29705       6       Removal/Revis of Cast W/Exam                                    38.00
53670       7       Catheterization Including Supplies                              45.00
70210       4       X-Ray Sinuses Complete                                          40.00
71020       4       X-Ray Chest Pa & Lat                                            58.00
72050       4       X-Ray Spine. Cerv (4 views)                                    150.00
72110       4       Spine, lumbosacral' a/p & Lat                                   48.00
75552       4       Cardiac Magnetic Resonance Imaging                           1,500.00
76088       4       Mammary Ductogram Complete                                     125.00
78465       4       MYOCARDIAL PERFUSION IMAGING-SPECT                           2,000.00
81000       4       Urinalysis                                                       8.00
82951       4       Glucose Tolerance Test                                          40.00
84550       4       Uric Acid: Blood Chemistry                                      15.00
85014       4       Hematocrit                                                      18.00
85031       4       Hemogram, Complete Blood Work                                   15.00
87070       4       Culture                                                         31.00
90701       5       Immunization -DTP                                               14.00
90749       5       Immunization - Unlisted                                         12.00
90782       5       Injection - Intramuscular                                       12.00
90843       2       Counseling - 25 Minutes                                         65.00
90844       2       Counseling - 50 Minutes                                        120.00
93000       4       Electrocardiogram                                               57.00
99080       1       Special Reports Of Medical Records                               0.00
99201       1       Office New:Focused Hx-Exam/Strgt-Fw                             25.00
99202       1       Office New:Expanded Hx-Exam/Str-Fwd                             40.00
99211       1       Office Estb:Min/None Hx-Exam/St-Fwd                             25.00
99212       1       Office Estb:Focused Hx-Exam/Str-Fwd                             30.00
99213       1       Office Estb: Expanded Hx-Exam / Low                             40.00
99214       1       Office Estb:Detailed Hx-Exam/Modera                             50.00
99215       1       Office Estb:Comprhn Hx-Exam / High                              85.00
99221       3       Hospital Initial:Comprh Hx-Exam/S-F                             72.00
99223       3       Hospital Initial:Comprh Hx-Exam/ Hi                             94.00
99231       3       Hosp.Subsequent:Comprh Hx-Ex/S-Fwd                             72.00
99232       3       Hosp.Subsequent:Comprhn Hx-Exam/Mod                             94.00
99233       3       Hosp. Subsequent:Comprhn Hx-Exam/Hi                             94.00
99238       3       Hospital Visit Discharge Exam                                   38.00
ADJUST CLM  0       COMPENSATE FOR COLLAPSED CLAIM                                   0.00
ALLER       17      `Allergy                                                         0.00
CARD        17      `Cardiovascular Disease                                          0.00
COPAY       1       Visit Copay                                                      0.00
IMCARD      17      `Internal Medicine - Card Work                                 250.00
MAT         17      `Maternity Care & Delivery                                       0.00
ORTH        17      `Orthopaedic                                                     0.00
PSY         17      `Psychiatry                                                      0.00
RAD         17      `Diagnostic Radiology                                            0.00
SURG        17      `Surgery                                                         0.00


                    ****  Number Printed : 47  ****
```

A backup is a complete copy of the practice's files.

A backup file refers to a floppy disk or tape that contains all the data you have entered about patients, insurance companies, procedures and treatments, appointments, and other related information. In the event of system difficulties, the backup file permits the practice to recover data needed to maintain updated patient records and other important practice-related information.

The Backup Process

To perform a daily backup you must first exit properly out of **The Medical Manager** software. Once you have exited the system, make sure your Student Data Disk is still in the computer's floppy drive and double-click on the Student Backup Icon (Figure 1-34) on your desktop.

Figure 1-34 Student Backup Icon

Follow the instructions shown on the Student Edition Backup window, shown in Figure 1-35, to perform a backup of your data. **The Medical Manager** files containing the work from your exercises will be copied onto the computer.

Figure 1-35 Student Edition Backup Window

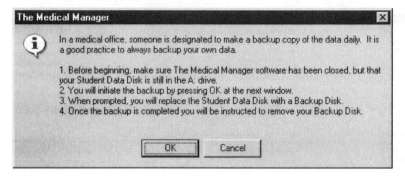

Then, when prompted (Figure 1-36), insert a formatted diskette for backup and the files will be copied onto the backup diskette.

Figure 1-36 Prompt to Insert Backup Disk

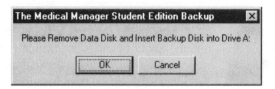

If you forget to remove your Student Data Disk and try to complete the backup process, the message shown in Figure 1-37 will appear. If this occurs, remove your Student Disk, insert your Backup Disk, and click on the 'Retry' button to continue.

Figure 1-37 Incorrect Disk Error Message

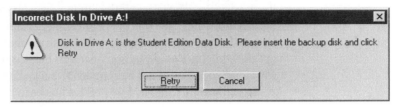

A message, shown in Figure 1-38, will indicate when the backup is complete.

Figure 1-38 Successful Backup Confirmation

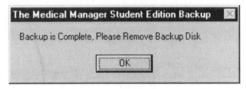

If you get any message indicating that the backup did not complete, reinsert your Student Disk and try again. A second failure may indicate a more serious problem, so notify your instructor immediately if the backup fails on the second try. Failure to maintain current backups could result in having to reenter part or all of your class work.

Returning to the Medical Manager System

When backup is complete, remove the backup disk and, if you plan to log back onto **The Medical Manager** system, reinsert your Student Disk. Then, double-click on **The Medical Manager** icon on your desktop to continue with the next section of the text.

If you forget to remove the backup disk, the following message (as shown in Figure 1-39) will appear:

Figure 1-39 Incorrect Disk Error Message

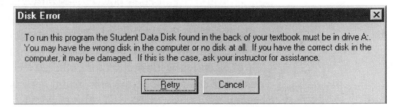

Remove the backup disk you just made, reinsert your Student Disk, and press the 'Retry' button to return to **The Medical Manager** system.

Canceling the Backup Routine

If you accidentally clicked on the Student backup icon and did not intend to do a backup, you may cancel the Daily Files Backup by clicking on the 'Cancel' button on the dialog box that appears. See Figure 1-35 for an example of the 'Cancel' option. You should not click on the 'Cancel' button once you have begun the Backup process because this will cause your files to not be completely backed up.

To confirm that the Backup process has been cancelled, the figure shown in Figure 1-40 will appear.

Figure 1-40 Operation Cancelled Message

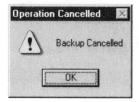

To cancel the Backup process, click 'OK' and you will be returned to the desktop.

FATAL ERROR MESSAGES

Always back up your work.

Fatal errors indicate that something is wrong with the data you are using with your program. If you ever see a message that says "Fatal Error," write down the complete message and contact your instructor immediately. Your instructor has access to a "hotline" telephone number where an individual can be reached to correct a problem. **Do not continue working if you get a Fatal Error Message**.

The most common fatal errors students encounter are:

114: Unexpected Language Level Error

115: Unexpected B-Tree Error

143: Synchronization Error in Log-On File

The most common cause of these errors is shutting off the computer or removing your Student Disk before you have properly exited **The Medical Manager** system. Errors can also be caused by power going off while you are working. In either case, this can cause data to be only partially written, or copied, to the disk. The fatal error message is the way in which **The Medical Manager** software detects and reports to you that the data may not have been complete when the system was shut off.

If these errors occur in a doctor's office, a technician is sent in to repair the files. In a classroom environment, the most usual remedy will be for your instructor to restore a backup disk for you to work on. Therefore, it is very important to prevent these errors by always exiting **The Medical Manager** system correctly before you shut off the computer. As a safety measure, it is very important to perform the backup process (described earlier) every time you use your Student Disk.

UNIT 1 SUMMARY

Information flow in a physician's office usually begins with the patient scheduling an appointment and concludes, at the end of the patient visit, with the patient making arrangements for payment or scheduling a return appointment, or both.

The scheduling of appointments in the physician's office is important because if too many appointments are made for the same time, the doctor's schedule will become overloaded and patients will be inconvenienced by having to wait. If too few patients are scheduled in time slots, the doctor will not be able to make productive use of the day.

An *encounter form* is a printed list of the most common procedures and treatments performed by the doctor. An encounter form serves as a communication device between the doctor and the front office and is typically generated the night before the patient's appointment. Another step that is usually taken the night before or the day of the patient's appointment is verification of insurance eligibility. This is to ensure that the patient's insurance coverage is in effect.

Many of the patients seen in the physician's office will have at least a portion of their health care cost paid by an insurance program. These insurance programs may be private health insurance; employer sponsored health insurance; managed care programs; or government programs such as Medicare, Medicaid, and Tricare. Managed care programs are also called Health Maintenance Organizations (HMO's). In a managed care program, a patient usually pays a small copay with the remainder of the costs covered by the HMO plan. In turn, the patient is usually restricted to visiting only physicians who are participating with the HMO. Some HMO plans assign each patient to a primary care physician (PCP) who they must see in order to receive a referral to a specialist.

Regardless of the type of insurance coverage, most physician practices receive the larger portion of their revenue from the patient's insurance and a smaller portion from the patient. The amount the patient pays is sometimes called the patient copay amount. Physicians who participate in managed care plans may receive payment in advance from the HMO as a monthly capitation. However, physician payments from government and private insurance plans are a result of the physician's office billing the insurance company.

Computers are widely used in physician's practices for insurance billing, patient accounting, record keeping, and appointment scheduling, as well as for electronic medical records such as laboratory orders and results, prescription writing, and word processing.

The Medical Manager software is a sophisticated computer program that helps the practice manage every aspect of scheduling, billing, and medical records. In this course, you will learn to use **The Medical Manager** software, and more about the routine medical office functions such as working with patients, filing insurance claims, and maintaining up-to-date records.

You will start **The Medical Manager** system by clicking on **The Medical Manager** icon on your desktop. When logging into the system, you will provide the User **#1** and the Password '**ICAN.**' Once you have successfully logged in, the Main Menu (Menu 1) will be displayed. You can navigate through **The Medical Manager** software using the menu system by keying a menu item number or moving the lightbar and pressing ENTER. You may also move through **The Medical Manager** by using short mnemonics called *direct chain commands*. A table of these commands is provided on the Quick Reference Guide (located at the back of this book.)

In addition to navigating **The Medical Manager** software, you will find a number of useful features that help speed data entry and reduce the amount of work. These include on-screen Help windows that appear when you enter a '?' in a field, pop-up calculators that let you perform mathematical calculations and store the value in a numeric field, and pop-up calendars that appear when you press a question mark in a date field. **The Medical Manager** also uses an extensive array of support files.

When information is stored in **The Medical Manager** software, it is stored in files. Support files are typically codified information that will be used many times throughout the day in the practice and seldom changes. Examples of support files include procedure codes, diagnosis codes, names and addresses of insurance plans, names of referring physicians, and other related information that will be used frequently.

In working on your Student Edition software, you should back up your files daily in order to protect your work. Similarly, in a medical office, the office manager makes a backup daily to protect all the practice's files. Technical difficulties, power failures, and a variety of other factors could cause you to lose information stored on your Student Disk. To perform a daily backup properly, you must first exit **The Medical Manager** software. Once you have exited the software, you will click an icon on your desktop and follow the instructions that are presented on the screen. Always make sure that you fully exit **The Medical Manager** before removing your Student Edition disk. Always take your Student Edition disk with you at the end of each class.

TESTING YOUR KNOWLEDGE

1. What generally takes place from the time a patient comes into the office for an appointment to the time he or she checks out? How can the flow of information in a medical office be described as circular?

2. In what ways is the appointment schedule important to the medical office? How does the appointment schedule affect the medical practice?

3. What items of information are necessary for scheduling an appointment?

4. Name and describe three methods of collecting insurance payments.

5. Briefly explain three types of health insurance coverage patients may have.

6. In **The Medical Manager**, what are software menus used for? How can these software menus be compared to restaurant menus?

(continues)

7. In **The Medical Manager** software, how does a user return to a previous screen? How does a user return to the Main Menu (Menu 1)?

8. Provide an example of a direct chaining command, and explain how it is used in **The Medical Manager** software.

9. How do you perform a daily backup? Why is backing up your data important?

10. Why are default options included in a software program? In what ways can default options be more efficient that manually keying responses?

11. How are CPT-4 and ICD-9 codes related?

They're related b/c they're both necessary 2 Insurance claim info.

12. Why would insurance plans carefully review CPT-4 and ICD-9 codes? Why should this be of concern to the practice?

Building Your Patient File

LEARNING OUTCOMES

After completing this unit, you should be able to:

◆ Enter patient account information.

◆ Enter data into supplemental screens.

◆ Discuss the importance of entering data correctly.

◆ Describe the relationship of the guarantor and patient.

◆ Explain the relevance of extended information.

◆ Discuss how help windows may be used.

Each time a new patient visits the medical office, information about the patient, the guarantor of the account, insurance plans, and dependents must be stored in the system so it can be retrieved when the patient returns for future visits. In addition, changes are constantly being made to update insurance plans, add dependents, indicate a change of employment, or for other reasons. This is how a medical office builds its patient files.

Accounts are posted with charges (generated by specific procedures and diagnoses) and credits (created by payments) each time a patient visits. This allows the system to maintain a current balance of each account as well as to build patients' medical and financial records.

NEW PATIENT ENTRY

New accounts are added to the Guarantor File from information on the patient registration form.

The guarantor agrees to be financially responsible for the account.

The patient completes the patient registration form, illustrated in Figure 2-1, when he or she arrives at the medical office for the first visit. Information requested on the form includes personal data about the patient; the name, address, and telephone number of the guarantor's employer; the names, addresses, and policy numbers of all health insurance plans covering the patient; the name of the referring physician; and information about any dependents.

The *guarantor* is the person who guarantees to pay the doctor for all charges incurred on an account, including charges for himself or herself and all dependents. The Guarantor File holds information about all patient accounts. Every time a new account is opened, **The Medical Manager** system automatically adds information about the account to the Guarantor File.

When adding an account, you may add up to 99 dependents, 99 insurance plans, and extended information about the patient, such as alternate address or legal representative. Patient records are stored under both the patient's name and patient number, which is the account number, followed by a decimal point and the patient's dependent number (e.g. Steven Carlson is account number 10 and he is the guarantor; his patient record would be 10.0; Sharon Carlson is Steven Carlson's wife, her patient record would be 10.1).

Figure 2-1 Patricia Evans—Patient Registration Form

Patient Registration Form

Sydney Carrington & Associates
34 Sycamore Street ● Madison, CA 95653

TODAY'S DATE: _01/10/2003_

FOR OFFICE USE ONLY	
ACCOUNT NO.:	**110**
DOCTOR:	**#3**
BILL TYPE:	**11**
EXTENDED INFO.:	**0**

PATIENT INFORMATION

Evans   *Patricia*   *G.*
PATIENT LAST NAME   FIRST NAME   MI

Self
RELATIONSHIP TO GUARANTOR

F | *12/13/1951* | *Single* | *908-23-6457*
SEX (M/F) DATE OF BIRTH MARITAL STATUS SOC. SEC. #

EMPLOYER OR SCHOOL NAME

ADDRESS OF EMPLOYER OR SCHOOL

CITY   STATE   ZIP CODE

    Leland Groves, M.D.
EMPLOYER OR SCHOOL PHONE   REFERRED BY

E-MAIL

GUARANTOR INFORMATION

Evans,   *Patricia*   *G.* | *F*
RESPONSIBLE PARTY LAST NAME FIRST NAME MI SEX (M/F)

8907 Harbor Drive
MAILING ADDRESS   STREET ADDRESS (IF DIFFERENT)

Madison   *CA* | *95653*
CITY   STATE   ZIP CODE

(916) 544-8275
(AREA CODE) HOME PHONE   (AREA CODE) WORK PHONE

12/13/1951 | *Single* | *908-23-6457*
DATE OF BIRTH MARITAL STATUS SOC. SEC. #

EMPLOYER NAME

EMPLOYER ADDRESS

CITY   STATE   ZIP CODE

PRIMARY INSURANCE

Epsilon Life & Casualty
NAME OF PRIMARY INSURANCE COMPANY

P.O. Box 189
ADDRESS

Macon   *GA* | *31298*
CITY   STATE   ZIP CODE

756575675
IDENTIFICATION #   GROUP NAME AND/OR #

Same
INSURED PERSON'S NAME (IF DIFFERENT FROM THE RESPONSIBLE PARTY)

Same
ADDRESS (IF DIFFERENT)

Same
CITY   STATE   ZIP CODE

(800) 908-7654   *908-23-6457*
PRIMARY INSURANCE PHONE NUMBER   SOC. SEC. #

Self
WHAT IS THE RESPONSIBLE PARTY'S RELATIONSHIP TO THE INSURED?

SECONDARY INSURANCE

NAME OF SECONDARY INSURANCE COMPANY

ADDRESS

CITY   STATE   ZIP CODE

IDENTIFICATION #   GROUP NAME AND/OR #

INSURED PERSON'S NAME (IF DIFFERENT FROM THE RESPONSIBLE PARTY)

ADDRESS (IF DIFFERENT)

CITY   STATE   ZIP CODE

SECONDARY INSURANCE PHONE NUMBER   SOC. SEC. #

WHAT IS THE RESPONSIBLE PARTY'S RELATIONSHIP TO THE INSURED?

I hereby consent for Sydney Carrington & Associates, P.A. to use or disclose my health information to carry out treatment, payment, and health care operations. I authorize the use of this signature on all insurance submissions. I understand that I am financially responsible for all charges whether or not paid by the insurance. I acknowledge receipt of the practice's privacy policy.

Patricia G. Evans   *01/10/2003*
PATIENT SIGNATURE   DATE

When several members of the same family arrive at a medical office for the first time, each patient completes a patient registration form. A feature of **The Medical Manager** Patient Entry allows you to add quickly several members of the same family in one session. In subsequent exercises, when adding multiple family members in New

Patient Entry, you will be provided with several registration forms, each of which has the same guarantor information.

Always begin a new account with the guarantor information. The guarantor information for these exercises is found in the box on the right of the form. Patient information, in the box on the left of the form, will differ from the guarantor information when patients are dependents.

New Patient Entry is used only to create new guarantor accounts.

Use the New Patient Entry screen only when a new guarantor account is opened. A different screen is used when names of dependents or insurance companies are added to an existing account, or when patient extended information such as an employer's name or address is needed. Edit Patient Entry will be explained in Unit 4 in the Student Edition course.

Practice patient entry procedures.

Start **The Medical Manager** system, if this is a new class session, and advance to the Main Menu (Menu 1).

Follow the steps below to practice the New Patient Entry procedure. Key in the examples shown in boldface taken from the patient registration form in Figure 2-1, for this practice exercise.

Note: All information on an account must be completed in one session. You cannot EXIT during account entry or all of your information entered will be lost and you will have to start over. Do not begin an exercise in Unit 2 if there is not enough class time to complete the entire exercise.

STEP 1

At the Main Menu (Menu 1), key option '1,' NEW Patient Entry, and press **ENTER**. (Remember that you may replace both of these steps by simply using the mouse to double-click on option 1.) The screen shown in Figure 2-2 will appear.

Figure 2-2 New Patient Entry Screen

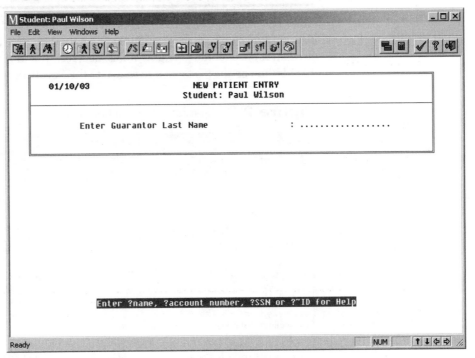

Note the prompt at the bottom of the screen: "Enter ?name, ?account number, ?SSN or ?~ID for Help." To check whether a name is already on file, you should first enter a question mark ('**?**') plus the last name of the guarantor and press **ENTER**. You can also click on the Help button ('**?**') on the top toolbar, then scroll through the names of any patients listed to see if the guarantor's name is already in the system. Accounts will be displayed in the name folder with the full name, date of birth, Social Security number, and Patient ID #. You would normally review the list to determine whether this patient's name is shown. However, because this is the first patient you will enter into the system, none will be listed.

♦   a. Enter Guarantor Last Name: **Evans**
     TIP: Required field, 18 alphanumeric characters allowed.

     The Medical Manager system requires you to complete this entry before you can move forward.

♦   b. Enter Patient Account #: **110**
     TIP: Required field, 6 numeric characters allowed.

All guarantors must be assigned a patient account number. Because last names may be the same, the account number must be different for each guarantor. **Once entered, the account number can never be changed.** Be sure to use the exact account numbers designated for each patient.

The patient account number can be automatically assigned by **The Medical Manager** software; however, this feature has been turned off in the Student Edition, so you should key each account number exactly as instructed (all patient account numbers are listed on the individual patient registration forms in the box labeled "For Office Use Only," along with the Doctor # and other information typically assigned by the practice).

An attempt to assign an account number that is already on file will result in this message: "30: Account Number Already on File." If this occurs, press ENTER and key in a valid account number.

GUARANTOR INFORMATION

The screen shown in Figure 2-3 will appear after you enter the guarantor's last name and patient number. Check the guarantor's last name at the top left side of the screen and the account number at the top right. If it is incorrect, you may press ESCAPE or click on the EXIT button on the top toolbar to return to the New Patient Entry screen and start over.

Figure 2-3 Guarantor Information Screen

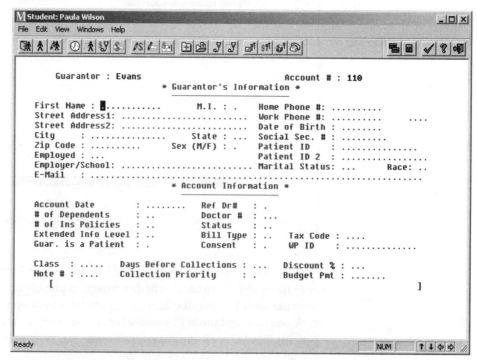

STEP 2   Use the information shown in Figure 2-1 to complete the fields as indicated below.

◆   a.   Enter First Name: **Patricia**
         TIP: Required field, 12 alphanumeric characters allowed

Enter the first name of the guarantor as you would like it to appear on all billings and reports.

◆   b.   Enter Middle Initial: **G**
         TIP: Optional field, 1 alphanumeric character allowed

Note: Entering a period ('.') after the guarantor's middle initial is not necessary.

◆   c.   Enter Street Address1: **8907 Harbor Drive**
         TIP: Optional field, 25 alphanumeric characters allowed

This is the guarantor's entire street address.

◆   d.   Enter Street Address2: (Press **ENTER** to leave blank)
         TIP: Optional field, 25 alphanumeric characters allowed

Enter any additional address information such as a route number or post office box number. You will press ENTER to leave this space blank if there is no additional information.

◆   e.   Enter City: **Madison**
         TIP: Optional field, 15 alphanumeric characters allowed

This is the city where the guarantor resides. Remember that Madison is the default city so you can simply press ENTER.

Note: A help window is available for this field. See Unit 1 for details.

◆   f.   Enter State (Abbreviation): **CA**
         TIP: Optional field, 3 alphanumeric characters allowed

CA is the two-letter post office code for the guarantor's state. Remember that CA is the default. In other words, if you press ENTER, 'CA' will automatically be entered into this field by the system.

◆   g.   Enter Zip Code: **95653**
         TIP: Optional field, 10 alphanumeric characters allowed

This field contains the zip code for the guarantor's state. Make sure that you do not press ENTER to accept the default for this field.

◆   h.   Enter Sex (M/F): **F**
         TIP: Required field, 1 alphanumeric character allowed

Use the letter code (M)ale or (F)emale for the gender of the guarantor.

◆   i.   Enter Employed: (Press **ENTER** to leave blank)
         TIP: Optional field, 3 alphanumeric characters allowed

Options for this field are (E)mployed, (P)art-Time Student, and (F)ull-Time Student. Because Ms. Evans is not employed, you will press ENTER to leave this blank.

◆   j.   Enter Employer/School: (Press **ENTER** to leave blank)
         TIP: Optional field, 26 alphanumeric characters allowed

This is the name of the guarantor's employer or school.

◆　k.　Enter Home Phone #: **9165448275**
　　　TIP: Optional field, 10 numeric characters allowed

This is the guarantor's home telephone number. Remember that this field in **The Medical Manager** system is self-formatting and parentheses and hyphens will automatically be added to this entry.

Note: In an actual practice situation, if only 7 digits are entered, the area code will default to the default area code set for the practice when The Medical Manager software was installed.

◆　l.　Enter Work Phone #: (Press **ENTER** to leave blank)
　　　TIP: Optional field, 10 numeric characters allowed

These fields are for the guarantor's work telephone number and extension. Press **ENTER** to bypass the work extension field since none is listed.

◆　m.　Enter Date of Birth: **12131951**
　　　TIP: Optional field, 8 numeric characters allowed.

This is the guarantor's date of birth. **The Medical Manager** software adds slashes between the numbers. Always use two numbers to indicate for each, the month and the day, and four digits for the year of birth. Add a zero to the front of one-digit months or days; for example, January 1, 2000, should be keyed '01012000'.

Note: To prevent a future date from being entered, it is strongly recommended that the eight-digit format (i.e., 'MMDDYYYY') always be used when entering dates of birth.

◆　n.　Enter Social Security #: **908236457**
　　　TIP: Optional field, 9 numeric characters accepted

This is the Social Security number of the guarantor. This field in **The Medical Manager** system is self-formatting and will automatically place hyphens where they are needed. For example, although you will key '908236457,' this will appear as '908-23-6457' when ENTER is pressed.

◆　o.　Enter Patient ID: (Press **ENTER** to leave blank)
　　　TIP: Optional field, 15 alphanumeric characters allowed

The Patient ID # is an optional field used to identify the guarantor for office use (a chart number, for example). For some insurance billing such as in the case of managed care plans, Patient ID # can be used to retrieve the patient's account.

◆　p.　Enter Patient ID 2: (Press **ENTER** to leave blank)
　　　TIP: Optional field, 17 alphanumeric characters allowed

The Patient ID # is used to identify the guarantor for either internal office use or for insurance billing information.

◆　q.　Enter Marital Status: (**S**)ingle
　　　TIP: Optional field, 3 alphanumeric characters allowed

This is the marital status of the guarantor. Valid entries are (S)ingle, (M)arried, or (O)ther.

◆　r.　Enter Race: (Press **ENTER** to leave blank)
　　　TIP: Optional field, 3 alphanumeric characters allowed

This is the race of the guarantor. For the purposes of the Student Edition, all race fields will be bypassed by pressing ENTER to leave the fields blank.

◆　s.　E-mail: (Press **ENTER** to leave blank)

Account Information

STEP 3

Enter information about the account.

You will need account information to complete this screen. Continue to complete each field by adding the information shown below. Beginning with this section, fields will no longer be designated as optional or required. Therefore, it is necessary that you complete every field for which information is provided.

◆ a. Enter Account Date: (Press **ENTER** for default)
TIP: 6 numeric characters allowed

Enter the date the guarantor's account was added to **The Medical Manager** system. This will generally be the current date. Press ENTER to accept the default date (the system date set in **The Medical Manager** software).

◆ b. Enter # of Dependents: **0**
TIP: 2 numeric characters allowed

Because no dependents are shown on Ms. Evans's registration form, enter '0' at this field. Remember that you can always add dependent information using option 1, EDIT Patient Records, on the File Maintenance Menu (Menu 2). (See Unit 4.)

◆ c. Enter # of Insurance Policies: **1**
TIP: 2 numeric characters allowed

Enter only the number of insurance policies that have been or will be covering the patients in this account. *Note that there is a limit of seven policies per patient.* You will be asked to enter information about each plan. If the guarantor has no insurance, you would press ENTER to accept the default of '0' insurance policies.

◆ d. Enter Extended Information Level: 0
TIP: 2 numeric characters

Extended information refers to helpful, optional facts.

The extended information option is a special feature that permits you to keep patient information that is not required, such as the name and address of an employer. Extended information questions can be set up, or customized, to fit the needs of an individual practice. If you press ENTER, **The Medical Manager** system will default to 0 for 'None.'

Refer to the chart shown below for an understanding of the levels of extended information. You will learn more about extended information levels later in this unit of the Student Edition.

Extended Information Levels

0   No patient extended information.

1   Comments only. These lines will appear on the Patient Retrieval Screen (discussed later in this unit).

2   Comments plus information lines. The comment lines will appear on the Patient Retrieval Screen.

◆ e. Enter Guarantor Is a Patient (Y/N): **Y**
TIP: 1 alphabetic character allowed

The guarantor is the financially responsible party.

This field determines whether or not the guarantor is a patient. (Y)es and (N)o are the only valid responses. A patient is the guarantor when he or she is financially responsible for medical services received. However, the patient may not be the guarantor of the account. For example, when a child is the patient, his parent or guardian would be listed as the guarantor.

◆ f. Enter Referring Doctor #: **2**
   TIP: 4 numeric characters allowed

Physicians refer their patients to other doctors when they think a specialist is needed to treat a more severe condition or medical problem. Each referring doctor is identified by a separate number. Enter the doctor number representing the physician who referred the patient, or press ENTER to default to no referring physician.

If you do not know a referring physician's number or wish to add a new referring physician's name and number, type '?' and press ENTER #1 or simply click on the Help button ('?') on the top toolbar. The following message will appear asking whether you want to add a referring doctor, go to the next page of names in the list, go to the previous page of names in the list, or search for an existing referring doctor: "(A)dd Ref Dr; (N)ext, (P)rev, (S)earch." You could also use the highlight bar to select the appropriate referring physician number 2, Leland W. Groves, M.D., and press ENTER to select the physician OR using the mouse, double-click on Dr. Groves to both highlight and select him as the Referring Doctor.

◆ g. Enter Doctor #: **3**
   TIP: 3 numeric characters

Each physician in the practice has been assigned a number. Key the doctor number representing the doctor who is primarily responsible for the patient. If you press ENTER, **The Medical Manager** software will default to Doctor #1.

You may type '?' in this field and press ENTER or click on the Help button ('?') on the top toolbar to search for the doctor's name. The highlight bar or the mouse pointer can then be used to select the appropriate doctor, in this case physician number 3, Sydney J. Carrington M.D.

◆ h. Enter Status: **1**
   TIP: 2 numeric characters allowed

This lets you specify whether the account is active or inactive. If the account is active, press ENTER to default to '1'. Other statuses such as '0' for an inactive account or '2' for an account referred to a collection agency, etc., are available.

Note: A help window is available for this field.

◆ i. Enter Bill Type: **11**
   TIP: 2 numeric characters allowed

The bill type is a two-part code that defines the type of walkout receipt and statement the patient is to receive. For Ms. Evans's account, key '11'; or press ENTER, and **The Medical Manager** system will default to '11.' The first 1 identifies the walkout receipt type, and the second 1 identifies the statement type. *Note that a help window is available for this field.*

◆ j. Enter Tax Code: (Press **ENTER** to bypass this field)
   TIP: 4 alphanumeric characters allowed

This field is reserved for future use by an external tax system.

◆ k. Enter Consent:
   TIP: The cursor moves to this field only if the Guarantor is a Patient Field above set to (**Y**)es.

This field indicates that the patient has signed a consent form or an acknowledgment that they received a copy of the practice privacy policy. Patient Privacy and Consent is discussed further in Unit 9.

Options for this field are (**Y**)es the patient has signed a consent form or acknowledges receipt of the privacy policy; (**N**)o the patient has not signed a consent form; (**R**)evoked, which indicates the patient has revoked a previously signed consent form; or (**U**)nknown, which indicates that the practice is not aware of the status of the patient's consent. You will notice that the consent information at the bottom of the patient registration form has been signed by Ms. Evans. Press **ENTER** to accept the default (**Y**)es.

◆ l. Enter the Word Processing (WP) ID: (Press **ENTER** to default to 'C:wp110.0')
TIP: 14 alphanumeric characters allowed

A medical practice may use a word processing system in conjunction with **The Medical Manager** software. In this field, you will enter the name of the word processing file that you will use with this account. For the purposes of the Student Edition, you may press ENTER to default this field to WP (Account Number).

◆ m. Enter Class: (Press **ENTER** to bypass this field)
TIP: 5 alphanumeric characters allowed

Some practices like to identify an account further in the class type field. Ms. Evans's physician does not use this designation, so press ENTER to bypass this field.

Note: A help window is available for this field.

◆ n. Enter Note #: **0**
TIP: 4 numeric characters allowed

The Medical Manager system allows notes and messages to be added to an account when needed. Many accounts do not require notes. Press ENTER to default to '0' or 'No' messages. You may type '?' in the field and press ENTER or click on the Help button ('?') on the top toolbar to search the list of available notes. The first five notes are reserved for printing and running messages regarding patient statements.

◆ o. Enter Days Before Collection: (Press **ENTER** to bypass this field)
TIP: 3 numeric characters allowed

This field is used in conjunction with the Collections System in **The Medical Manager** system.

◆ p. Enter Collection Priority: (Press **ENTER** to bypass this field)
TIP: 1 numeric character allowed

This field is also used in conjunction with the Collections System in **The Medical Manager** system.

◆ q. Enter Discount %: (Press **ENTER** to accept default percentage)
TIP: 3 numeric characters allowed

Some accounts are discounted for special reasons; for example, a discount may be given when another physician or a staff member's family receives care from a doctor. The percent of discount could be entered in this field, and **The Medical Manager** system would automatically reduce all procedure charges by the amount of the discount. Press ENTER to default to '0' (zero) percent discount.

◆ r. Enter Budget Payment: (Press **ENTER** to accept default amount)
TIP: 7 numeric characters allowed

Doctors often make special arrangements for patients to pay large amounts over time. These are called *budget payment accounts*. For budget payment accounts, enter the regular monthly payment required of the patient and press ENTER. To default to monthly payment, press ENTER.

STEP 4

PROCESS stores information; EXIT leaves the screen without saving.

After all fields on the Guarantor's Information screen are entered and edited, your screen should be similar to Figure 2-4. Review all information carefully and press **F1** or click the PROCESS button ('√') on the top toolbar to process and save your work. The PROCESS key (**F1**) or PROCESS button ('√') is used to store the information you have entered on the screen. The ESCAPE key (the 'Esc' key is generally located on the top left corner of the keyboard) or EXIT button (located in the rightmost corner of the top toolbar) is used when you want to leave a screen without processing or storing the information. **Do not EXIT before you PROCESS unless you want to discard the information you entered and start over**.

Figure 2-4 Completed Guarantor Screen

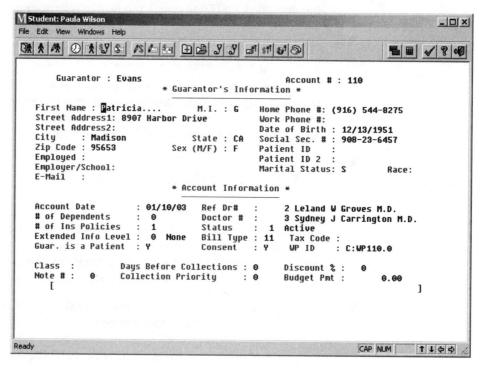

ADDITIONAL SCREENS

You will be asked to provide additional information about the account if you selected the patient extended information option, if the patient has dependents or insurance plans. If none of these options were selected, **The Medical Manager** system will allow you to add another new guarantor or other insurance plans.

Ms. Evans's account indicated one insurance plan. Therefore, the software will continue by displaying a screen asking for insurance information. Complete the fields in each screen by entering the information given below.

Insurance Policy Information

STEP 1

Medical offices need to have complete information about a patient's health insurance coverage. Note that a separate Insurance Policy Information screen will be completed

Figure 2-5 Insurance Policy Information Screen

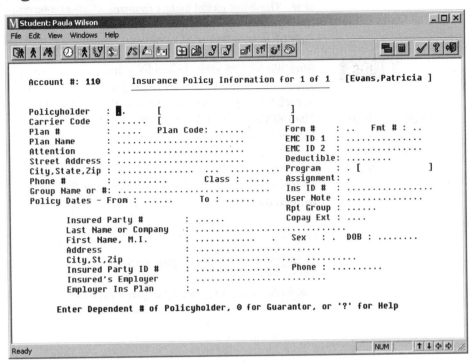

for each of the guarantor's plans. A blank Insurance Policy Screen Information is shown in Figure 2-5.

Before proceeding with the remainder of this exercise, review the information below for determining whether the patient is the (G)uarantor, (P)olicyholder, or (N)ew Insured Party.

Option	When to Choose This Option
(G)uarantor	Choose (G)uarantor when the name of the insurance subscriber is the same name as the guarantor's (e.g., Ms. Evans owns his Medicare policy and is also the guarantor for the account).
(P)olicyholder	Choose (P)olicyholder when the name of the insurance subscriber is the same as anyone else (besides the guarantor) in the account.
(N)ew Insured Party	Choose (N)ew Insured Party when the name of the insurance subscriber is not the same as anyone else in the account. (This will be illustrated in Exercise 6.)

Use the information shown below to complete the screens needed for Ms. Evans's account.

◆ a. Enter Policyholder: **0**
TIP: Required field, 2 numeric characters allowed

The Policyholder owns the insurance policy.

The Policyholder is the person who brings the insurance policy to the family account. This person must be the guarantor or one of the dependents on the account.

Valid responses for this field are '0' for guarantor, or a dependent number. Because this policy belongs to Patricia Evans, a '0' should be entered here.

Note: A help window of dependent numbers is available for this field.

◆   b.   Enter Carrier Code: **EPSLON**

A carrier code is a grouping of insurance companies. This field may be left blank because when the next field, Plan #, is completed, the system will automatically enter the appropriate carrier code.

If a carrier code was entered in the previous field, a help window will automatically display showing only the insurance plans associated with the carrier. Using the keyboard or mouse, you could then select the plan from the list shown.

A new insurance plan may also be added at this point. However, since this insurance plan already exists in the system, simply highlight EPSILON and press ENTER to select it OR using the mouse, double-click on the plan to both highlight and select it. The information stored in the support file will display.

Note: Because you already selected EPSILON as the insurance plan, The Medical Manager software will automatically complete the plan number field.

◆   c.   Enter Assignment (Y/N): (**Y**)es

Some physicians accept assignment of claims. For government programs, this means that they agree to accept an amount determined to be reasonable by the insurance carrier. For other types of insurance, this means the patient has assigned benefits to the doctor. Valid responses are (Y)es and (N)o.

Finding an existing carrier code. Enter '?' at the Carrier Code field and **The Medical Manager** will search for an existing carrier code number. A prompt will appear with the message: "(N)ext, (P)rev, (S)earch." If you press (S)earch, you will be asked to enter the starting name. **The Medical Manager** will list all carrier codes in alphabetical order, beginning with the name you entered. You may select (N)ext or (P)revious to view other claim centers in the file. EXIT to return to the Carrier Code field, then enter the number you located in the list for the carrier code.

Entering a New Carrier Code. Enter '0' as a carrier code number and **The Medical Manager** will permit you to add a new insurance carrier code to the file. A prompt will ask: "Do You Wish to Open New Carrier Code? (Y/N)." Select '**Y**' and key the correct information at Name of Carrier. The system will automatically number this new carrier code, and the information entered in this section will be added to the carrier code file.

◆   d.   Enter Group Name or #: (Press **ENTER** to leave blank)

This is the name of the group purchasing the insurance. Often, this is the person's employer.

◆   e.   Enter Policy Dates - From: (Press **ENTER** to bypass this field)
                          To: (Press **ENTER** to bypass this field)

The policy beginning and/or end dates of coverage can be entered here if they are known.

◆   f.   Enter Insurance ID #: **75675675**

This is the number of the patient's insurance policy. Enter the information given above about the first insurance carrier. Remember to key the ID as shown.

◆ g. Enter User Note: (Press **ENTER** to bypass this field)

This field can be any note about the insurance policy for this account.

◆ h. Enter Report Group: (Press **ENTER** to bypass this field)

Reporting Groups are user-defined categories that can be used on custom reports.

Note: A help window is available for this field.

◆ i. Enter Copay Ext: (Press **ENTER** to bypass this field)

◆ j. Enter Insured Party #: **0**

The insured party is the person who is named as the primary holder of the insurance policy. The insured party is called the subscriber by many insurance plans. When you key '0' and press ENTER, the following prompt will appear:

(**N**)ew Insured Party, (**G**)uarantor, or (**P**)olicyholder

Because Ms. Evans is both the insured party and the guarantor of the account, key '**G**.' The system will automatically fill in all necessary Insured Party Information using the information you have previously entered for Ms. Evans. The cursor will move to the field labeled Employer Ins Plan (Y/N).

◆ k. Enter Employer Insurance Plan: (**N**)o

Type '**N**' because Ms. Evans is not insured through an employer. Press **ENTER**. Compare your screen with Figure 2-6. Once you are sure the information is correct, press the **F1** key or click on the PROCESS button ('√') on the top toolbar to process.

Figure 2-6 Completed Insurance Policy Information Screen

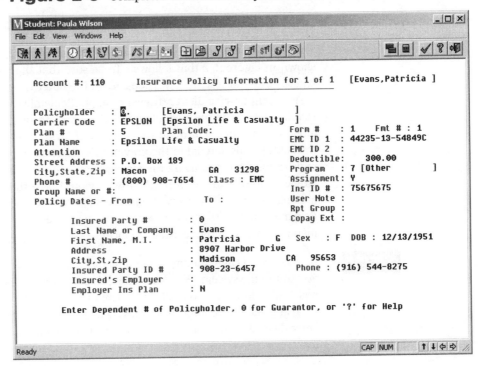

STEP 2

The next screen that will display automatically is the Insurance Coverage Priority screen. Because Ms. Evans has only one insurance policy that is listed as her primary plan, press the **F1** key or click on the PROCESS button ('√') to process this screen.

Press **ESCAPE** or click on the **EXIT** button to return to the Main Menu (Menu 1).

APPLYING YOUR KNOWLEDGE

Press ENTER to bypass fields for which no information is provided

Patient registration forms are provided for seven new patients on the following pages. These are patients with whom you will work for the remainder of the course. You will be transferring data from the patient registration forms into **The Medical Manager** system by applying the knowledge you gained and the same steps you used while entering Patricia Evans's account.

All information must be completed correctly for a patient in one session. If you exit during account entry, you will have to go to Edit Patient to complete the Patient Entry. Similarly, you should carefully check each screen before pressing 'F1' or clicking the PROCESS ('√') button because you cannot go back to a screen once you leave it. If you process a screen with errors, you will correct the errors in Edit Patient. Edit Patient is covered in Unit 4. Ask your instructor before proceeding to Unit 4 out of sequence to correct errors.

The patient registration forms used as examples in the Student Edition course are similar to those you might encounter in any medical office. Be sure to enter the exact account numbers provided in the forms because they will be required during the remainder of this course. When there is no information given to complete a field, press ENTER to bypass the field and continue with the remaining information. When each section of information is completed, remember to press the F1 key or click on the PROCESS button ('√') on the top toolbar to process and to advance to the next screen.

Remember that some fields, such as the Account Date field, are default fields; therefore, correct information can be entered automatically, simply by pressing ENTER at each field location.

EXERCISE 1: Claire E. League

Adding a Patient with Multiple Insurance Plans

The next account you will enter is for Mrs. Claire League. Her account information is shown in Figure 2-7 that follows. To be sure that the patient has not already been entered into the system, key '**?League**' in the Enter Guarantor Last Name field at the New Patient Entry patient retrieval prompt. Remember that you can also click on the Help button ('?') on the top toolbar and then scroll through the list of patients who have already been entered into the system to see if Mrs. League is on file. Progress through the fields just as you did in the previous exercise, taking information from the patient registration form and using the appropriate help windows if necessary. The only difference between this account and the previous one is that Mrs. League has two insurance plans. Follow the instructions below to add Claire League's account to the system. Remember to key '0' for extended information level since no Employer or School information appears on the registration form.

STEP 1

Because Mrs. League's name is not already on file, press **ENTER** to proceed and add her account to the system. Key Mrs. League's patient number, '**30**,' shown on her patient registration form and press **ENTER**. The Guarantor Information screen will appear.

Using the information from Mrs. League's patient registration form (Figure 2-7), enter the additional information to create her account in **The Medical Manager** system.

Figure 2-7 Claire League—Patient Registration Form

Patient Registration Form

Sydney Carrington & Associates
34 Sycamore Street ● Madison, CA 95653

FOR OFFICE USE ONLY	
ACCOUNT NO.:	30
DOCTOR:	#1
BILL TYPE:	11
EXTENDED INFO.:	0

TODAY'S DATE: _01/10/2003_

PATIENT INFORMATION

League	_Claire_	_E._
PATIENT LAST NAME	FIRST NAME	MI

Self
RELATIONSHIP TO GUARANTOR

_F_	_06/11/1929_	_Married_	_738-76-4128_
SEX (M/F)	DATE OF BIRTH	MARITAL STATUS	SOC. SEC. #

EMPLOYER OR SCHOOL NAME

ADDRESS OF EMPLOYER OR SCHOOL

CITY	STATE	ZIP CODE

Lucinda A. Fredericks, M.D.

EMPLOYER OR SCHOOL PHONE	REFERRED BY

E-MAIL

GUARANTOR INFORMATION

League	_Claire_	_E._	_F_
RESPONSIBLE PARTY LAST NAME	FIRST NAME	MI	SEX (M/F)

800 Illagas Road	
MAILING ADDRESS	STREET ADDRESS (IF DIFFERENT)

Morgan Hill	_CA_	_98076_
CITY	STATE	ZIP CODE

_(408)907-4352_	
(AREA CODE) HOME PHONE	(AREA CODE) WORK PHONE

_06/11/1929_	_Married_	_738-76-4128_
DATE OF BIRTH	MARITAL STATUS	SOC. SEC. #

EMPLOYER NAME

EMPLOYER ADDRESS

CITY	STATE	ZIP CODE

PRIMARY INSURANCE

Medicare
NAME OF PRIMARY INSURANCE COMPANY

Claims Dept. Box 443A, 760 University Street
ADDRESS

Washington	_DC_	_17654-1234_
CITY	STATE	ZIP CODE

_738764128D_	
IDENTIFICATION #	GROUP NAME AND/OR #

Claire E. League
INSURED PERSON'S NAME (IF DIFFERENT FROM THE RESPONSIBLE PARTY)

Same
ADDRESS (IF DIFFERENT)

Same

CITY	STATE	ZIP CODE

_(800) 879-6789_	_738-76-4128_
PRIMARY INSURANCE PHONE NUMBER	SOC. SEC. #

Self
WHAT IS THE RESPONSIBLE PARTY'S RELATIONSHIP TO THE INSURED?

SECONDARY INSURANCE

Medicare Plus
NAME OF SECONDARY INSURANCE COMPANY

34567 Arvor Avenue
ADDRESS

Madison	_CA_	_95653_
CITY	STATE	ZIP CODE

_328948929299_	
IDENTIFICATION #	GROUP NAME AND/OR #

Claire E. League
INSURED PERSON'S NAME (IF DIFFERENT FROM THE RESPONSIBLE PARTY)

Same
ADDRESS (IF DIFFERENT)

Same

CITY	STATE	ZIP CODE

_(800) 675-4354_	_738-76-4128_
SECONDARY INSURANCE PHONE NUMBER	SOC. SEC. #

Self
WHAT IS THE RESPONSIBLE PARTY'S RELATIONSHIP TO THE INSURED?

I hereby consent for Sydney Carrington & Associates, P.A. to use or disclose my health information to carry out treatment, payment, and health care operations. I authorize the use of this signature on all insurance submissions. I understand that I am financially responsible for all charges whether or not paid by the insurance. I acknowledge receipt of the practice's privacy policy.

Claire E. League	_01/10/2003_
PATIENT SIGNATURE	DATE

Note: Remember to enter the patient number correctly, because it may never be changed.

First Name: **Claire**

M.I.: **E**

Street Address1: **800 Illagas Road**

Street Address2: (Press **ENTER** to leave blank)

City: **Morgan Hill**

State: **CA**

Zip Code: **98076**

Sex (M/F): (**F**)emale

Employed: (Press **ENTER** to leave blank)

Employer/School: (Press **ENTER** to leave blank)

Home Phone #: **4089074352**

Work Phone #: (Press **ENTER** to leave blank)

Work Ext #: (Press **ENTER** to leave blank)

Date of Birth: **06111929**

Social Sec. #: **738764128**

Patient ID: (Press **ENTER** to leave blank)

Patient ID 2: (Press **ENTER** to leave blank)

Marital Status: (**M**)arried

Race: (Press **ENTER** to leave blank)

E-mail: (Press **ENTER** to leave blank)

Account Date: (Press **ENTER** to default to current system date of 01/10/03)

# of Dependents: **0**

# of Ins. Policies: **2**

Extended Info. Level: **0** (None)

Guar. Is a Patient: (**Y**)es

Ref. Dr. #: **3** (Dr. Lucinda Fredericks)

Doctor #: **1** (Dr. James Monroe)

Status: (Press **ENTER** to accept default of '1')

Bill Type: (Press **ENTER** to accept default of '11')

Tax Code: (Press **ENTER** to leave blank)

Consent: (Press **ENTER** to accept the default of (**Y**)es)

WP ID: (Press **ENTER** to accept default of 'C:wp30.0')

Class: (Press **ENTER** to leave blank)

Note: (Press **ENTER** to accept default of '0')

Days Before Collections: (Press **ENTER** to accept default of '0')

Collection Priority: (Press **ENTER** to accept default of '0')

Discount %: (Press **ENTER** to accept default of '0')

Budget Payment: (Press **ENTER** to accept default of '0.00')

Carefully check your screen against the information shown on Mrs. League's patient registration form. When you are sure all information has been entered correctly, press F1 or click on the PROCESS button ('√') on the top toolbar to process. Your screen should resemble Figure 2-8.

Figure 2-8 Completed Guarantor Information Screen

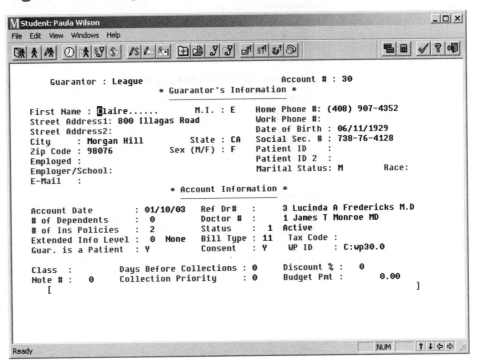

```
M Student: Paula Wilson                                              _ □ ×
File  Edit  View  Windows  Help

[toolbar icons]                                              [toolbar icons]

        Guarantor : League                      Account # : 30
                            * Guarantor's Information *

    First Name : Claire......      M.I. : E   Home Phone #: (408) 907-4352
    Street Address1: 800 Illagas Road         Work Phone #:
    Street Address2:                          Date of Birth : 06/11/1929
    City     : Morgan Hill        State : CA  Social Sec. # : 738-76-4128
    Zip Code : 98076          Sex (M/F) : F   Patient ID   :
    Employed :                                Patient ID 2 :
    Employer/School:                          Marital Status: M      Race:
    E-Mail   :
                             * Account Information *

    Account Date       : 01/10/03   Ref Dr#  :   3 Lucinda A Fredericks M.D
    # of Dependents    :  0         Doctor # :   1 James T Monroe MD
    # of Ins Policies  :  2         Status   :  1 Active
    Extended Info Level :  0  None  Bill Type : 11   Tax Code :
    Guar. is a Patient :  Y         Consent  : Y    WP ID    : C:wp30.0

    Class  :             Days Before Collections : 0   Discount % :   0
    Note # :   0         Collection Priority     : 0   Budget Pmt :     0.00
       [                                                               ]

Ready                                                    NUM     ↑↓⇐⇒
```

STEP 2

Once you have processed the Guarantor Information entered for Mrs. League, the first of two screens for Insurance Policy Information will appear. Mrs. League has a basic Medicare plan and a Medicare supplement plan. Mrs. League is the policyholder and the insured party for both insurance policies, so choose '**0**.' Choose the carrier code **MEDI**. Then, select the appropriate plan (there is only one) from the help window that automatically displays. Press **ENTER** to accept the default of 'Y' for the Assignment field. Press **ENTER** to leave the Group Name or # field blank and at both of the Policy Dates fields. Enter Mrs. League's Ins. ID #, **738764128D**, from her patient registration form. Press **ENTER** to leave the User Note, Rpt. Group, and Copay Ext. fields blank. Enter '**0**' then choose '**G**' for Guarantor at the Insured Party # field and the system will complete the relevant guarantor information for you. Choose '**N**' at the Employer Ins. Plan field because *Mrs. League's insurance is not provided by* an employer. Finally, press **F1** or click on the PROCESS button ('√') on the top toolbar to process and the Insurance Policy Information screen for Mrs. League's second policy will appear.

Enter '**0**' again at the Policyholder field. Then enter the carrier code for Mrs. League's second policy, a supplemental policy through Medicare Plus (**MEDIP**). Select the appropriate plan (there is only one) from the help window that automatically displays. Press **ENTER** to accept the default of 'Y' for the Assignment field. Press **ENTER** to leave the Group Name or # field blank and at both of the Policy Dates fields. Enter Mrs. League's Ins. ID #, **328948929299**, from her patient registration form. Press **ENTER** to leave the User Note, Rpt. Group, and Copay Ext. fields blank. Enter '**0**' then choose (**G**)uarantor at the Insured Party # field and the system will complete the relevant guarantor information for you. Choose '**N**' at the Employer Ins. Plan field since Mrs. League's insurance is not through an employer. Finally, press **F1** or click on the Process button ('√') on the top toolbar and the Insurance Policy Information screen for Mrs. League's second policy will be processed.

Figure 2-9 Adding Primary Insurance, Medicare

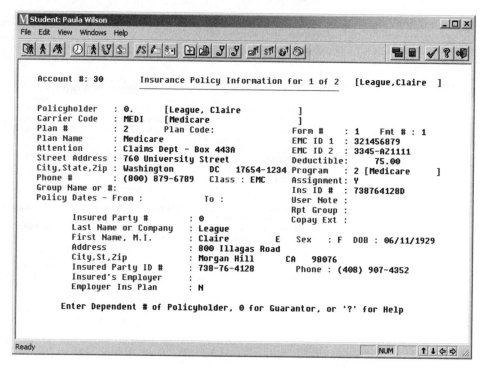

Your screens should be similar to Figures 2-9 and 2-10. Once you have processed both Insurance Policy Information screens, the Insurance Coverage Priority screen will appear. This screen tells the system the order in which the insurance plans should be billed for each patient. This first screen is used to set the coverage priority for the guarantor. Priorities are displayed in the order the policies were entered, as shown in Figure 2-11. *Note that Medicare is the primary policy and Medicare Plus is the secondary policy.*

Figure 2-10 Adding Secondary Insurance, Medicare Plus

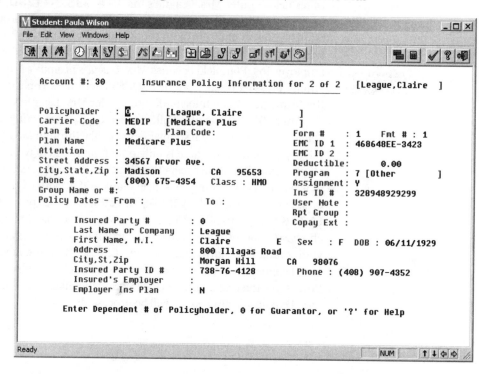

Figure 2-11 Insurance Coverage Priority—Guarantor List

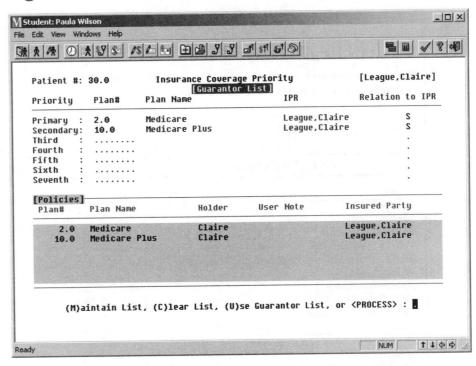

Press **F1** or click on the PROCESS button ('√') to process the Coverage Priority screen. The system will return to the New Patient Entry screen.

EXERCISE 2: Wayne R. Dudley

Adding a Patient with Extended Information

The next account is for Mr. Wayne Dudley. Complete the fields as you did in previous accounts, using the information shown in Figure 2-12 that follows. To be sure that Mr. Dudley has not already been entered into the system, key '**?Dudley**' in the Guarantor Last Name field at New Patient Entry and press **ENTER**. Remember that you can also click on the Help button ('?') on the top toolbar and then scroll through the list of patients who have already been entered into the system to see if Mr. Dudley is on file.

STEP 1

Because Mr. Dudley's name is not already on file, press **ESCAPE** then press **ENTER** to proceed and add his account to the system. Key Mr. Dudley's patient number, '**34**', shown on his patient registration form and press **ENTER**. The Guarantor Information screen will appear. Progress through the fields just as you did in the previous exercise, taking information from the patient registration form (Figure 2-12) and using the appropriate help windows, if necessary.

Note: Remember to key '2' for extended information because Mr. Dudley completed information concerning his employer that needs to be entered in the Extended Information screen.

First Name: **Wayne**
M.I.: **R**
Street Address1: **Route 1, Box 23**
Street Address2: (Press **ENTER** to leave blank)
City: **Woodside**
State: **CA**
Zip Code: **98076**

Figure 2-12 Wayne Dudley—Patient Registration Form

Patient Registration Form

Sydney Carrington & Associates
34 Sycamore Street ● Madison, CA 95653

TODAY'S DATE: _01/10/2003_

FOR OFFICE USE ONLY	
ACCOUNT NO.:	**34**
DOCTOR:	**#3**
BILL TYPE:	**11**
EXTENDED INFO.:	**2**

PATIENT INFORMATION

Dudley | _Wayne_ | _R._
PATIENT LAST NAME | FIRST NAME | MI

Self
RELATIONSHIP TO GUARANTOR

_M_ | _08/28/1965_ | _Single_ | _678-75-4343_
SEX (M/F) | DATE OF BIRTH | MARITAL STATUS | SOC. SEC. #

Hudson Construction
EMPLOYER OR SCHOOL NAME

Route 1, Box 23
ADDRESS OF EMPLOYER OR SCHOOL

Woodside | _CA_ | _98076_
CITY | STATE | ZIP CODE

_(408) 789-3209_ | _David Barrett, M.D._
EMPLOYER OR SCHOOL PHONE | REFERRED BY

E-MAIL

GUARANTOR INFORMATION

Dudley | _Wayne_ | _R._ | _M_
RESPONSIBLE PARTY LAST NAME | FIRST NAME | MI | SEX (M/F)

Route 1, Box 23
MAILING ADDRESS | STREET ADDRESS (IF DIFFERENT)

Woodside | _CA_ | _98076_
CITY | STATE | ZIP CODE

_(408) 789-6654_ | _(408) 789-3209_
(AREA CODE) HOME PHONE | (AREA CODE) WORK PHONE

_08/28/1965_ | _Single_ | _678-75-4343_
DATE OF BIRTH | MARITAL STATUS | SOC. SEC. #

Hudson Construction
EMPLOYER NAME

Route 1, Box 23
EMPLOYER ADDRESS

Woodside | _CA_ | _98076_
CITY | STATE | ZIP CODE

PRIMARY INSURANCE

Cross and Shield Ins. Plus
NAME OF PRIMARY INSURANCE COMPANY

435 Embarcadero
ADDRESS

Madison | _CA_ | _95653_
CITY | STATE | ZIP CODE

_8678754343_ | _Hudson Construction_
IDENTIFICATION # | GROUP NAME AND/OR #

Wayne R. Dudley
INSURED PERSON'S NAME (IF DIFFERENT FROM THE RESPONSIBLE PARTY)

Same
ADDRESS (IF DIFFERENT)

Same
CITY | STATE | ZIP CODE

_(800) 345-7689_ | _678-75-4343_
PRIMARY INSURANCE PHONE NUMBER | SOC. SEC. #

Self
WHAT IS THE RESPONSIBLE PARTY'S RELATIONSHIP TO THE INSURED?

SECONDARY INSURANCE

NAME OF SECONDARY INSURANCE COMPANY

ADDRESS

CITY | STATE | ZIP CODE

IDENTIFICATION # | GROUP NAME AND/OR #

INSURED PERSON'S NAME (IF DIFFERENT FROM THE RESPONSIBLE PARTY)

ADDRESS (IF DIFFERENT)

CITY | STATE | ZIP CODE

SECONDARY INSURANCE PHONE NUMBER | SOC. SEC. #

WHAT IS THE RESPONSIBLE PARTY'S RELATIONSHIP TO THE INSURED?

I hereby consent for Sydney Carrington & Associates, P.A. to use or disclose my health information to carry out treatment, payment, and health care operations. I authorize the use of this signature on all insurance submissions. I understand that I am financially responsible for all charges whether or not paid by the insurance. I acknowledge receipt of the practice's privacy policy.

Wayne R. Dudley | _01/10/2003_
PATIENT SIGNATURE | DATE

Sex (M/F): (**M**)ale
Employed: (**E**)mployed
Employer/School: **Hudson Construction**
Home Phone #: **4087896654**

Work Phone #: **4087893209**
Work Ext #: (Press **ENTER** to leave blank)
Date of Birth: **08281965**
Social Sec. #: **678754343**
Patient ID: (Press **ENTER** to leave blank)
Patient ID 2: (Press **ENTER** to leave blank)
Marital Status: (**S**)ingle
Race: (Press **ENTER** to leave blank)
E-mail: (Press **ENTER** to leave blank)
Account Date: (Press **ENTER** to default to current system date of 01/10/03)
# of Dependents: **0**
# of Ins. Policies: **1**
Extended Info. Level: **2** (Full)
Guar. Is a Patient: (**Y**)es
Ref. Dr #: **1** (Dr. David Barrett)
Doctor #: **3** (Dr. Sydney Carrington)
Status: (Press **ENTER** to accept default of '1')
Bill Type: (Press **ENTER** to accept default of '11')
Tax Code: (Press **ENTER** to leave blank)
Consent: (Press **ENTER** to accept the default of (**Y**)es)
WP ID: (Press **ENTER** to accept default of 'C:wp34.0')
Class: (Press **ENTER** to leave blank)
Note: (Press **ENTER** to accept default of '0')
Days Before Collections: (Press **ENTER** to accept default of '0')
Collection Priority: (Press **ENTER** to accept default of '0')
Discount %: (Press **ENTER** to accept default of '0')
Budget Payment: (Press **ENTER** to accept default of '0.00')

Compare your screen with Figure 2-13. When you are sure all information has been entered correctly, press **F1** or click on the PROCESS button ('√') on the top toolbar to process.

Figure 2-13 Completed Guarantor Information

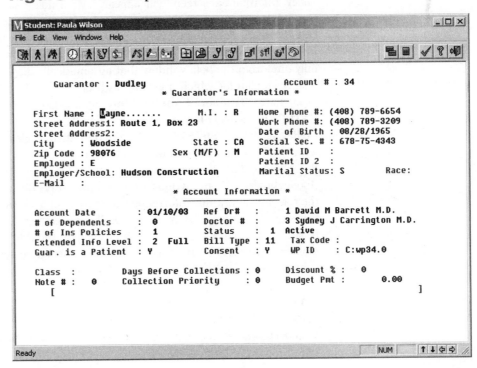

Figure 2-14 Completed Extended Information Screen

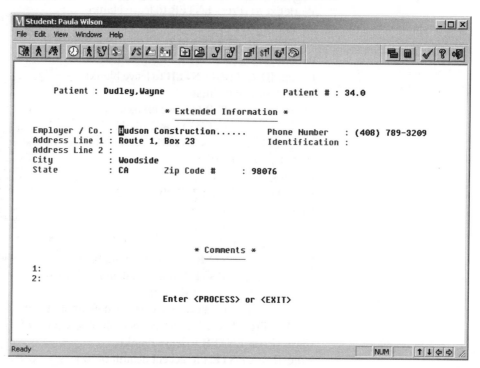

```
M Student: Paula Wilson                                                    _□×
File  Edit  View  Windows  Help

 ▨▯▯  ▯▯▯  ▯▯▯  ▯▯▯  ▯▯▯  ▯▯▯  ▯▯▯  ▯▯▯              ▯▯  ▯▯▯

        Patient : Dudley,Wayne                  Patient # : 34.0

                         * Extended Information *
                         ───────────────────────
     Employer / Co. : Hudson Construction......    Phone Number   : (408) 789-3209
     Address Line 1 : Route 1, Box 23             Identification :
     Address Line 2 :
     City           : Woodside
     State          : CA        Zip Code #   : 98076




                            * Comments *
                            ────────────
       1:
       2:

                       Enter <PROCESS> or <EXIT>




Ready                                                      NUM       ↑↓⇦⇨
```

STEP 2

Once you have processed the Guarantor Information entered for Mr. Dudley, the Extended Information screen will appear. Enter the information listed on Mr. Dudley's patient registration form regarding his employer, Hudson Construction. Press **ENTER** to bypass the Identification and both Comment fields. Compare your screen with the Extended Information screen shown in Figure 2-14. When you are sure the information you entered is correct, press the **F1** key or click on the PROCESS button ('√') on the top toolbar to process.

After processing the Extended Information screen for Mr. Dudley, the Insurance Policy Information screen will appear. Mr. Dudley has basic insurance coverage through his employer, Hudson Construction. Mr. Dudley is the policyholder so you will enter '**O**' at the Policyholder field. Use the help window to find the correct carrier code. Choose the carrier code **CASA**. Then, select the appropriate insurance plan (there is only one) from the help window that automatically displays. Mr. Dudley's is the first insurance plan for which a group has been listed. Press **ENTER** at the Assignment Field. Enter '**Hudson Construction**' in the Group Name or # field, then press **ENTER**. Press **ENTER** at both of the Policy Dates fields to leave them blank. Enter Mr. Dudley's Ins. ID #, **S678754343**, from his patient registration form. Press **ENTER** to leave the User Note, Rpt. Group, and Copay Ext. fields blank. Key '**O**' at the Insured Party field and the prompt will appear asking for (N)ew Insured Party, (G)uarantor, or (P)olicyholder. Choose (**G**)uarantor and press **ENTER** and the system will complete the relevant guarantor information for you. Enter (**Y**)es at the Employer Insurance field since his employer provides Mr. Dudley's coverage. Your completed screen should be similar to Figure 2-15. Press **F1** or click on the PROCESS button ('√') on the top toolbar to process first the Insurance Plan Information screen, then again to process the Coverage Priority screen.

Figure 2-15 Completed Insurance Plan Information Screen

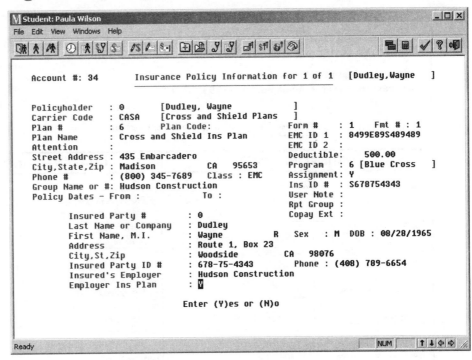

EXERCISE 3: Deborah A. Evans

Adding an Account with a Dependent

In this exercise, you will add an account for Deborah and Gene Evans. You will have two patient registration forms. Begin with the form for Deborah (Figure 2-17) because she is the guarantor. Note that the name Evans has been entered previously. If you key '**?Evans**' in the Enter Guarantor Last Name field and press **ENTER**, the screen shown in Figure 2-16 will appear, indicating that an account with that last name is on file

Figure 2-16 Check for Existing Account

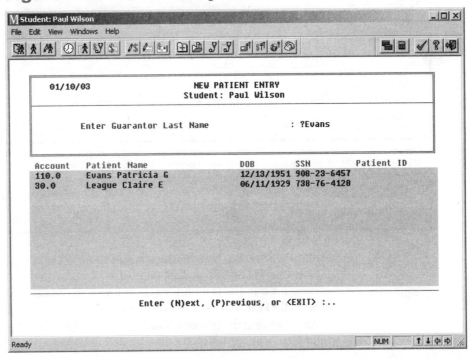

Figure 2-17 Deborah Evans—Patient Registration Form

Patient Registration Form

Sydney Carrington & Associates
34 Sycamore Street ● Madison, CA 95653

TODAY'S DATE: _01/10/2003_

FOR OFFICE USE ONLY	
ACCOUNT NO.:	**14**
DOCTOR:	**#3**
BILL TYPE:	**11**
EXTENDED INFO.:	**2**

PATIENT INFORMATION

Evans   _Deborah_   _A._
PATIENT LAST NAME   FIRST NAME   MI
Self
RELATIONSHIP TO GUARANTOR
_F_   _11/27/1969_   _Married_   _908-78-5674_
SEX (M/F)   DATE OF BIRTH   MARITAL STATUS   SOC. SEC. #
Bell Labs
EMPLOYER OR SCHOOL NAME
374 S. Grange Street
ADDRESS OF EMPLOYER OR SCHOOL
Madison   _CA_   _95642_
CITY   STATE   ZIP CODE
_(916) 665-3456_   _Leland Groves, M.D._
EMPLOYER OR SCHOOL PHONE   REFERRED BY

E-MAIL

GUARANTOR INFORMATION

Evans   _Deborah_   _A._ | _F_
RESPONSIBLE PARTY LAST NAME   FIRST NAME   MI   SEX (M/F)
1901 NW 2nd Street
MAILING ADDRESS   STREET ADDRESS (IF DIFFERENT)
Madison   _CA_   _95653_
CITY   STATE   ZIP CODE
_(916) 678-5674_   _(916) 665-3456_
(AREA CODE) HOME PHONE   (AREA CODE) WORK PHONE
_11/27/1969_   _Married_   _908-78-5674_
DATE OF BIRTH   MARITAL STATUS   SOC. SEC. #
Bell Labs
EMPLOYER NAME
374 S. Grange Street
EMPLOYER ADDRESS
Madison   _CA_   _95642_
CITY   STATE   ZIP CODE

PRIMARY INSURANCE

Pan American Health Ins.
NAME OF PRIMARY INSURANCE COMPANY
4567 Newberry Road
ADDRESS
Los Angeles   _CA_   _98706_
CITY   STATE   ZIP CODE
_908785674_   _Bell Labs_
IDENTIFICATION #   GROUP NAME AND/OR #
Deborah A. Evans
INSURED PERSON'S NAME (IF DIFFERENT FROM THE RESPONSIBLE PARTY)
Same
ADDRESS (IF DIFFERENT)
Same
CITY   STATE   ZIP CODE
_(213) 456-7654_   _908-78-5674_
PRIMARY INSURANCE PHONE NUMBER   SOC. SEC. #
Self
WHAT IS THE RESPONSIBLE PARTY'S RELATIONSHIP TO THE INSURED?

SECONDARY INSURANCE

NAME OF SECONDARY INSURANCE COMPANY

ADDRESS

CITY   STATE   ZIP CODE

IDENTIFICATION #   GROUP NAME AND/OR #

INSURED PERSON'S NAME (IF DIFFERENT FROM THE RESPONSIBLE PARTY)

ADDRESS (IF DIFFERENT)

CITY   STATE   ZIP CODE

SECONDARY INSURANCE PHONE NUMBER   SOC. SEC. #

WHAT IS THE RESPONSIBLE PARTY'S RELATIONSHIP TO THE INSURED?

I hereby consent for Sydney Carrington & Associates, P.A. to use or disclose my health information to carry out treatment, payment, and health care operations. I authorize the use of this signature on all insurance submissions. I understand that I am financially responsible for all charges whether or not paid by the insurance. I acknowledge receipt of the practice's privacy policy.

Deborah A. Evans   _01/10/2003_
PATIENT SIGNATURE   DATE

already. However, because the account you want to add has nothing to do with Patricia Evans, press **ESCAPE** or click on the EXIT button on the top toolbar and the cursor will move back to the Guarantor Last Name field. Because this is the correct last name, press **ENTER** to accept it. The cursor will then move to the Account Number field. After entering the proper account number, '**14**', enter the data shown in Figure 2-17 for Mrs. Evans by following the instructions below.

Before attempting data entry, study the patient registration form shown in Figures 2-17 and 2-20 (page 80) and answer the following questions:

1. Where does Mrs. Evans work?

2. What is Mrs. Evans's husband's name?

3. Where does Mrs. Evans's husband work?

4. Who holds the insurance policy listed, Deborah or her husband?

5. Is the insurance policy offered through an employer? If so, whose?

STEP 1

Continue posting Mrs. Evans's account using the information provided in her patient registration form (Figure 2-17). Because Mrs. Evans's employer information is provided, be sure to enter '2' in the Extended Info Level field of the Guarantor Information screen. Also, since Mrs. Evans's husband is considered a dependent (for data entry purposes), be sure to enter '1' in the # Dependents field of the Guarantor Information screen.

First Name: **Deborah**
M.I.: **A**
Street Address1: **1901 NW 2nd Street**
Street Address2: (Press **ENTER** to leave blank)
City: **Madison**
State: **CA**
Zip Code: **95653**
Sex (M/F): (**F**)emale
Employed: (**E**)mployed
Employer/School: **Bell Labs**
Home Phone #: **9166785674**
Work Phone #: **9166653456**
Work Ext #: (Press **ENTER** to leave blank)
Date of Birth: **11271969**
Social Sec. #: **908785674**
Patient ID: (Press **ENTER** to leave blank)
Patient ID 2: (Press **ENTER** to leave blank)
Marital Status: (**M**)arried
Race: (Press **ENTER** to leave blank)
E-mail: (Press **ENTER** to leave blank)
Account Date: (Press **ENTER** to default to current system date of 01/10/03)
# of Dependents: **1**
# of Ins. Policies: **1**
Extended Info. Level: **2** (Full)
Guar. Is a Patient: (**Y**)es
Ref. Dr. #: **2** (Dr. Leland Groves)
Doctor #: **3** (Dr. Sydney Carrington)
Status: (Press **ENTER** to accept default of '1')
Bill Type: (Press **ENTER** to accept default of '11')
Tax Code: (Press **ENTER** to leave blank)
Consent: (Press **ENTER** to accept the default of (**Y**)es)
WP ID: (Press **ENTER** to accept default of 'C:wp14.0')
Class: (Press **ENTER** to leave blank)
Note: (Press **ENTER** to accept default of '0')
Days Before Collections: (Press **ENTER** to accept default of '0')
Collection Priority: (Press **ENTER** to accept default of '0')
Discount %: (Press **ENTER** to accept default of '0')
Budget Payment: (Press **ENTER** to accept default of '0.00')

Figure 2-18 Completed Guarantor Information Screen

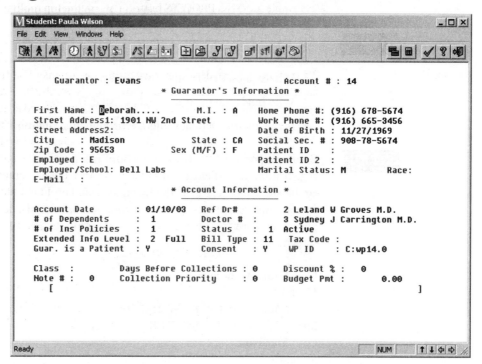

Check your screen against Figure 2-18. When you are sure all information has been entered correctly, press **F1** or click on the PROCESS button ('√') on the top toolbar to process.

STEP 2

When the information you entered above is processed, the Extended Information screen will appear so that you can enter additional employment information for Mrs. Evans. Use the information shown in her patient registration form to complete this screen. You may also use Figure 2-19 as a guide. Remember to complete all fields for

Figure 2-19 Completed Extended Information Screen

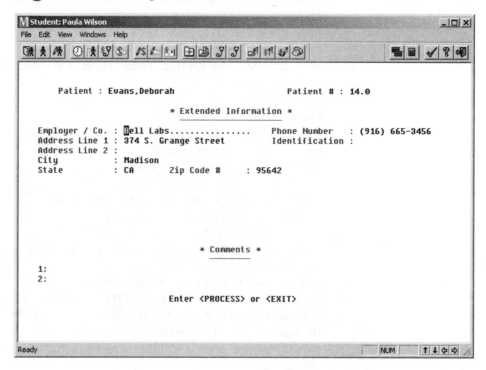

which you have information. Compare your screen to Figure 2-19, then press the **F1** key or click on the PROCESS button ('√') on the top toolbar.

STEP 3 After you have processed the Extended Information screen for Mrs. Evans, the Dependent Information screen will appear so that you may enter information about Mrs. Evans's dependent, her husband, Gene Evans. Use the information provided on his patient registration form as shown in Figure 2-20. Even though two patients are entered in the one account, each patient has completed a separate form. When you are completing the Dependent Information screen, remember to press **ENTER** at any field for which no information is provided on the patient registration form. Because employment information is provided for Mr. Evans, be sure to enter '**2**' in the Extended Information Level field of the Dependent Information screen. Once processed, you will be provided with a separate screen in which you may enter Extended Information for Mr. Evans.

Dependent Information

Enter the dependent information for Mrs. Evans's husband Gene using the information provided on Mr. Evans's patient registration form (Figure 2-20). Because the dependent's last name is the same as the guarantor's last name, press **ENTER** to accept the default last name for this account, 'Evans.'

Remember that the Dependent # is assigned automatically by **The Medical Manager** system.

Dependent Last Name: **Evans**
Dependent First Name: **Gene**
M.I.: **S**
Dependent Date of Birth: **12121968**
Dependent Sex: (**M**)ale
Relationship to Guarantor: (**H**)usband
Social Security #: **652874136**
Patient ID: (Press **ENTER** to leave blank)
Patient ID 2: (Press **ENTER** to leave blank)
Default Doctor #: (Press **ENTER** to default to '0' – Use Guarantor's Doctor)
Referring Doctor #: (Press **ENTER** to default to '0')
Extended Information Level: **2** (Full)
WP File ID: (Press **ENTER** to default to 'C:wp14.1')
Marital Status: (**M**)arried
Race: (Press **ENTER** to leave blank)
Employment/Student Status: (**E**)mployed
Date Became a Patient: (Press **ENTER** to default to system date)
Consent Info.: (Press **ENTER**) to accept default of (**Y**)es)
E-mail: (Press **ENTER** to leave blank)

Your screen should be similar to Figure 2-21. Press **F1** or click on the PROCESS button ('√') when you are ready to process and save the information you entered.

Figure 2-20 Gene Evans—Patient Registration Form

Patient Registration Form

Sydney Carrington & Associates
34 Sycamore Street ● Madison, CA 95653

TODAY'S DATE: _01/10/2003_

FOR OFFICE USE ONLY	
ACCOUNT NO.:	**14**
DOCTOR:	**#3**
BILL TYPE:	**11**
EXTENDED INFO.:	**2**

PATIENT INFORMATION

Evans   _Gene_   _A._
PATIENT LAST NAME   FIRST NAME   MI

Husband
RELATIONSHIP TO GUARANTOR

_M_ | _12/12/1968_ | _Married_ | _652-87-4136_
SEX (M/F)   DATE OF BIRTH   MARITAL STATUS   SOC. SEC. #

Elton Printing Co.
EMPLOYER OR SCHOOL NAME

2357 W. Fulton Avenue
ADDRESS OF EMPLOYER OR SCHOOL

Madison | _CA_ | _95642_
CITY   STATE   ZIP CODE

_(916) 561-0042_ | _Leland Groves, M.D._
EMPLOYER OR SCHOOL PHONE   REFERRED BY

E-MAIL

GUARANTOR INFORMATION

Evans   _Deborah_   _A._ | _F_
RESPONSIBLE PARTY LAST NAME   FIRST NAME   MI   SEX (M/F)

1901 NW 2nd Street
MAILING ADDRESS   STREET ADDRESS (IF DIFFERENT)

Madison | _CA_ | _95653_
CITY   STATE   ZIP CODE

_(916) 678-5674_ | _(916) 665-3456_
(AREA CODE) HOME PHONE   (AREA CODE) WORK PHONE

_11/27/1969_ | _Married_ | _908-78-5674_
DATE OF BIRTH   MARITAL STATUS   SOC. SEC. #

Bell Labs
EMPLOYER NAME

374 S. Grange Street
EMPLOYER ADDRESS

Madison | _CA_ | _95642_
CITY   STATE   ZIP CODE

PRIMARY INSURANCE

Pan American Health Ins.
NAME OF PRIMARY INSURANCE COMPANY

4567 Newberry Road
ADDRESS

Los Angeles | _CA_ | _98706_
CITY   STATE   ZIP CODE

_908785674_ | _Bell Labs_
IDENTIFICATION #   GROUP NAME AND/OR #

Deborah A. Evans
INSURED PERSON'S NAME (IF DIFFERENT FROM THE RESPONSIBLE PARTY)

1901 NW 2nd Street
ADDRESS (IF DIFFERENT)

Madison | _CA_ | _95653_
CITY   STATE   ZIP CODE

_(213) 456-7654_ | _908-78-5674_
PRIMARY INSURANCE PHONE NUMBER   SOC. SEC. #

Self
WHAT IS THE RESPONSIBLE PARTY'S RELATIONSHIP TO THE INSURED?

SECONDARY INSURANCE

NAME OF SECONDARY INSURANCE COMPANY

ADDRESS

CITY   STATE   ZIP CODE

IDENTIFICATION #   GROUP NAME AND/OR #

INSURED PERSON'S NAME (IF DIFFERENT FROM THE RESPONSIBLE PARTY)

ADDRESS (IF DIFFERENT)

CITY   STATE   ZIP CODE

SECONDARY INSURANCE PHONE NUMBER   SOC. SEC. #

WHAT IS THE RESPONSIBLE PARTY'S RELATIONSHIP TO THE INSURED?

I hereby consent for Sydney Carrington & Associates, P.A. to use or disclose my health information to carry out treatment, payment, and health care operations. I authorize the use of this signature on all insurance submissions. I understand that I am financially responsible for all charges whether or not paid by the insurance. I acknowledge receipt of the practice's privacy policy.

Gene S. Evans   _01/10/2003_
PATIENT SIGNATURE   DATE

Figure 2-21 Completed Dependent Information Screen

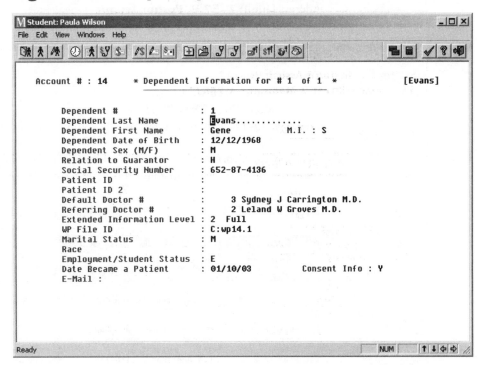

Dependent Extended Information

STEP 4

Because the encounter form shows employment information for Mr. Evans, and you chose extended information level 2, a screen requesting dependent extended information will appear as in Figure 2-22. Complete the fields using the information given below. When there is no information available for a field, remember to press **ENTER** to leave the field blank.

Figure 2-22 Completed Dependent Extended Information Screen

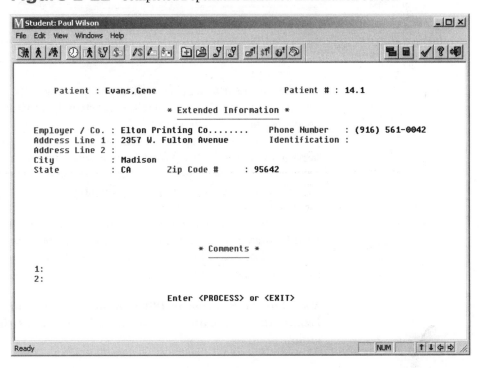

Employer/Co.: **Elton Printing Co.**
Address Line 1: **2357 W. Fulton Avenue**
Address Line 2: (Press **ENTER** to leave blank)
City: **Madison**
State: **CA**
Zip Code #: **95642**
Phone Number: **9165610042**
Identification: (Press **ENTER** to leave blank)
Press **ENTER** twice to bypass each of the comment fields.

After you process all dependent information, the Insurance Policy Information screen will appear for you to complete. Your screen should resemble Figure 2-23.

Figure 2-23 Completed Insurance Policy Information Screen

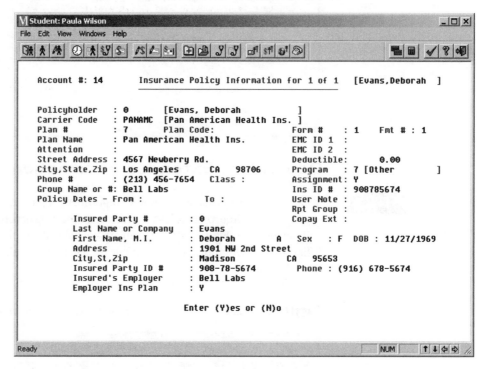

After the insurance policy is added and processed, the Insurance Coverage Priority screen will display. This screen tells the system the order in which the insurance plans should be billed for each patient.

This first screen is used to set the coverage priority for the guarantor. Priorities are displayed in the order the policies were entered, as shown in Figure 2-24. Make sure your screen looks like Figure 2-24 then press the **F1** key or click on the PROCESS button ('√') on the top toolbar to process the screen.

The next screen that will display is the Coverage Priority By Dependent screen. Mr. Evans's coverage priority is not currently set. Position the light bar on Gene Evans and press **ENTER**. Select the (**U**)se Guarantor List option to set Gene Evans's coverage the same as his wife's. Your screen should look like Figure 2-25.

Note that the Relation to IPR field has been automatically set to (H)usband because the system understands the relationship of the dependent to the guarantor.

Figure 2-27 Portia Edwards—Patient Registration Form

Patient Registration Form

Sydney Carrington & Associates
34 Sycamore Street ● Madison, CA 95653

TODAY'S DATE: _01/10/2003_

PATIENT INFORMATION

Edwards	Portia	D.
PATIENT LAST NAME	FIRST NAME	MI

Self
RELATIONSHIP TO GUARANTOR

F	11/25/1955	Married	766-54-4378
SEX (M/F)	DATE OF BIRTH	MARITAL STATUS	SOC. SEC. #

Portia Property Mgmt.
EMPLOYER OR SCHOOL NAME

487 James Road
ADDRESS OF EMPLOYER OR SCHOOL

Madison	CA	95653
CITY	STATE	ZIP CODE

(916) 899-9384
EMPLOYER OR SCHOOL PHONE   REFERRED BY

E-MAIL

GUARANTOR INFORMATION

Edwards	Portia	D.	F
RESPONSIBLE PARTY LAST NAME	FIRST NAME	MI	SEX (M/F)

235 Mandolin Court
MAILING ADDRESS   STREET ADDRESS (IF DIFFERENT)

Madison	CA	95653-0235
CITY	STATE	ZIP CODE

(916) 899-7800	(916) 899-9384
(AREA CODE) HOME PHONE	(AREA CODE) WORK PHONE

11/25/1955	Married	766-54-4378
DATE OF BIRTH	MARITAL STATUS	SOC. SEC. #

Portia Property Management
EMPLOYER NAME

487 James Road
EMPLOYER ADDRESS

Madison	CA	95653
CITY	STATE	ZIP CODE

PRIMARY INSURANCE

Epsilon Life & Casualty
NAME OF PRIMARY INSURANCE COMPANY

P.O. Box 189
ADDRESS

Macon	GA	31298
CITY	STATE	ZIP CODE

19FV293D01F	Watton Realty
IDENTIFICATION #	GROUP NAME AND/OR #

Edwards E. Edwards
INSURED PERSON'S NAME (IF DIFFERENT FROM THE RESPONSIBLE PARTY)

235 Mandolin Court
ADDRESS (IF DIFFERENT)

Madison	CA	95653-0235
CITY	STATE	ZIP CODE

(800) 908-7654	343-22-8898
PRIMARY INSURANCE PHONE NUMBER	SOC. SEC. #

Self
WHAT IS THE RESPONSIBLE PARTY'S RELATIONSHIP TO THE INSURED?

SECONDARY INSURANCE

NAME OF SECONDARY INSURANCE COMPANY

ADDRESS

CITY	STATE	ZIP CODE

IDENTIFICATION #	GROUP NAME AND/OR #

INSURED PERSON'S NAME (IF DIFFERENT FROM THE RESPONSIBLE PARTY)

ADDRESS (IF DIFFERENT)

CITY	STATE	ZIP CODE

SECONDARY INSURANCE PHONE NUMBER	SOC. SEC. #

WHAT IS THE RESPONSIBLE PARTY'S RELATIONSHIP TO THE INSURED?

I hereby consent for Sydney Carrington & Associates, P.A. to use or disclose my health information to carry out treatment, payment, and health care operations. I authorize the use of this signature on all insurance submissions. I understand that I am financially responsible for all charges whether or not paid by the insurance. I acknowledge receipt of the practice's privacy policy.

Portia D. Edwards	01/10/2003
PATIENT SIGNATURE	DATE

Complete the fields as you did in previous accounts, using the information shown in Figure 2-27. To be sure that Mrs. Edwards has not already been entered into the system, key '**?Edwards**' in the Enter Guarantor Last Name field at Patient Retrieval prompt of New Patient Entry and press **ENTER**. Remember that you can also click on the Help button ('?') on the top toolbar and then scroll through the list of patients who have already been entered into the system to see if Mrs. Edwards is on file.

STEP 1

Because Mrs. Edwards's name is not already on file, Press **ESCAPE** then press **ENTER** to proceed and add her account to the system. Key Mrs. Edwards' patient number, '**21**', shown on her patient registration form and press **ENTER**. The Guarantor Information screen will appear. Progress through the fields just as you did in the previous exercise, taking information from the patient registration form and using the appropriate help windows, if necessary. Be sure to enter the number of dependents as 2.

First Name: **Portia**
M.I.: **D**
Street Address1: **235 Mandolin Court**
Street Address2: (Press **ENTER** to leave blank)
City: **Madison**
State: **CA**
Zip Code: **95653-0235**
Sex (M/F): (**F**)emale
Employed: (**E**)mployed
Employer/School: **Portia Property Mgmt**.
Home Phone #: **9168997800**
Work Phone #: **9168999384**
Work Ext. #: (Press **ENTER** to leave blank)
Date of Birth: **11251955**
Social Sec. #: **766544378**
Patient ID: (Press **ENTER** to leave blank)
Patient ID 2: (Press **ENTER** to leave blank)
Marital Status: (**M**)arried
Race: (Press **ENTER** to leave blank)
E-mail: (Press **ENTER** to leave blank)
Account Date: (Press **ENTER** to default to current system date of 01/10/03)
# of Dependents: **2**
# of Ins. Policies: **1**
Extended Info. Level: **2** (Full)
Guar. Is a Patient: (**Y**)es
Ref. Dr. #: (Press **ENTER** to accept default of '0')
Doctor #: **3** (Dr. Sydney Carrington)
Status: (Press **ENTER** to accept default of '1')
Bill Type: (Press **ENTER** to accept default of '11')
Tax Code: (Press **ENTER** to leave blank)
Consent: (Press **ENTER** to accept the default of (**Y**)es)
WP ID: (Press **ENTER** to default to 'C:wp21.0')
Class: (Press **ENTER** to leave blank)
Note: (Press **ENTER** to accept default of '0')
Days Before Collections: (Press **ENTER** to accept default of '0')
Collection Priority: (Press **ENTER** to accept default of '0')
Discount %: (Press **ENTER** to accept default of '0')
Budget Payment: (Press **ENTER** to accept default of '0.00')

Check your screen against Mrs. Edwards's patient registration form. When you are sure all information has been entered correctly, press **F1** or click on the PROCESS button ('√') on the top toolbar to process.

STEP 2

When the information you entered above is processed, the Extended Information screen will appear so that you can enter additional employment information for Mrs. Edwards. Use the information shown in her patient registration form to complete this screen. When you are sure that you have completed all fields for which you have information, press the **F1** key or click on the PROCESS button ('√') on the top toolbar.

 STEP 3 After you have processed the Extended Information screen for Mrs. Edwards, the Dependent Information screen will appear so that you may enter information about

Figure 2-28 Edward Edwards—Patient Registration Form

Patient Registration Form

Sydney Carrington & Associates
34 Sycamore Street • Madison, CA 95653

FOR OFFICE USE ONLY	
ACCOUNT NO.:	21
DOCTOR:	#3
BILL TYPE:	11
EXTENDED INFO.:	2

TODAY'S DATE: _01/10/2003_

PATIENT INFORMATION

Edwards	_Edward_	_E._
PATIENT LAST NAME	FIRST NAME	MI

Husband
RELATIONSHIP TO GUARANTOR

_M_	_07/20/1954_	_Married_	_343-22-8898_
SEX (M/F)	DATE OF BIRTH	MARITAL STATUS	SOC. SEC. #

Watton Realty
EMPLOYER OR SCHOOL NAME

410 NW Rainbow Avenue
ADDRESS OF EMPLOYER OR SCHOOL

Madison	_CA_	_95653_
CITY	STATE	ZIP CODE

_(916) 899-7800_
EMPLOYER OR SCHOOL PHONE   REFERRED BY

E-MAIL

GUARANTOR INFORMATION

Edwards	_Portia_	_D._	_F_
RESPONSIBLE PARTY LAST NAME	FIRST NAME	MI	SEX (M/F)

235 Mandolin Court
MAILING ADDRESS   STREET ADDRESS (IF DIFFERENT)

Madison	_CA_	_95653-0235_
CITY	STATE	ZIP CODE

_(916) 899-7800_	_(916) 899-9384_
(AREA CODE) HOME PHONE	(AREA CODE) WORK PHONE

_11/25/1955_	_Married_	_766-54-4378_
DATE OF BIRTH	MARITAL STATUS	SOC. SEC. #

Portia Property Management
EMPLOYER NAME

487 James Road
EMPLOYER ADDRESS

Madison	_CA_	_95653_
CITY	STATE	ZIP CODE

PRIMARY INSURANCE

Epsilon Life & Casualty
NAME OF PRIMARY INSURANCE COMPANY

P.O. Box 189
ADDRESS

Macon	_GA_	_31298_
CITY	STATE	ZIP CODE

_19FV293D01F_	_Watton Realty_
IDENTIFICATION #	GROUP NAME AND/OR #

Edwards E. Edwards
INSURED PERSON'S NAME (IF DIFFERENT FROM THE RESPONSIBLE PARTY)

235 Mandolin Court
ADDRESS (IF DIFFERENT)

Madison	_CA_	_95653-0235_
CITY	STATE	ZIP CODE

_(800) 908-7654_	_343-22-8898_
PRIMARY INSURANCE PHONE NUMBER	SOC. SEC. #

Wife
WHAT IS THE RESPONSIBLE PARTY'S RELATIONSHIP TO THE INSURED?

SECONDARY INSURANCE

NAME OF SECONDARY INSURANCE COMPANY

ADDRESS

CITY	STATE	ZIP CODE

IDENTIFICATION #	GROUP NAME AND/OR #

INSURED PERSON'S NAME (IF DIFFERENT FROM THE RESPONSIBLE PARTY)

ADDRESS (IF DIFFERENT)

CITY	STATE	ZIP CODE

SECONDARY INSURANCE PHONE NUMBER	SOC. SEC. #

WHAT IS THE RESPONSIBLE PARTY'S RELATIONSHIP TO THE INSURED?

I hereby consent for Sydney Carrington & Associates, P.A. to use or disclose my health information to carry out treatment, payment, and health care operations. I authorize the use of this signature on all insurance submissions. I understand that I am financially responsible for all charges whether or not paid by the insurance. I acknowledge receipt of the practice's privacy policy.

Edward E. Edwards	_01/10/2003_
PATIENT SIGNATURE	DATE

Figure 2-29 First Dependent's Information Screen

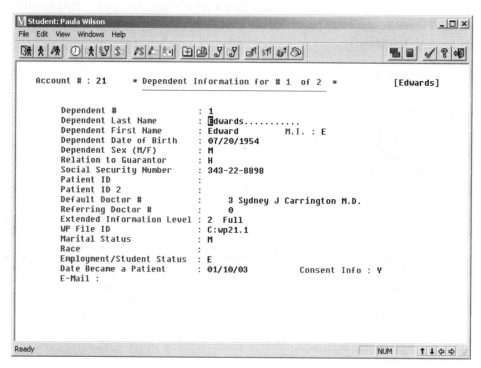

her first dependent, who is her husband, Edward. When you are completing the Dependent Information screen, remember that you may press ENTER at any field for which no information is provided on the patient registration form. Your screens should be similar to Figures 2-29 and 2-30.

Figure 2-30 First Dependent's Extended Information Screen

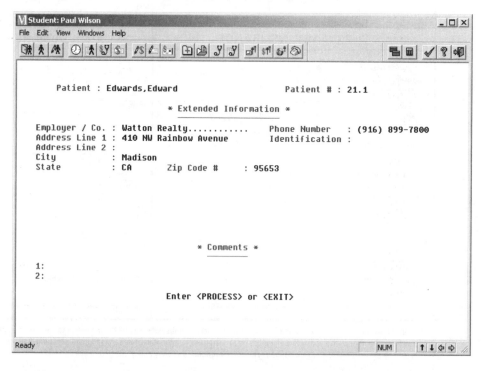

STEP 4   After you have processed the Extended Information screen for Mr. Edwards, the Dependent Information screen will appear again so that you may enter information

about the second dependent, their daughter Andrea. When you are completing the Dependent Information screen, remember to refer to Andrea's patient registration form as shown in Figure 2-31.

Figure 2-31 Andrea Edwards—Patient Registration Form

Patient Registration Form

Sydney Carrington & Associates
34 Sycamore Street ● Madison, CA 95653

TODAY'S DATE: _01/10/2003_

FOR OFFICE USE ONLY	
ACCOUNT NO.:	**21**
DOCTOR:	**#3**
BILL TYPE:	**11**
EXTENDED INFO.:	**2**

PATIENT INFORMATION

Edwards	Andrea	L.
PATIENT LAST NAME	FIRST NAME	MI

Daughter
RELATIONSHIP TO GUARANTOR

F	02/02/1988	Single	525-22-9314
SEX (M/F) DATE OF BIRTH	MARITAL STATUS		SOC. SEC. #

Madison High School
EMPLOYER OR SCHOOL NAME

ADDRESS OF EMPLOYER OR SCHOOL

Madison	CA	95642
CITY	STATE	ZIP CODE

EMPLOYER OR SCHOOL PHONE   REFERRED BY

E-MAIL

GUARANTOR INFORMATION

Edwards	Portia	D.	F
RESPONSIBLE PARTY LAST NAME	FIRST NAME	MI	SEX (M/F)

235 Mandolin Court
MAILING ADDRESS   STREET ADDRESS (IF DIFFERENT)

Madison	CA	95653-0235
CITY	STATE	ZIP CODE

(916)899-7800	(916) 899-9384
(AREA CODE) HOME PHONE	(AREA CODE) WORK PHONE

11/25/1955	Married	766-54-4378
DATE OF BIRTH	MARITAL STATUS	SOC. SEC. #

Portia Property Management
EMPLOYER NAME

487 James Road
EMPLOYER ADDRESS

Madison	CA	95653
CITY	STATE	ZIP CODE

PRIMARY INSURANCE

Epsilon Life & Casualty
NAME OF PRIMARY INSURANCE COMPANY

P.O. Box 189
ADDRESS

Macon	GA	31298
CITY	STATE	ZIP CODE

19FV293D01F	Watton Realty
IDENTIFICATION #	GROUP NAME AND/OR #

Edwards E. Edwards
INSURED PERSON'S NAME (IF DIFFERENT FROM THE RESPONSIBLE PARTY)

235 Mandolin Court
ADDRESS (IF DIFFERENT)

Madison	CA	95653-0235
CITY	STATE	ZIP CODE

(800)908-7654	343-22-8898
PRIMARY INSURANCE PHONE NUMBER	SOC. SEC. #

Wife
WHAT IS THE RESPONSIBLE PARTY'S RELATIONSHIP TO THE INSURED?

SECONDARY INSURANCE

NAME OF SECONDARY INSURANCE COMPANY

ADDRESS

CITY	STATE	ZIP CODE

IDENTIFICATION #	GROUP NAME AND/OR #

INSURED PERSON'S NAME (IF DIFFERENT FROM THE RESPONSIBLE PARTY)

ADDRESS (IF DIFFERENT)

CITY	STATE	ZIP CODE

SECONDARY INSURANCE PHONE NUMBER	SOC. SEC. #

WHAT IS THE RESPONSIBLE PARTY'S RELATIONSHIP TO THE INSURED?

I hereby consent for Sydney Carrington & Associates, P.A. to use or disclose my health information to carry out treatment, payment, and health care operations. I authorize the use of this signature on all insurance submissions. I understand that I am financially responsible for all charges whether or not paid by the insurance. I acknowledge receipt of the practice's privacy policy.

Portia D. Edwards (Mother)	01/10/2003
PATIENT SIGNATURE	DATE

Figure 2-32 Second Dependent's Information

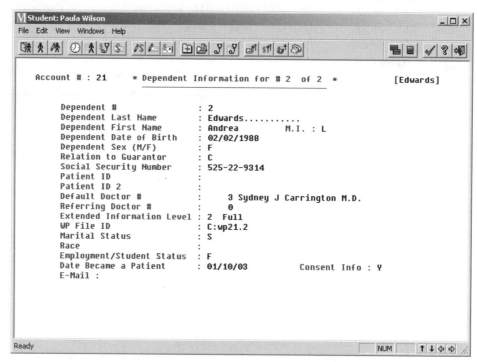

Figure 2-33 Second Dependent's Extended Information Screen

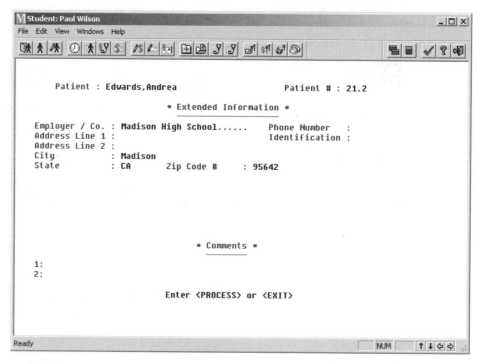

STEP 5   After you process all dependent information, the Insurance Policy Information Screen will appear for you to complete. Note that Mrs. Edwards is the guarantor of the account; however, the insurance plan is owned by her husband. When the cursor reaches the Insured Party # field, key (**P**)olicyholder (instead of (G)uarantor as you have done in previous exercises. In this exercise, the guarantor and the policyholder are two different people). Then answer (**Y**)es to create a new IPR (Insured Party Record). Do not type an insured party number yourself, because it will automatically be assigned by **The Medical Manager** system. Under some conditions, the number assigned may not

Insured party numbers are automatically assigned. Your number may be different from Figure 2-34.

match the number shown in Figure 2-34. Key in all remaining information. Be sure to include the insured's (Mr. Edwards's) ID number. Compare your screen with Figure 2-34, and press **F1** or click on the PROCESS button ('√') on the top toolbar to process.

Figure 2-34 Completed Insurance Policy Information Screen

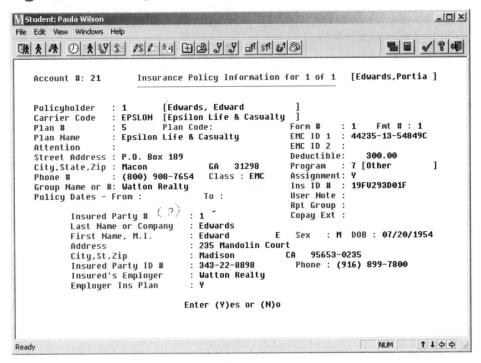

STEP 6 When the Coverage Priority screen displays, choose (**M**)aintain the list. Modify the list so that Epsilon is the primary policy. The two dependents will use the guarantor list. Your screen should be similar to Figure 2-35.

Figure 2-35 Coverage Priority By Dependent Screen

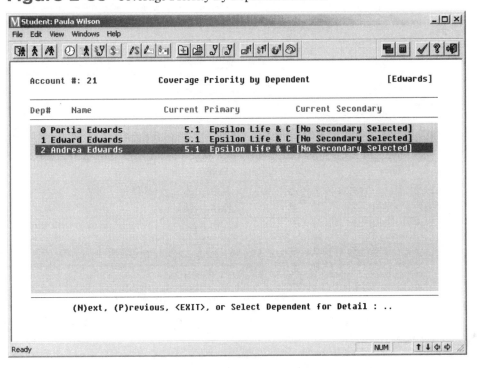

Complete all screens presented.

From now on, the repetitive screens, such as Guarantor Information, Extended Information, and others, will not be shown in the remaining exercises. Only new screens will be illustrated. However, you should complete all screens presented to you by the system during data entry. Remember to press ENTER to bypass any fields for which no information is provided.

Figure 2-36   Timothy Davis—Patient Registration Form

Patient Registration Form

Sydney Carrington & Associates
34 Sycamore Street ● Madison, CA 95653

TODAY'S DATE: _01/10/2003_

FOR OFFICE USE ONLY	
ACCOUNT NO.:	**80**
DOCTOR:	**#2**
BILL TYPE:	**11**
EXTENDED INFO.:	**2**

PATIENT INFORMATION

Davis   *Timothy*   *R.*
PATIENT LAST NAME   FIRST NAME   MI

Self
RELATIONSHIP TO GUARANTOR

M | *04/15/1959* | *Married* | *835-17-5465*
SEX (M/F)   DATE OF BIRTH   MARITAL STATUS   SOC. SEC. #

Bob Clark Construction
EMPLOYER OR SCHOOL NAME

P.O. Box 356
ADDRESS OF EMPLOYER OR SCHOOL

Madison | *CA* | *95653*
CITY   STATE   ZIP CODE

(916) 908-6479 | *Jason K. Detrasnik, M.D.*
EMPLOYER OR SCHOOL PHONE   REFERRED BY

E-MAIL

GUARANTOR INFORMATION

Davis   *Timothy*   *R.* | *M*
RESPONSIBLE PARTY LAST NAME   FIRST NAME   MI   SEX (M/F)

113 NE 22nd Avenue
MAILING ADDRESS   STREET ADDRESS (IF DIFFERENT)

Madison | *CA* | *95653*
CITY   STATE   ZIP CODE

(916) 908-7657 | *(916) 908-6479*
(AREA CODE) HOME PHONE   (AREA CODE) WORK PHONE

04/15/1959 | *Married* | *835-17-5465*
DATE OF BIRTH   MARITAL STATUS   SOC. SEC. #

Bob Clark Construction
EMPLOYER NAME

P.O. Box 356
EMPLOYER ADDRESS

Madison | *CA* | *95653*
CITY   STATE   ZIP CODE

PRIMARY INSURANCE

Fringe Benefits Center
NAME OF PRIMARY INSURANCE COMPANY

123 Mission Corners
ADDRESS

San Mateo | *TX* | *78723*
CITY   STATE   ZIP CODE

835175465
IDENTIFICATION # | *Bob Clark Construction*
          GROUP NAME AND/OR #

Bob Clark Construction
INSURED PERSON'S NAME (IF DIFFERENT FROM THE RESPONSIBLE PARTY)

P.O. Box 356
ADDRESS (IF DIFFERENT)

Madison | *CA* | *95653*
CITY   STATE   ZIP CODE

(800) 999-1234 | *835-17-5465*
PRIMARY INSURANCE PHONE NUMBER   SOC. SEC. #

Other
WHAT IS THE RESPONSIBLE PARTY'S RELATIONSHIP TO THE INSURED?

SECONDARY INSURANCE

NAME OF SECONDARY INSURANCE COMPANY

ADDRESS

| |
CITY   STATE   ZIP CODE

IDENTIFICATION #   GROUP NAME AND/OR #

INSURED PERSON'S NAME (IF DIFFERENT FROM THE RESPONSIBLE PARTY)

ADDRESS (IF DIFFERENT)

| |
CITY   STATE   ZIP CODE

| |
SECONDARY INSURANCE PHONE NUMBER   SOC. SEC. #

WHAT IS THE RESPONSIBLE PARTY'S RELATIONSHIP TO THE INSURED?

I hereby consent for Sydney Carrington & Associates, P.A. to use or disclose my health information to carry out treatment, payment, and health care operations. I authorize the use of this signature on all insurance submissions. I understand that I am financially responsible for all charges whether or not paid by the insurance. I acknowledge receipt of the practice's privacy policy.

Timothy R. Davis   *01/10/2003*
PATIENT SIGNATURE   DATE

EXERCISE 5: Timothy R. Davis

Adding an Account with Different Coverage Priorities

Mr. Timothy Davis is the guarantor on this account. His wife, Elizabeth, and daughter, Mindy, are also patients. Set up the account and dependent information using the information provided in Mr. Davis's patient registration forms (Figures 2-36, 2-37, page 95, and 2-39 on page 97). Note that Mindy has extended information, but Mrs. Davis does not. Therefore, be sure to enter '2' for Mindy to indicate that she has extended information. You will enter '0' for Mrs. Davis because there is no extended information provided for her on the patient registration form.

Complete the fields as you did in previous accounts, using the information shown in Figure 2-36. To be sure that Mr. Davis has not already been entered into the system, key '?**Davis**' in the Enter Guarantor Last Name field at New Patient Entry and press **ENTER**. Remember that you can also click on the Help button ('?') on the top toolbar and then scroll through the list of patients who have already been entered into the system to see if Mr. Davis is on file.

STEP 1 Since Mr. Davis's name is not already on file, press **ESCAPE** then press **ENTER** to proceed and add his account to the system. Key Mr. Davis's patient number, '**80**,' shown on his patient registration form and press **ENTER**. The Guarantor Information screen will appear. Progress through the fields just as you did in the previous exercise, taking information from the patient registration form and using the appropriate help windows, if necessary.

First Name: **Timothy**

M.I.: **R**

Street Address1: **113 NE 22nd Avenue**

Street Address2: (Press **ENTER** to leave blank)

City: **Madison**

State: **CA**

Zip Code: **95653**

Sex (M/F): **M**

Employed: **E**

Employer/School: **Bob Clark Construction**

Home Phone #: **9169087657**

Work Phone #: **9169086479**

Work Ext. #: (Press **ENTER** to leave blank)

Date of Birth: **04151959**

Social Sec. #: **835175465**

Patient ID: (Press **ENTER** to leave blank)

Patient ID 2: (Press **ENTER** to leave blank)

Marital Status: (**M**)arried

Race: (Press **ENTER** to leave blank)

E-mail: (Press **ENTER** to leave blank)

Account Date: (Press **ENTER** to default to current system date of 01/10/03)

# of Dependents: **2**

# of Ins. Policies: **1**

Extended Info. Level: **2** (Full)

Guar. Is a Patient: (**Y**)es

Ref. Dr. #: **4** (Dr. Jason Detrasnik)

Doctor #: **2** (Dr. Frances Simpson)

Status: (Press **ENTER** to accept default of '1')

Bill Type: (Press **ENTER** to accept default of '11')

Tax Code: (Press **ENTER** to leave blank)

Consent: (Press **ENTER** to accept the default of (**Y**)es)

WP ID: (Press **ENTER** to default to 'C:wp80.0')

Class: (Press **ENTER** to leave blank)

Note: (Press **ENTER** to accept default of '0')

Days Before Collections: (Press **ENTER** to accept default of '0')

Collection Priority: (Press **ENTER** to accept default of '0')

Discount %: (Press **ENTER** to accept default of '0')

Budget Payment: (Press **ENTER** to accept default of '0.00')

Check your screen against Mr. Davis's patient registration form. When you are sure all information has been entered correctly, press **F1** or click on the PROCESS button ('√') on the top toolbar to process.

STEP 2　When the information you entered above is processed, the Extended Information screen will appear so that you can enter additional employment information for Mr. Davis. Use the information shown on his patient registration form to complete this screen. When you are sure that you have completed all fields for which you have information, press the **F1** key or click on the PROCESS button ('√') on the top toolbar.

STEP 3　After you have processed the Extended Information screen for Mr. Davis, the Dependent Information screen will appear so that you may enter information about his dependents: his wife and daughter. Remember that you may press **ENTER** at any field for which no information is provided on the patient registration form. Use the patient registration form (Figure 2-37) to add the information for Elizabeth.

Dependent #: **1**

Dependent Last Name: **Davis**

Dependent First Name: **Elizabeth**

M.I.: **S.**

Dependent Date of Birth: **11251961**

Figure 2-37 Elizabeth Davis—Patient Registration Form

Patient Registration Form

Sydney Carrington & Associates
34 Sycamore Street ● Madison, CA 95653

FOR OFFICE USE ONLY	
ACCOUNT NO.:	**80**
DOCTOR:	**#2**
BILL TYPE:	**11**
EXTENDED INFO.:	**0**

TODAY'S DATE: _01/10/2003_

PATIENT INFORMATION

Davis   Elizabeth   S.
PATIENT LAST NAME   FIRST NAME   MI

Wife
RELATIONSHIP TO GUARANTOR

F | 11/25/1961 | Married | 764-65-7988
SEX (M/F) DATE OF BIRTH MARITAL STATUS SOC. SEC. #

EMPLOYER OR SCHOOL NAME

ADDRESS OF EMPLOYER OR SCHOOL

CITY   STATE   ZIP CODE

Jason K. Detrasnik, M.D.
EMPLOYER OR SCHOOL PHONE   REFERRED BY

E-MAIL

GUARANTOR INFORMATION

Davis   Timothy   R. | M
RESPONSIBLE PARTY LAST NAME FIRST NAME MI SEX (M/F)

113 NE 22nd Avenue
MAILING ADDRESS   STREET ADDRESS (IF DIFFERENT)

Madison   CA | 95653
CITY   STATE ZIP CODE

(916) 908-7657   (916) 908-6479
(AREA CODE) HOME PHONE   (AREA CODE) WORK PHONE

04/15/1959 | Married | 835-17-5465
DATE OF BIRTH MARITAL STATUS SOC. SEC. #

Bob Clark Construction
EMPLOYER NAME

P.O. Box 356
EMPLOYER ADDRESS

Madison   CA | 95653
CITY   STATE ZIP CODE

PRIMARY INSURANCE

NAME OF PRIMARY INSURANCE COMPANY

ADDRESS

CITY   STATE   ZIP CODE

IDENTIFICATION #   GROUP NAME AND/OR #

INSURED PERSON'S NAME (IF DIFFERENT FROM THE RESPONSIBLE PARTY)

ADDRESS (IF DIFFERENT)

CITY   STATE   ZIP CODE

PRIMARY INSURANCE PHONE NUMBER   SOC. SEC. #

WHAT IS THE RESPONSIBLE PARTY'S RELATIONSHIP TO THE INSURED?

SECONDARY INSURANCE

NAME OF SECONDARY INSURANCE COMPANY

ADDRESS

CITY   STATE   ZIP CODE

IDENTIFICATION #   GROUP NAME AND/OR #

INSURED PERSON'S NAME (IF DIFFERENT FROM THE RESPONSIBLE PARTY)

ADDRESS (IF DIFFERENT)

CITY   STATE   ZIP CODE

SECONDARY INSURANCE PHONE NUMBER   SOC. SEC. #

WHAT IS THE RESPONSIBLE PARTY'S RELATIONSHIP TO THE INSURED?

I hereby consent for Sydney Carrington & Associates, P.A. to use or disclose my health information to carry out treatment, payment, and health care operations. I authorize the use of this signature on all insurance submissions. I understand that I am financially responsible for all charges whether or not paid by the insurance. I acknowledge receipt of the practice's privacy policy.

Elizabeth S. Davis   01/10/2003
PATIENT SIGNATURE   DATE

Dependent Sex: **F**

Relation to Guarantor: **W**

Social Security #: **764657988**

Patient ID: (Press **ENTER** to leave blank)

Patient ID 2: (Press **ENTER** to leave blank)

Default Doctor #: (Press **ENTER** to default to '0' - use Guarantor's Doctor)

Referring Doctor #: (Press **ENTER** to default to '0')

Extended Information Level: **0**

WP File ID: (Press **ENTER** to default to C:wp80.1)

Marital Status: **M**

Race: (Press **ENTER** to leave blank)

Employment/Student Status: (Press **ENTER** to leave blank)

Date Became a Patient: (Press **ENTER** to default to system date)

Consent Info.: (Press **ENTER** to accept default of (**Y**)es)

E-mail: (Press **ENTER** to leave blank)

When you have completed entering information for the first dependent, your screen should be similar to Figure 2-38. Press **F1** or click on the PROCESS button ('√') on the top toolbar.

Figure 2-38 First Dependent's Information Screen

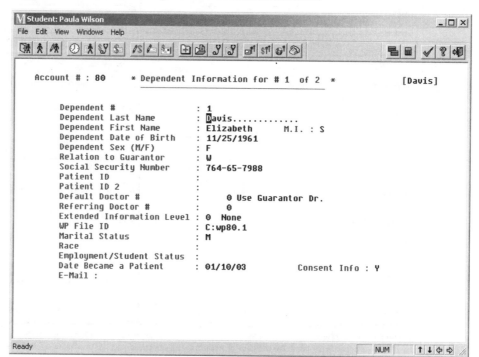

Now add the second dependent. Use the patient registration form in Figure 2-39 to add the information for Mindy Davis. Your screen should be similar to Figure 2-40. Press **F1** or click on the PROCESS button ('√') on the top toolbar.

Figure 2-39 Mindy Davis—Patient Registration Form

Patient Registration Form

Sydney Carrington & Associates
34 Sycamore Street ● Madison, CA 95653

TODAY'S DATE: _01/10/2003_

PATIENT INFORMATION	GUARANTOR INFORMATION
Davis *Mindy* *A.*	*Davis* *Timothy* *R.* *M*
PATIENT LAST NAME FIRST NAME MI	RESPONSIBLE PARTY LAST NAME FIRST NAME MI SEX (M/F)
Child	*113 NE 22nd Avenue*
RELATIONSHIP TO GUARANTOR	MAILING ADDRESS STREET ADDRESS (IF DIFFERENT)
F *06/18/1984* *Single* *968-64-6543*	*Madison* *CA* *95653*
SEX (M/F) DATE OF BIRTH MARITAL STATUS SOC. SEC. #	CITY STATE ZIP CODE
Madison Community College	*(916) 908-7657* *(916) 908-6479*
EMPLOYER OR SCHOOL NAME	(AREA CODE) HOME PHONE (AREA CODE) WORK PHONE
Jentsen Blvd.	*04/15/1959* *Married* *835-17-5465*
ADDRESS OF EMPLOYER OR SCHOOL	DATE OF BIRTH MARITAL STATUS SOC. SEC. #
Madison *CA* *95653*	*Bob Clark Construction*
CITY STATE ZIP CODE	EMPLOYER NAME
(916) 472-6315 *Jason K. Detrasnik, M.D.*	*P.O. Box 356*
EMPLOYER OR SCHOOL PHONE REFERRED BY	EMPLOYER ADDRESS
	Madison *CA* *95653*
E-MAIL	CITY STATE ZIP CODE

PRIMARY INSURANCE	SECONDARY INSURANCE
NAME OF PRIMARY INSURANCE COMPANY	NAME OF SECONDARY INSURANCE COMPANY
ADDRESS	ADDRESS
CITY STATE ZIP CODE	CITY STATE ZIP CODE
IDENTIFICATION # GROUP NAME AND/OR #	IDENTIFICATION # GROUP NAME AND/OR #
INSURED PERSON'S NAME (IF DIFFERENT FROM THE RESPONSIBLE PARTY)	INSURED PERSON'S NAME (IF DIFFERENT FROM THE RESPONSIBLE PARTY)
ADDRESS (IF DIFFERENT)	ADDRESS (IF DIFFERENT)
CITY STATE ZIP CODE	CITY STATE ZIP CODE
PRIMARY INSURANCE PHONE NUMBER SOC. SEC. #	SECONDARY INSURANCE PHONE NUMBER SOC. SEC. #
WHAT IS THE RESPONSIBLE PARTY'S RELATIONSHIP TO THE INSURED?	WHAT IS THE RESPONSIBLE PARTY'S RELATIONSHIP TO THE INSURED?

I hereby consent for Sydney Carrington & Associates, P.A. to use or disclose my health information to carry out treatment, payment, and health care operations. I authorize the use of this signature on all insurance submissions. I understand that I am financially responsible for all charges whether or not paid by the insurance. I acknowledge receipt of the practice's privacy policy.

Mindy A. Davis   *01/10/2003*

PATIENT SIGNATURE   DATE

Dependent #: **2**
Dependent Last Name: **Davis**
Dependent First Name: **Mindy**
M.I.: **A.**
Dependent Date of Birth: **06181984**
Dependent Sex: **F**
Relation to Guarantor: **C**
Social Security #: **968646543**
Patient ID: (Press **ENTER** to leave blank)
Patient ID 2: (Press **ENTER** to leave blank)
Default Doctor #: (Press **ENTER** to default to '0' - use Guarantor's Doctor)
Referring Doctor #: (Press **ENTER** to default to '0')
Extended Information Level: **2**
WP File ID: (Press **ENTER** to default to C:wp80.2)
Marital Status: **S**
Race: (Press **ENTER** to leave blank)
Employment/Student Status: **F**
Date Became a Patient: (Press **ENTER** to accept default system date)
Consent Info.: (Press **ENTER** to accept default of (**Y**)es)
E-mail: (Press **ENTER** to leave blank)

Figure 2-40 Second Dependent's Information Screen

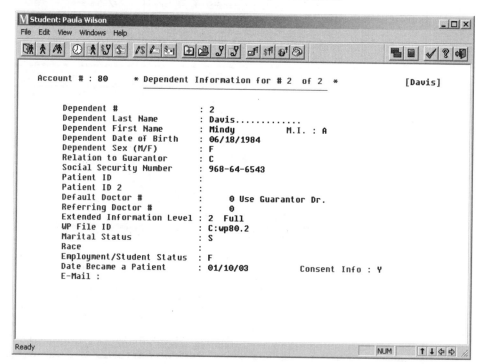

The Extended Information screen will appear. Enter Mindy's school information and compare your screen to Figure 2-41. Press **F1** or click on the PROCESS button ('√') on the top toolbar.

STEP 4

After you process all dependent information, the Insurance Policy Information screen will appear for you to complete. The Davises do not have insurance coverage on the family, but Mr. Davis has coverage for a Worker's Compensation injury through his employer. You should indicate in the User Note that the insurance policy on this account is for Mr. Davis's Worker's Compensation injury only. Mr. Davis's employer will be the (**N**)ew Insured Party. Refer back to Figure 2-36 for Mr. Davis's insurance information

Figure 2-41 Second Dependent's Extended Information Screen

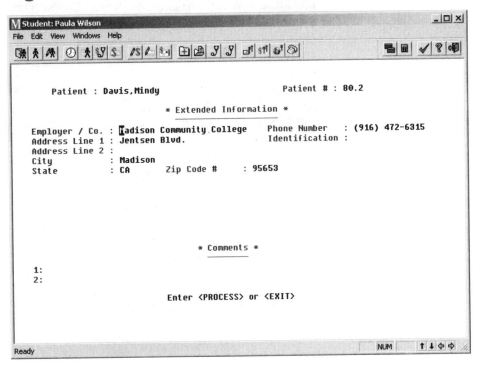

Note: Insured party numbers are automatically assigned by The Medical Manager system. Under certain conditions the numbers may not match those shown in Figure 2-42. All other fields in the figure should match your screen. When your screen is correct, press F1 or click on the PROCESS button ('√') on the top toolbar.

Figure 2-42 Insurance Policy Information for Coverage through Worker's Compensation

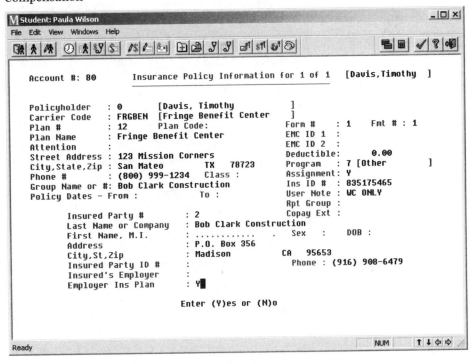

Next, the Insurance Coverage Priority list for the guarantor will display. Press **ENTER** to move to the Relation to IPR field. Choose (**O**)ther for Mr. Davis's relationship to the Insured Party (in this case, Bob Clark Construction). See Figure 2-43.

Figure 2-43 Insurance Coverage Priority Screen

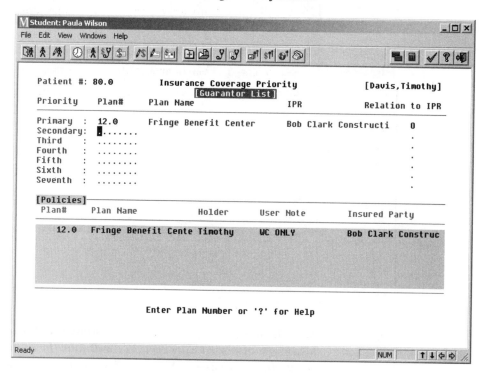

The next screen displayed will be the Coverage Priority By Dependent screen. Your screen should be similar to Figure 2-44. Press ESCAPE

Figure 2-44 Coverage Priority By Dependent Screen

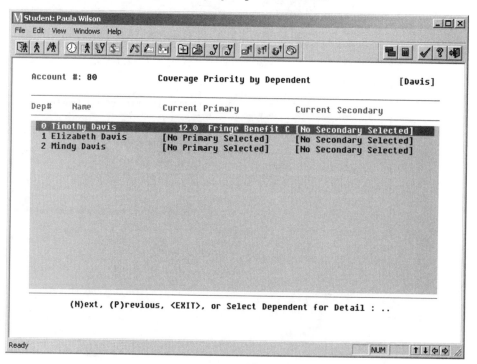

Before attempting data entry, study the patient registration form shown in Figures 2-45 and 2-50 (page 106); answer the following questions:

1. How many children does Ms. Williams have?

Figure 2-45 Laura Simmons—Patient Registration Form

Patient Registration Form

Sydney Carrington & Associates
34 Sycamore Street ● Madison, CA 95653

TODAY'S DATE: _01/10/2003_

<table>
<tr><td colspan="2">FOR OFFICE USE ONLY</td></tr>
<tr><td>ACCOUNT NO.:</td><td>120</td></tr>
<tr><td>DOCTOR:</td><td>#1</td></tr>
<tr><td>BILL TYPE:</td><td>11</td></tr>
<tr><td>EXTENDED INFO.:</td><td>2</td></tr>
</table>

PATIENT INFORMATION

Simmons	Laura	S.
PATIENT LAST NAME	FIRST NAME	MI

Daughter
RELATIONSHIP TO GUARANTOR

F	03/24/1987	Single	928-74-9412
SEX (M/F)	DATE OF BIRTH	MARITAL STATUS	SOC. SEC. #

JFK High School
EMPLOYER OR SCHOOL NAME

ADDRESS OF EMPLOYER OR SCHOOL

Wallace	CA	95039
CITY	STATE	ZIP CODE

	Leland Groves, M.D.
EMPLOYER OR SCHOOL PHONE	REFERRED BY

E-MAIL

GUARANTOR INFORMATION

Williams	Terry	L.	F
RESPONSIBLE PARTY LAST NAME	FIRST NAME	MI	SEX (M/F)

P.O. Box 609	207 Chestnut Street
MAILING ADDRESS	STREET ADDRESS (IF DIFFERENT)

Wallace	CA	95039
CITY	STATE	ZIP CODE

(916) 875-3256	(916) 875-3963
(AREA CODE) HOME PHONE	(AREA CODE) WORK PHONE

01/04/1960	Single	972-65-8971
DATE OF BIRTH	MARITAL STATUS	SOC. SEC. #

Comptech Research
EMPLOYER NAME

693 Industrial Park Road
EMPLOYER ADDRESS

Palo Alto	CA	94033
CITY	STATE	ZIP CODE

PRIMARY INSURANCE

Health Maintenance Organization
NAME OF PRIMARY INSURANCE COMPANY

6632 3rd Avenue
ADDRESS

New York	NY	10017
CITY	STATE	ZIP CODE

2289669820	Comptech Research
IDENTIFICATION #	GROUP NAME AND/OR #

Terry Williams
INSURED PERSON'S NAME (IF DIFFERENT FROM THE RESPONSIBLE PARTY)

P.O. Box 609
ADDRESS (IF DIFFERENT)

Wallace	CA	95039
CITY	STATE	ZIP CODE

(800) 999-1234	972-65-8971
PRIMARY INSURANCE PHONE NUMBER	SOC. SEC. #

Self
WHAT IS THE RESPONSIBLE PARTY'S RELATIONSHIP TO THE INSURED?

SECONDARY INSURANCE

NAME OF SECONDARY INSURANCE COMPANY

ADDRESS

CITY	STATE	ZIP CODE

IDENTIFICATION #	GROUP NAME AND/OR #

INSURED PERSON'S NAME (IF DIFFERENT FROM THE RESPONSIBLE PARTY)

ADDRESS (IF DIFFERENT)

CITY	STATE	ZIP CODE

SECONDARY INSURANCE PHONE NUMBER	SOC. SEC. #

WHAT IS THE RESPONSIBLE PARTY'S RELATIONSHIP TO THE INSURED?

I hereby consent for Sydney Carrington & Associates, P.A. to use or disclose my health information to carry out treatment, payment, and health care operations. I authorize the use of this signature on all insurance submissions. I understand that I am financially responsible for all charges whether or not paid by the insurance. I acknowledge receipt of the practice's privacy policy.

Terry L. Williams (Mother)	01/10/2003
PATIENT SIGNATURE	DATE

2. Who holds the primary insurance policy?

3. Is the primary insurance policy offered through an employer? If so, whose?

4. Who holds the secondary insurance policy?

5. Is the secondary insurance policy offered through an employer? If so, whose?

6. Does the secondary insurance policy cover both children?

7. Is extended information provided for each of the children?

8. Is extended information provided for Ms. Williams?

The guarantor of this account is Terry Williams. She is divorced and has children with different last names. Ms. Williams is not a patient in the practice, so remember to answer (**N**)o to the Guarantor is a Patient field. This will cause the consent field to default to (**N**)o as well. Her signature on the registration form is consent on behalf of her daughter not herself. Her children are both patients of Dr. James Monroe. Note that extended information is provided for each of the children, and that the insurance is different for one of the children. Begin working on Laura Simmons's form by entering her mother's information from the guarantor box on the right side of the form.

STEP 1   Since Ms. Williams's name is not already on file, press **ENTER** to proceed and add her account to the system. Key Ms. Williams's patient number, '**120**,' shown on her patient registration form and press **ENTER**. The Guarantor Information screen will appear. Progress through the fields just as you did in the previous exercises, taking information from the patient registration form and using the appropriate help windows, if necessary.

First Name: **Terry**

M.I.: **L**

Street Address1: **P.O. Box 609**

Street Address2: **207 Chestnut Street**

City: **Wallace**

State: **CA**

Zip Code: **95039**

Sex (M/F): (**F**)emale

Employed: (**E**)mployed

Employer/School: **Comptech Research**

Home Phone #: **9168753256**

Work Phone #: **9168753963**

Work Ext. #: (Press **ENTER** to leave blank)

Date of Birth: **01041960**

Social Sec. #: **972658971**

Patient ID: (Press **ENTER** to leave blank)

Patient ID 2: (Press **ENTER** to leave blank)

Marital Status: (**S**)ingle

Race: (Press **ENTER** to leave blank)

E-mail: (Press **ENTER** to leave blank)

Account Date: (Press **ENTER** to default to current system date of 01/10/03)

# of Dependents: **2**

# of Ins. Policies: **2**

Extended Info. Level: **2** (Full)

Guar. Is a Patient: (**N**)o

Ref. Dr. #: **2** (Dr. Leland Groves)

Doctor #: **1** (Dr. James Monroe)

Status: (Press **ENTER** to accept default of '1')

Bill Type: (Press **ENTER** to accept default of '11')

Tax Code: (Press **ENTER** to leave blank)

Consent: (Press **ENTER** to accept the default of (**N**)o)

WP ID: (Press **ENTER** to default to 'C:wp:120.0')

Class: (Press **ENTER** to leave blank)

Note: (Press **ENTER** to accept default of '0')

Days Before Collections: (Press **ENTER** to accept default of '0')

Collection Priority: (Press **ENTER** to accept default of '0')

Discount %: (Press **ENTER** to accept default of '0')

Budget Payment: (Press **ENTER** to accept default of '0.00')

Compare your screen with Figure 2-46. When you are sure all information has been entered correctly, press **F1** or click on the PROCESS button ('√') on the top tool-bar to process.

Figure 2-46 Guarantor's Information Screen

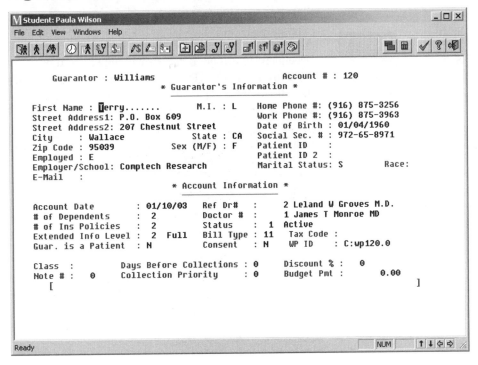

Figure 2-47 Extended Information—Terry Williams

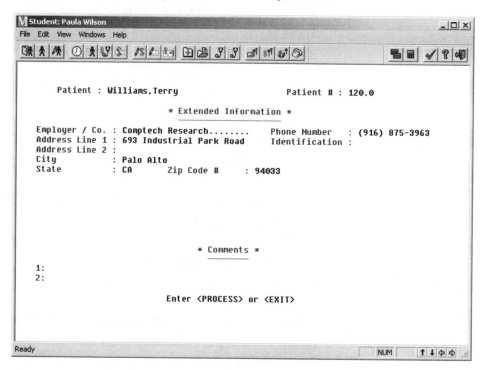

```
M Student: Paula Wilson                                               _ | □ | x |
File  Edit  View  Windows  Help

┌────────────────────────────────────────────────────────────────────────────┐
│ [toolbar icons]                                           [toolbar icons]    │
├────────────────────────────────────────────────────────────────────────────┤
│                                                                              │
│          Patient : Williams,Terry                  Patient # : 120.0         │
│                                                                              │
│                        * Extended Information *                              │
│                                                                              │
│    Employer / Co. : Comptech Research........    Phone Number  : (916) 875-3963 │
│    Address Line 1 : 693 Industrial Park Road     Identification :            │
│    Address Line 2 :                                                          │
│    City           : Palo Alto                                                │
│    State          : CA        Zip Code #    : 94033                          │
│                                                                              │
│                                                                              │
│                                                                              │
│                             * Comments *                                     │
│                                                                              │
│    1:                                                                        │
│    2:                                                                        │
│                                                                              │
│                        Enter <PROCESS> or <EXIT>                             │
│                                                                              │
├────────────────────────────────────────────────────────────────────────────┤
│ Ready                                              NUM        ↑ ↓ ⇦ ⇨        │
└────────────────────────────────────────────────────────────────────────────┘
```

STEP 2

When the information you entered above is processed, the Extended Information screen will appear so that you can enter additional employment information for Ms. Williams. Use the information shown in her patient registration form to complete this screen. When you are sure that you have completed all fields for which you have information, compare your screen with Figure 2-47, then press **F1** or click on the PROCESS button ('√') on the top toolbar.

STEP 3

After you have processed the Extended Information screen for Ms. Williams, the Dependent Information screen will appear so that you may enter information about her daughter Laura. Enter Laura's information from the patient information box on the left side of the patient registration form shown in Figure 2-45. Compare your screens with Figures 2-48 and 2-49. Remember to press **ENTER** at any field for which no information is provided on the patient registration form. When you are finished completing the Dependent Information screens, press **F1** or click on the PROCESS button ('√') on the top toolbar.

Figure 2-48 First Dependent's Information Screen

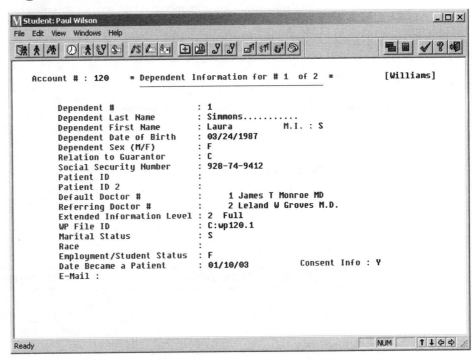

Figure 2-49 Extended Information—Laura Simmons

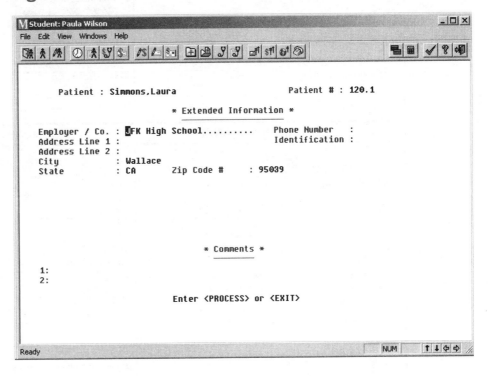

STEP 4

After you have processed the extended information for Laura Simmons, the dependent information screen will appear again so that you may enter information about her sister, Alice Spivey. Enter Alice's information from the patient information box on the left side of her registration form shown in Figure 2-50. Compare your screens to those shown in Figures 2-51 and 2-52.

Figure 2-50 Alice Spivey—Patient Registration Form

Patient Registration Form

Sydney Carrington & Associates
34 Sycamore Street ● Madison, CA 95653

TODAY'S DATE: _01/10/2003_

FOR OFFICE USE ONLY	
ACCOUNT NO.:	**120**
DOCTOR:	**#1**
BILL TYPE:	**11**
EXTENDED INFO.:	**2**

PATIENT INFORMATION

Spivey	_Alice_	_J._
PATIENT LAST NAME	FIRST NAME	MI
Daughter		
RELATIONSHIP TO GUARANTOR		
_F_ _05/01/1991_	_Single_	_928-64-5012_
SEX (M/F) DATE OF BIRTH	MARITAL STATUS	SOC. SEC. #
Wallace Jr. High		
EMPLOYER OR SCHOOL NAME		
Wallace	_CA_	_95039_
ADDRESS OF EMPLOYER OR SCHOOL		
CITY	STATE	ZIP CODE
	Leland Groves, M.D.	
EMPLOYER OR SCHOOL PHONE	REFERRED BY	
E-MAIL		

GUARANTOR INFORMATION

Williams	_Terry_	_L._	_F_
RESPONSIBLE PARTY LAST NAME	FIRST NAME	MI	SEX (M/F)
P.O. Box 609	_207 Chestnut Street_		
MAILING ADDRESS	STREET ADDRESS (IF DIFFERENT)		
Wallace	_CA_	_95039_	
CITY	STATE	ZIP CODE	
_(916) 875-3256_	_(916) 875-3963_		
(AREA CODE) HOME PHONE	(AREA CODE) WORK PHONE		
_01/04/1960_	_Single_	_972-65-8971_	
DATE OF BIRTH	MARITAL STATUS	SOC. SEC. #	
Comptech Research			
EMPLOYER NAME			
693 Industrial Park Road			
EMPLOYER ADDRESS			
Palo Alto	_CA_	_94033_	
CITY	STATE	ZIP CODE	

PRIMARY INSURANCE

Health Maintenance Organization		
NAME OF PRIMARY INSURANCE COMPANY		
6632 3rd Avenue		
ADDRESS		
New York	_NY_	_10017_
CITY	STATE ZIP CODE	
_2289669820_	_Comptech Research_	
IDENTIFICATION #	GROUP NAME AND/OR #	
Terry Williams		
INSURED PERSON'S NAME (IF DIFFERENT FROM THE RESPONSIBLE PARTY)		
P.O. Box 609	_207 Chestnut Street_	
ADDRESS (IF DIFFERENT)		
Wallace	_CA_	_95039_
CITY	STATE	ZIP CODE
_(800) 999-1234_	_972-65-8971_	
PRIMARY INSURANCE PHONE NUMBER	SOC. SEC. #	
Self		
WHAT IS THE RESPONSIBLE PARTY'S RELATIONSHIP TO THE INSURED?		

SECONDARY INSURANCE

Epsilon Life & Casualty (Insurance for Alice Spivey Only)		
NAME OF SECONDARY INSURANCE COMPANY		
P.O. Box 189		
ADDRESS		
Macon	_GA_	_31298_
CITY	STATE ZIP CODE	
_76432079_	_McDonnell-Douglas_	
IDENTIFICATION #	GROUP NAME AND/OR #	
William Spivey		
INSURED PERSON'S NAME (IF DIFFERENT FROM THE RESPONSIBLE PARTY)		
P.O. Box 2780		
ADDRESS (IF DIFFERENT)		
San Jose	_CA_	_94064_
CITY	STATE	ZIP CODE
_(800) 908-7654_	_276-84-9037_	
SECONDARY INSURANCE PHONE NUMBER	SOC. SEC. #	
Ex-wife		
WHAT IS THE RESPONSIBLE PARTY'S RELATIONSHIP TO THE INSURED?		

I hereby consent for Sydney Carrington & Associates, P.A. to use or disclose my health information to carry out treatment, payment, and health care operations. I authorize the use of this signature on all insurance submissions. I understand that I am financially responsible for all charges whether or not paid by the insurance. I acknowledge receipt of the practice's privacy policy.

Terry L. Williams (Mother)	_01/10/2003_
PATIENT SIGNATURE	DATE

Figure 2-51 Second Dependent's Information Screen

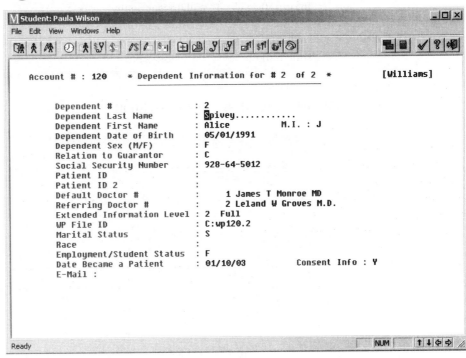

Figure 2-52 Second Dependent's Extended Information Screen

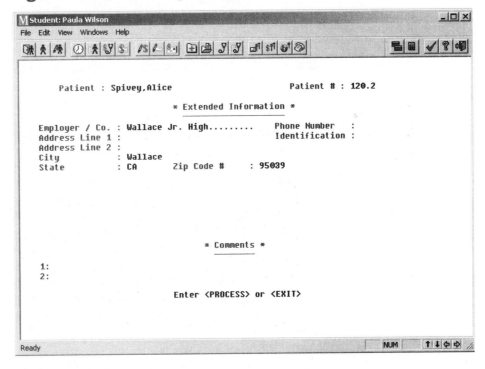

After you process all dependent information, the Insurance Policy Information screen for the first plan will appear for you to complete. Ms. Williams has insurance coverage on her family with an HMO that she participates in through her employer therefore she will be the insured party on the policy. However, in addition to her mother's plan, Alice is also covered by her father's group policy. While adding the second policy, you will create a (N)ew insured party and enter information about Alice's father,

William Spivey. Since the second policy covers only Alice and not Laura, each child will need a separate coverage list.

Enter the primary insurance policy first, using the information on the patient registration form shown in Figure 2-45 or 2-50. Compare your screen with Figure 2-53, and press **F1** or click the PROCESS button ('√') on the top toolbar.

Figure 2-53 Primary First Insurance Plan Screen

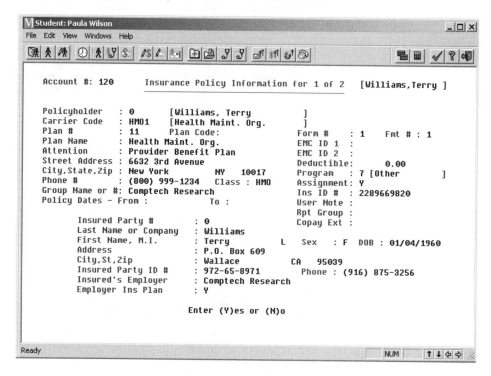

Enter the secondary insurance plan found on the patient registration form shown in Figure 2-50.

*Reminder: The Policyholder is the person who brings the insurance policy to the family account. For the second policy, it is not the Guarantor, Terry Williams, who has the policy but rather Alice Spivey who brings her father's insurance into the account. Valid responses for the Policyholder field are 'O' for the guarantor or a dependent number. Because Alice was assigned dependent number **2** in the previous step, enter a '2' into the Policyholder field.*

Compare your screen with Figure 2-54. Remember **The Medical Manager** automatically assigns a number to a New Insured Party, and the number on your screen may vary from that shown in Figure 2-54. Press **F1** or click the PROCESS button ('√') on the top toolbar.

Press (**M**)aintain to maintain the Coverage Priority List for the guarantor (use only the HMO for the guarantor). Each dependent except Alice may use the guarantor's list. Select Alice and modify her list appropriately to include her father's insurance plan as her secondary coverage.

When you add the second policy, you will fill in the name of Alice's father since he is the (**N**)ew Insured Party. For the Insured Party ID, enter William Spivey's Social

Figure 2-54 Insurance Plan for Alice Only Screen

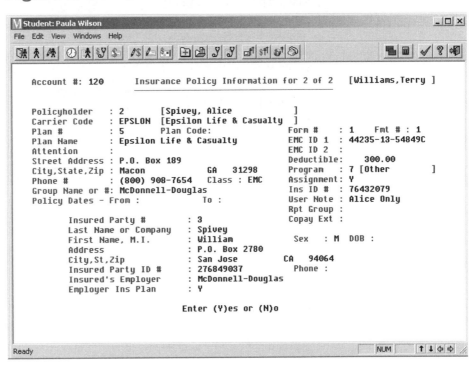

Security number since this is how this policy is identified through his employer. Remember to add hyphens, as needed, since this field is not self-formatting. Your screens should be similar to Figures 2-53 through 2-54.

When both plans have been added, The Set Coverage screen will display the Guarantor List as shown in Figure 2-55. Press **F1** or click the PROCESS button ('√') on the top toolbar. A list of the account family members will then display. Select Laura

Figure 2-55 Family Coverage Screen

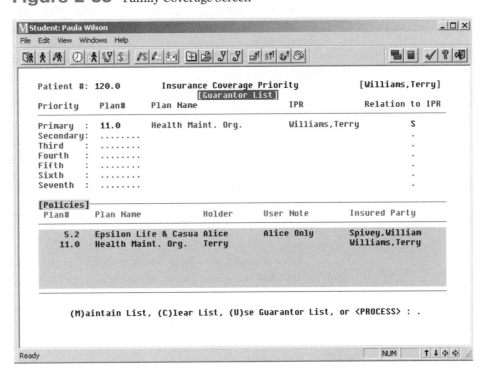

Figure 2-56 Laura's Coverage List

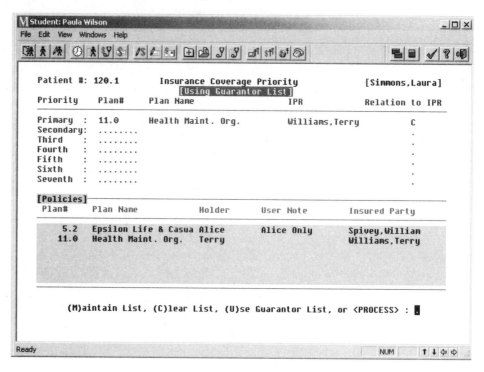

Simmons and press **ENTER**. Choose (**U**)se Guarantor List for Laura, and Press **F1** or click the PROCESS button ('√') on the top toolbar (Figure 2-56).

Select Alice Spivey and press **ENTER**. Choose (**M**)aintain List. From this window, you will set the order in which insurance policies should be billed and the order they will default in Procedure Entry. Press '?' (question mark) to display a list of the policies on the account. Select 11.0 Health Maintenance Organization as Alice's Primary. Enter the relationship of Alice to the Insured Party in The Relation to IPR field. Press **ENTER** to accept the default of "**C**" for child. The cursor will automatically move to the field for the Secondary Insurance Policy. Key **5.2** into the field or press '?' to redisplay the help window and select Epsilon as the secondary plan for Alice. *Do not* accept the default relation to IPR as (**O**)ther, key a (**C**)hild . Press the **F1** key twice or click the PROCESS button ('√') on the top toolbar twice to complete the coverage list and patient registration for Terry Williams' family.

> **Tip:** The relationship field is sometimes a point of confusion. The insurance plan wishes to know the relationship of the patient to the insured party. When the insured party is a spouse or a parent, **The Medical Manager** automatically defaults to the correct response based on the patient's relationship to the guarantor. However when the insured party is a business or someone not on the account, the default is (**O**)ther, because the relationship cannot be calculated.

Once you have processed all of the above-mentioned screens, press **ESCAPE** or click on the **EXIT** button on the top toolbar until you return to the Main Menu (Menu 1).

Figure 2-57 Alice's Coverage List

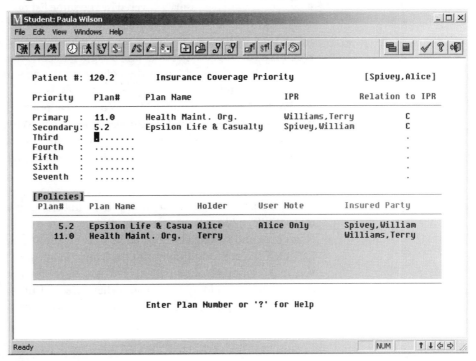

UNIT 2 SUMMARY

Accuracy in setting up patient guarantor and insurance information is of the utmost importance. In modern computer systems like **The Medical Manager,** this information is maintained in a central patient file and is used over and over again for many purposes. Failing to record accurately the information could result in lost or misdirected mail affecting billing, payment, and even important medical notices that are being mailed to the patient.

Patients typically complete a patient registration form; one for each member of the family. The information from the form is then keyed into the computer. This includes the patient's name, date of birth, employer, and so on, as well as account information about the guarantor, billing address, health insurance and policy numbers, the insured party or subscriber in whose name the policy is registered, and additional extended information such as the employer name and address.

The *guarantor* is the person who guarantees to pay the doctor for all charges incurred on the account, including charges for all dependents. In some medical practices, all members of the family are recorded in one account with the person in whose name the account is set up listed as guarantor of the account. Additional family members are listed as dependents on the account. Other medical practices may put each patient in their own separate account. **The Medical Manager** supports both methods.

When adding insurance policy information, each insurance policy will be identified with a *policyholder*, the member of the account who is primarily associated with that particular policy. The policyholder number is a combination of the number of the insurance plan and the number of the dependent. The policyholder will always be a member of the account.

Insured Party indicates the subscriber (person or company) to whom the insurance policy is issued. The insured party may be the same as the guarantor of the account, the same as the policyholder, or even another person or a business such as an employer or ex-spouse.

An insurance *coverage list* handles situations in which not all members of a family-style account are necessarily covered by the same list of insurance policies (e.g., a husband and wife who both work may each be covered by their own employer's policy rather than by their spouse's policy). Once insurance policies have been added to the account a coverage list is set up and assigned to each member of the family. The coverage list determines which of the policies on the account are available for use with each family member.

Typically, when a family comes to a medical practice, each member of the family will fill out his or her own patient registration form. When entering multiple forms for a family that shares the same guarantor, you will set up a family-style account by first entering the guarantor's information then the subsequent registration forms for each additional family member.

When adding new accounts through New Patient Entry you should always use the Patient Help window to ensure that you are not creating a duplicate account in the system. While adding new patients, the screens automatically move through the Guarantor and Extended Information screens, the Dependent screens, the Dependent Extended screens, and finally, the Insurance Policy and Set Coverage List screens. If you make an error on a patient and you have already moved past that particular screen, continue adding the account then refer to Unit 4 *Editing Patient Information* to correct your error. You cannot edit patient information in New Patient Entry.

COMPREHENSIVE EXERCISE

This comprehensive exercise will enable you and your instructor to evaluate your understanding of new patient entry. Using the patient registration forms provided on the following pages, you will add a new account that has two patients, each with extended information; there are three insurance plans, and each patient will have his or her own insurance coverage list. In completing this exercise, you will use each of the screens that you have learned in the previous exercises.

Before you begin, read through this exercise completely. Make sure you understand the concepts required of you, and if necessary, review any of the previous exercises in this unit.

Caution: Do not begin this exercise if there is not enough class time to complete the entire exercise. All information on the account must be completed in one session.

EXERCISE 7: Steven Carlson

Comprehensive Exercise

The next account is for Mr. and Mrs. Steven Carlson. Before attempting data entry study the patient registration form shown in Figures 2-58 and 2-59; answer the following questions:

1. Who is the patient responsible (the guarantor) for the account?

2. What is Mr. Carlson's wife's name?

3. Mr. Carlson is retired. Is his wife employed?

4. Is extended information provided for Mr. Carlson's wife?

5. Mr. Carlson and his wife each have separate insurance coverage. Mr. Carlson has primary coverage with Medicare and secondary coverage with Epsilon. What is

Complete the fields as you did in previous exercises using the information shown on Figure 2-58 for Mr. Carlson and Figure 2-59 for Mrs. Carlson. To be sure that the Carlsons are not already entered in the system, key '? **Carlson**' in the enter Guarantor Last Name field at the patient retrieval prompt of New Patient Entry and press **ENTER**.

Figure 2-58 Steven Carlson—Patient Registration Form

Patient Registration Form

Sydney Carrington & Associates
34 Sycamore Street • Madison, CA 95653

TODAY'S DATE: _01/10/2003_

FOR OFFICE USE ONLY	
ACCOUNT NO.:	**10**
DOCTOR:	**#3**
BILL TYPE:	**11**
EXTENDED INFO.:	**2**

PATIENT INFORMATION

Carlson	_Steven_	_W._
PATIENT LAST NAME	FIRST NAME	MI

Self
RELATIONSHIP TO GUARANTOR

_M_	_11/16/1931_	_Married_	_345-65-3434_
SEX (M/F)	DATE OF BIRTH	MARITAL STATUS	SOC. SEC. #

Hite Telecommunications (Retired)
EMPLOYER OR SCHOOL NAME

87 S. Main Street
ADDRESS OF EMPLOYER OR SCHOOL

Floral City	_CA_	_90083_
CITY	STATE	ZIP CODE

_(916) 988-6495_	_Leland Groves, M.D._
EMPLOYER OR SCHOOL PHONE	REFERRED BY

E-MAIL

GUARANTOR INFORMATION

Carlson	_Steven_	_W._	_M_
RESPONSIBLE PARTY LAST NAME	FIRST NAME	MI	SEX (M/F)

3456 West Palm #34

MAILING ADDRESS	STREET ADDRESS (IF DIFFERENT)	
Madison	_CA_	_95653_
CITY	STATE	ZIP CODE

_(916) 988-3293_

(AREA CODE) HOME PHONE	(AREA CODE) WORK PHONE	
_11/16/1931_	_Married_	_345-65-3434_
DATE OF BIRTH	MARITAL STATUS	SOC. SEC. #

Hite Telecommunications
EMPLOYER NAME

87 S. Main Street
EMPLOYER ADDRESS

Floral City	_CA_	_90083_
CITY	STATE	ZIP CODE

PRIMARY INSURANCE

Medicare
NAME OF PRIMARY INSURANCE COMPANY

Claims Dept. Box 443A, 760 University Street
ADDRESS

Washington	_DC_	_17654-1234_
CITY	STATE	ZIP CODE

_345653434A_
IDENTIFICATION #   GROUP NAME AND/OR #

Same
INSURED PERSON'S NAME (IF DIFFERENT FROM THE RESPONSIBLE PARTY)

Same	_CA_	_95039_
ADDRESS (IF DIFFERENT)	STATE	ZIP CODE
CITY		

_(800) 879-6789_	_345-65-3434_
PRIMARY INSURANCE PHONE NUMBER	SOC. SEC. #

Self
WHAT IS THE RESPONSIBLE PARTY'S RELATIONSHIP TO THE INSURED?

SECONDARY INSURANCE

Epsilon Life & Casualty
NAME OF SECONDARY INSURANCE COMPANY

P.O. Box 189
ADDRESS

Macon	_GA_	_31298_
CITY	STATE	ZIP CODE

MSA876587665	_Hite Telecommunications_
IDENTIFICATION #	GROUP NAME AND/OR #

Same
INSURED PERSON'S NAME (IF DIFFERENT FROM THE RESPONSIBLE PARTY)

Same		
ADDRESS (IF DIFFERENT)	STATE	ZIP CODE
CITY		

_(800) 908-7654_	_345-65-3434_
SECONDARY INSURANCE PHONE NUMBER	SOC. SEC. #

Self
WHAT IS THE RESPONSIBLE PARTY'S RELATIONSHIP TO THE INSURED?

I hereby consent for Sydney Carrington & Associates, P.A. to use or disclose my health information to carry out treatment, payment, and health care operations. I authorize the use of this signature on all insurance submissions. I understand that I am financially responsible for all charges whether or not paid by the insurance. I acknowledge receipt of the practice's privacy policy.

Steven W. Carlson	_01/10/2003_
PATIENT SIGNATURE	DATE

Figure 2-59 Sharon Carlson—Patient Registration Form

Patient Registration Form

Sydney Carrington & Associates
34 Sycamore Street ● **Madison, CA 95653**

TODAY'S DATE: _01/10/2003_

PATIENT INFORMATION

Carlson	Sharon	A.
PATIENT LAST NAME	FIRST NAME	MI

Wife
RELATIONSHIP TO GUARANTOR

F	03/13/1936	Married	643-86-5639
SEX (M/F)	DATE OF BIRTH	MARITAL STATUS	SOC. SEC. #

Madison County Hospital
EMPLOYER OR SCHOOL NAME

234 Lincoln Road
ADDRESS OF EMPLOYER OR SCHOOL

Madison	CA	95651
CITY	STATE	ZIP CODE

(916) 436-5910	Leland Groves, M.D.
EMPLOYER OR SCHOOL PHONE	REFERRED BY

E-MAIL

GUARANTOR INFORMATION

Carlson	Steven	W.	M
RESPONSIBLE PARTY LAST NAME	FIRST NAME	MI	SEX (M/F)

3456 West Palm #34

MAILING ADDRESS	STREET ADDRESS (IF DIFFERENT)

Madison	CA	95653
CITY	STATE	ZIP CODE

_(916) 988-3293_
(AREA CODE) HOME PHONE   (AREA CODE) WORK PHONE

11/16/1931	Married	345-65-3434
DATE OF BIRTH	MARITAL STATUS	SOC. SEC. #

Hite Telecommunications
EMPLOYER NAME

87 S. Main Street
EMPLOYER ADDRESS

Floral City	CA	90083
CITY	STATE	ZIP CODE

PRIMARY INSURANCE

Pan American Health Ins.
NAME OF PRIMARY INSURANCE COMPANY

4567 Newberry Road
ADDRESS

Los Angeles	DC	98706
CITY	STATE	ZIP CODE

9876086546	Madison County Hospital
IDENTIFICATION #	GROUP NAME AND/OR #

Sharon A. Carlson
INSURED PERSON'S NAME (IF DIFFERENT FROM THE RESPONSIBLE PARTY)

3456 West Palm #34
ADDRESS (IF DIFFERENT)

Madison	CA	95653
CITY	STATE	ZIP CODE

(213) 456-7654	643-86-5639
PRIMARY INSURANCE PHONE NUMBER	SOC. SEC. #

Husband
WHAT IS THE RESPONSIBLE PARTY'S RELATIONSHIP TO THE INSURED?

SECONDARY INSURANCE

NAME OF SECONDARY INSURANCE COMPANY

ADDRESS

CITY	STATE	ZIP CODE

IDENTIFICATION #	GROUP NAME AND/OR #

INSURED PERSON'S NAME (IF DIFFERENT FROM THE RESPONSIBLE PARTY)

ADDRESS (IF DIFFERENT)

CITY	STATE	ZIP CODE

SECONDARY INSURANCE PHONE NUMBER	SOC. SEC. #

WHAT IS THE RESPONSIBLE PARTY'S RELATIONSHIP TO THE INSURED?

Sharon A. Carlson	_01/10/2003_
PATIENT SIGNATURE	DATE

STEP 1

Because Mr. Carlson's name is not already on file, press **ESCAPE** then press **ENTER** to proceed and add his account to the system. Key Mr. Carlson's patient number, '**10**', as shown on his patient registration form and press **ENTER**. The Guarantor Information screen will appear. Progress through the rest of the fields just as you did in previous exercises, taking the information from the patient registration form and using the appropriate help windows, if necessary.

Last Name: **Carlson**

First Name: **Steven**

M.I.: **W.**

Street Address1: **3456 West Palm #34**

Street Address2: (Press **ENTER** to leave blank)

City: **Madison**

State: **CA**

Zip Code: **95653**

Sex (M/F): **M**

Employed: (Press **ENTER** to leave blank)

Employer/School: **Hite Telecommunications**

Home Phone #: **9169883293**

Work Phone #: (Press **ENTER** to leave blank)

Work Ext #: (Press **ENTER** to leave blank)

Date of Birth: **11161931**

Social Sec. #: **345653434**

Patient ID: (Press **ENTER** to leave blank)

Patient ID 2: (Press **ENTER** to leave blank)

Marital Status: **M**

Race: (Press **ENTER** to leave blank)

E-mail: (Press **ENTER** to leave blank)

Account Date: (Press **ENTER** to default to current system date of 01/10/2003)

# of Dependents: **1**

# of Ins. Policies: **3**

Extended Info. Level: **2**

Guar. Is a Patient: **Y**

Ref. Dr. #: **2**

Doctor #: **3**

Status: (Press **ENTER** to accept default of '**1**')

Bill Type: (Press **ENTER** to accept default of '**11**')

Tax Code: (Press **ENTER** to leave blank)

Consent Info.: (Press **ENTER** to accept default of (**Y**)es)

WP ID: (Press **ENTER** to accept default of **C:wp10.0**)

Class: (Press **ENTER** to leave blank)

Note: (Press **ENTER** to accept default of '**0**')

Days Before Collections: (Press **ENTER** to accept default of '**0**')

Collection Priority: (Press **ENTER** to accept default of '**0**')

Discount %: (Press **ENTER** to accept default of '**0**')

Budget Payment: (Press **ENTER** to accept default of '**0.00**')

Check your screen against Mr. Carlson's patient preregistration form. When you are sure all information has been entered correctly, press '**F1**' or click on the PROCESS button ('√') on the top toolbar to process.

STEP 2   When the information you have entered above is processed, the Extended Information screen will appear so that you can enter additional employment information for Mr. Carlson. Even though Mr. Carlson is retired he is still receiving benefits from his previous employer.

Employer/Co.: **Hite Telecommunications**
Address Line 1: **87 S. Main Street**
Address Line 2: (Press **ENTER** to leave blank)
City: **Floral City**
State: **CA**
Zip Code #: **90083**
Phone Number: **9169886495**
Identification: **Retired**

When you are sure that you have completed all fields for which you have information, press the '**F1**' key or click on the PROCESS button ('√') on the top toolbar.

STEP 3   After you have processed the Extended Information screen for Mr. Carlson, the Dependent Information screen will appear so that you may enter information about his wife.

Dependent #: **1**
Dependent Last Name: **Carlson**
Dependent First Name: **Sharon**
M.I.: **A.**
Dependent Date of Birth: **03131936**
Dependent Sex: **F**
Relation to Guarantor: **W**
Social Security #: **643865639**
Patient ID: (Press **ENTER** to leave blank)
Patient ID 2: (Press **ENTER** to leave blank)
Default Doctor #: (Press **ENTER** to default to '**0**' - use Guarantor's Doctor)
Referring Doctor #: (Press **ENTER** to default to '0')
Extended Information Level: **2**
WP File ID: (Press **ENTER** to default to **C:wp10.1**)
Marital Status: **M**
Race: (Press **ENTER** to leave blank)
Employment/Student Status: **E**
Date Became a Patient: (Press **ENTER** to default to system date)
Consent Info.: (Press **ENTER** to accept default of (**Y**)es)
E-mail: (Press **ENTER** to leave blank)

After you have processed dependent information, the Extended Information screen will appear so that you can enter additional employment information for Mrs. Carlson.

Employer/Co.: **Madison County Hospital**
Address Line 1: **234 Lincoln Road**
Address Line 2: (Press **ENTER** to leave blank)
City: **Madison**
State: **CA**
Zip Code #: **95651**
Phone Number: **9164365910**
Identification: (Press **ENTER** to leave blank)

When you are sure that you have completed all the fields for which you have information, press the '**F1**' key or click on the PROCESS ('√') button on the top toolbar.

STEP 4 After you process the dependent information, the Insurance Policy Information screen will appear for you to complete. Note that Mr. and Mrs. Carlson have different insurance policies and different insurance coverage. Mrs. Carlson is her own insured party. Begin by referring to Figure 2-58 and entering the primary and secondary insurance information for Mr. Carlson. When you are sure that you have each policy's information complete, press the '**F1**' key or click on the PROCESS ('√') button on the top toolbar and the next policy information screen will display. When you have completed both policies for Mr. Carlson refer to Figure 2-59 and enter the insurance information for Mrs. Carlson.

STEP 5 Once the policies have been entered for both patients, the Patient Coverage Information screen will be displayed. Note that Mrs. Carlson has different insurance coverage from Mr. Carlson. Set the coverage for Mr. Carlson, then select Sharon Carlson from the coverage screen and create a separate coverage list for her. She will not use the guarantor coverage list.

Once you have processed all of the above screens, press **ESCAPE** or click on the **EXIT** button on the top toolbar until you have returned to the main menu.

Guarantor and Patient Reports

Guarantor reports present demographic and insurance information from the guarantor's file as well as custom defined patient extended information and insurance policy information. These reports can be generated at any time and may be used whenever the practice desires a hard copy for the doctor or office management purposes of patient demographic information.

EXERCISE 8: Generating a Guarantor File Report

STEP 1

From the Main Menu (Menu 1) using the keyboard or mouse, select option **5**, Report Generation, then option **1**, Guarantor File Reports. Then select option **2**, Guarantor's Full Report. The screen shown in Figure 2-60 will appear.

Figure 2-60 Guarantor File Report Screen

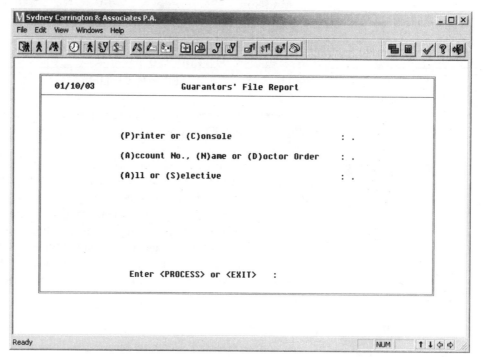

STEP 2

Enter the following selections for the Guarantor File Report: (**P**)rinter, (**A**)ccount, (**A**)ll. Then press '**F1**' or click on the PROCESS ('√') button on the top toolbar to process. Compare your printouts to Figures 2-61a and b and hand in to your instructor. Press **ESCAPE** or click on the **EXIT** button on the top toolbar until you return to the Main Menu (Menu 1).

Figure 2-61a Guarantor File Report

```
01/10/03                         GUARANTORS' FILE REPORT BY ACCOUNT                        Page    1
                                       Student: Paul Wilson
                                          All Accounts

Acct #  Name                  Soc.Sec. #   DOB         Patient ID      Patient ID2     Dr.  Ref  Rel Sex  Mar Emp Race
==============================================================================================================
10      Carlson, Steven W     345-65-3434  11/16/1931                                   3    2   S   M    M        ]
        [1   Sharon A Carlson  643-86-5639  03/13/1936                                   0    0   W   F    M   E    ]

        3456 West Palm #34          (916) 988-3293      Acct.Date: 01/10/03    Bill Type: 11       Status:1  Class:
                                                        DOL Visit:             Discount : 0%       Collection > days: 0
        Madison       CA  95653     Hite Telecommunicatio   Tax Code :         Budget:    0.00     Collection Priority: 0

          3 Ins.Plans: (7.1     Pan American Health Ins.) (5.0      Epsilon Life & Casualty)  (2.0      Medicare)
----------------------
14      Evans, Deborah A      908-78-5674  11/27/1969                                   3    2   S   F    M   E    ]
        [1   Gene S Evans      652-87-4136  12/12/1968                                   3    2   H   M    M   E    ]

        1901 NW 2nd Street          (916) 678-5674      Acct.Date: 01/10/03    Bill Type: 11       Status:1  Class:
                                    (916) 665-3456      DOL Visit:             Discount : 0%       Collection > days: 0
        Madison       CA  95653     Bell Labs           Tax Code :             Budget:    0.00     Collection Priority: 0

          1 Ins.Plan : (7.0     Pan American Health Ins.)
----------------------
21      Edwards, Portia D     766-54-4378  11/25/1955                                   3    0   S   F    M   E    ]
        [1   Edward E Edwards  343-22-8898  07/20/1954                                   3    0   H   M    M   E    ]
        [2   Andrea L Edwards  525-22-9314  02/02/1988                                   3    0   C   F    S   F    ]

        235 Mandolin Court          (916) 899-7800      Acct.Date: 01/10/03    Bill Type: 11       Status:1  Class:
                                    (916) 899-9384      DOL Visit:             Discount : 0%       Collection > days: 0
        Madison       CA  95653-0235  Portia Property Mgmt.  Tax Code :        Budget:    0.00     Collection Priority: 0

          1 Ins.Plan : (5.1     Epsilon Life & Casualty)
----------------------
30      League, Claire E      738-76-4128  06/11/1929                                   1    3   S   F    M        ]

        800 Illagas Road            (408) 907-4352      Acct.Date: 01/10/03    Bill Type: 11       Status:1  Class:
                                                        DOL Visit:             Discount : 0%       Collection > days: 0
        Morgan Hill    CA  98076                        Tax Code :             Budget:    0.00     Collection Priority: 0

          2 Ins.Plans: (10.0    Medicare Plus)          (2.0      Medicare)
----------------------
34      Dudley, Wayne R       678-75-4343  08/28/1965                                   3    1   S   M    S   E    ]

        Route 1, Box 23             (408) 789-6654      Acct.Date: 01/10/03    Bill Type: 11       Status:1  Class:
                                    (408) 789-3209      DOL Visit:             Discount : 0%       Collection > days: 0
        Woodside      CA  98076     Hudson Construction  Tax Code :            Budget:    0.00     Collection Priority: 0

          1 Ins.Plan : (6.0     Cross and Shield Ins Plan)
----------------------
```

Figure 2-61b Guarantor File Report

```
01/10/03                        GUARANTORS' FILE REPORT BY ACCOUNT                          Page   2
                                       Student: Paul Wilson

Acct #  Name                    Soc.Sec. #    DOB         Patient ID      Patient ID2     Dr.  Ref   Rel Sex Mar Emp Race
========================================================================================================================
80      Davis, Timothy R        835-17-5465  04/15/1959                                    2    4    S   M   M   E      ]
        [1   Elizabeth S Davis   764-65-7988  11/25/1961                                    0    0    W   F   M          ]
        [2   Mindy A Davis       968-64-6543  06/18/1984                                    0    0    C   F   S   F      ]

        113 NE 22nd Avenue           (916) 908-7657      Acct.Date: 01/10/03    Bill Type: 11      Status:1  Class:
                                     (916) 908-6479      DOL Visit:             Discount : 0%      Collection > days: 0
        Madison      CA  95653      Bob Clark Constructio Tax Code :            Budget:    0.00     Collection Priority: 0

        1 Ins.Plan : (12.0     Fringe Benefit Center)
---------------------
110     Evans, Patricia G       908-23-6457  12/13/1951                                    3    2    S   F   S          ]

        8907 Harbor Drive            (916) 544-8275      Acct.Date: 01/10/03    Bill Type: 11      Status:1  Class:
                                                         DOL Visit:             Discount : 0%      Collection > days: 0
        Madison      CA  95653                           Tax Code :             Budget:    0.00     Collection Priority: 0

        1 Ins.Plan : (5.0      Epsilon Life & Casualty)
---------------------
120     Williams, Terry L       972-65-8971  01/04/1960                                    1    2    S   F   S   E      ]
        [1   Laura S Simmons     928-74-9412  03/24/1987                                    1    2    C   F   S   F      ]
        [2   Alice J Spivey      928-64-5012  05/01/1991                                    1    2    C   F   S   F      ]

        P.O. Box 609                 (916) 875-3256      Acct.Date: 01/10/03    Bill Type: 11      Status:1  Class:
        207 Chestnut Street          (916) 875-3963      DOL Visit:             Discount : 0%      Collection > days: 0
        Wallace      CA  95039      Comptech Research     Tax Code :             Budget:    0.00     Collection Priority: 0

        2 Ins.Plans: (5.2      Epsilon Life & Casualty)  (11.0     Health Maint. Org.)
---------------------


                            ****  Number Printed : 8  ****
                            ****  Number Active  : 8  ****
```

TESTING YOUR KNOWLEDGE

1. How are new accounts entered in **The Medical Manager** software? How does the user check to make sure the patient isn't already on file?

2. Name and discuss the function of any three screens.

3. In what way can the guarantor and patient be related? Can the guarantor be the patient?

4. Why is it important to enter information accurately for patient accounts?

(continues)

5. What type of information could be included in a patient's extended information? Why is this information important for the practice to have?

6. What is a help window? How do you invoke a help window? Why are help windows important?

Posting Your Entries

LEARNING OUTCOMES

After completing this unit, you should be able to:

◆ Retrieve patient accounts.

◆ Post procedure codes and diagnosis codes under varying circumstances.

◆ Describe Ailment Information.

◆ Explain the process of posting accounts.

◆ Name three components of the Daily Report and discuss their purposes.

◆ Run the Daily Report.

PROCEDURE ENTRY

Each time a patient is examined or treated by a physician, the procedures performed by the doctor must be posted to the patient's account, along with any payment that the patient makes before leaving the office. In this unit, you will practice posting procedures and diagnoses. Posting payments (Payment Entry) will be demonstrated in Unit 6.

The encounter form shows procedures, charges, and diagnoses.

As you will see in this unit, when a procedure is posted, **The Medical Manager** software is designed to assign automatically a prearranged charge (a fee) for that procedure. You will know what procedures and diagnoses to post by studying the encounter form that is completed for each patient when they are seen by the doctor. The encounter form includes a listing of the most frequently performed procedures, the charges that accompany those procedures, and a list of the most common diagnoses treated by the physician.

Before you can post charges and credits, you must retrieve an account. Because you will frequently retrieve patient accounts, **The Medical Manager** system provides a convenient Patient Retrieval screen, which appears when you choose many of the options provided on the Main Menu (Menu 1) and other menus. At the appropriate time, when you choose option 2, PROCEDURE Entry, a Patient Retrieval screen will be presented in which you can enter a patient's last name or other identifying information to bring them up on the system.

However, before you retrieve an account and attempt data entry, study the encounter form for Steven Carlson, shown in Figure 3-1, and answer the following questions:

1. What is Steven Carlson's patient number?

2. What is the date the patient, Steven Carlson, was seen by the doctor?

3. What is the name of the doctor who saw Steven?

4. What procedure did the physician perform?

5. What is the charge for the procedure performed?

6. What diagnosis was assigned with this procedure?

Figure 3-1 Steven Carlson's Encounter Form—Voucher #1050

Sydney Carrington & Associates P.A.
34 Sycamore Street   Suite 300
Madison, CA 95653

Date: 01/10/2003

Voucher No.: 1050

Time: 08:30

Patient: Steven Carlson
Guarantor: Steven W. Carlson

Patient No.: 10.0
Doctor: 3 - S. Carrington

CPT	DESCRIPTION	FEE
OFFICE/HOSPITAL CONSULTS		
☐ 99201	Office New:Focused Hx-Exam	
☐ 99202	Office New:Expanded Hx-Exam	
☐ 99211	Office Estb:Min/None Hx-Exa	
☐ 99212	Office Estb:Focused Hx-Exam	
☐ 99213	Office Estb:Expanded Hx-Exa	
☒ 99214	Office Estb:Detailed Hx-Exa	$50.00
☐ 99215	Office Estb:Comprhn Hx-Exam	
☐ 99221	Hosp. Initial:Comprh Hx-	
☐ 99223	Hosp.Ini:Comprh Hx-Exam/Hi	
☐ 99231	Hosp. Subsequent: S-Fwd	
☐ 99232	Hosp. Subsequent: Comprhn Hx	
☐ 99233	Hosp. Subsequent: Ex/Hi	
☐ 99238	Hospital Visit Discharge Ex	
☐ 99371	Telephone Consult - Simple	
☐ 99372	Telephone Consult - Intermed	
☐ 99373	Telephone Consult - Complex	
☐ 90843	Counseling - 25 minutes	
☐ 90844	Counseling - 50 minutes	
☐ 90865	Counseling - Special Interview	
IMMUNIZATIONS/INJECTIONS		
☐ 90585	BCG Vaccine	
☐ 90659	Influenza Virus Vaccine	
☐ 90701	Immunization-DTP	
☐ 90702	DT Vaccine	
☐ 90703	Tetanus Toxoids	
☐ 90732	Pneumococcal Vaccine	
☐ 90746	Hepatitis B Vaccine	
☐ 90749	Immunization; Unlisted	

CPT	DESCRIPTION	FEE
LABORATORY/RADIOLOGY		
☐ 81000	Urinalysis	
☐ 81002	Urinalysis; Pregnancy Test	
☐ 82951	Glucose Tolerance Test	
☐ 84478	Triglycerides	
☐ 84550	Uric Acid: Blood Chemistry	
☐ 84830	Ovulation Test	
☐ 85014	Hematocrit	
☐ 85031	Hemogram, Complete Blood Wk	
☐ 86403	Particle Agglutination Test	
☐ 86485	Skin Test; Candida	
☐ 86580	TB Intradermal Test	
☐ 86585	TB Tine Test	
☐ 87070	Culture	
☐ 70190	X-Ray; Optic Foramina	
☐ 70210	X-Ray Sinuses Complete	
☐ 71010	Radiological Exam Ent Spine	
☐ 71020	X-Ray Chest Pa & Lat	
☐ 72050	X-Ray Spine, Cerv (4 views)	
☐ 72090	X-Ray Spine; Scoliosis Ex	
☐ 72110	Spine, lumbosacral; a/p & Lat	
☐ 73030	Shoulder-Comp, min w/ 2vws	
☐ 73070	Elbow, anteropost & later vws	
☐ 73120	X-Ray; Hand, 2 views	
☐ 73560	X-Ray, Knee, 1 or 2 views	
☐ 74022	X-Ray; Abdomen, Complete	
☐ 75552	Cardiac Magnetic Res Img	
☐ 76020	X-Ray; Bone Age Studies	
☐ 76088	Mammary Ductogram Complete	
☐ 78465	Myocardial Perfusion Img	

CPT	DESCRIPTION	FEE
PROCEDURES/TESTS		
☐ 00452	Anesthesia for Rad Surgery	
☐ 11100	Skin Biopsy	
☐ 15852	Dressing Change	
☐ 29075	Cast Appl. - Lower Arm	
☐ 29530	Strapping of Knee	
☐ 29705	Removal/Revis of Cast w/Exa	
☐ 53670	Catheterization Incl. Suppl	
☐ 57452	Colposcopy	
☐ 57505	ECC	
☐ 69420	Myringotomy	
☐ 92081	Visual Field Examination	
☐ 92100	Serial Tonometry Exam	
☐ 92120	Tonography	
☐ 92552	Pure Tone Audiometry	
☐ 92567	Tympanometry	
☐ 93000	Electrocardiogram	
☐ 93015	Exercise Stress Test (ETT)	
☐ 93017	ETT Tracing Only	
☐ 93040	Electrocardiogram - Rhythm	
☐ 96100	Psychological Testing	
☐ 99000	Specimen Handling	
☐ 99058	Office Emergency Care	
☐ 99070	Surgical Tray - Misc.	
☐ 99080	Special Reports of Med Rec	
☐ 99195	Phlebotomy	
☐		
☐		
☐		

ICD-9	CODE DIAGNOSIS
☐ 009.0	Ill-defined Intestinal Infect
☐ 133.2	Establish Baseline
☐ 174.9	Breast Cancer
☐ 185.0	Prostate Cancer
☐ 250	Diabetes Mellitus
☐ 272.4	Hyperlipidemia
☐ 282.5	Anemia - Sickle Trait
☐ 282.60	Anemia - Sickle Cell
☐ 285.9	Anemia, Unspecified
☐ 300.4	Neurotic Depression
☐ 340	Multiple Sclerosis
☐ 342.9	Hemiplegia - Unspecified
☐ 346.9	Migraine Headache
☐ 352.9	Cranial Neuralgia
☐ 354.0	Carpal Tunnel Syndrome
☐ 355.0	Sciatic Nerve Root Lesion
☐ 366.9	Cataract
☐ 386.0	Vertigo
☐ 401.1	Essential Hypertension
☐ 414.9	Ischemic Hearth Disease
☐ 428.0	Congestive Heart Failure

ICD-9	CODE DIAGNOSIS
☐ 435.0	Basilar Artery Syndrome
☐ 440.0	Atherosclerosis
☐ 442.81	Carotid Artery
☐ 460.0	Common Cold
☐ 461.9	Acute Sinusitis
☐ 474.0	Tonsillitis
☐ 477.9	Hay Fever
☐ 487.0	Flu
☐ 496	Chronic Airway Obstruction
☐ 522	Low Red Blood Count
☐ 524.6	Temporo-Mandibular Jnt Synd
☐ 538.8	Stomach Pain
☐ 553.3	Hiatal Hernia
☒ 564.1	Spastic Colon
☐ 571.4	Chronic Hepatitis
☐ 571.5	Cirrhosis of Liver
☐ 573.3	Hepatitis
☐ 575.2	Obstruction of Gallbladder
☐ 648.2	Anemia - Compl. Pregnancy
☐ 715.90	Osteoarthritis - Unspec
☐ 721.3	Lumbar Osteo/Spondylarthrit

ICD-9	CODE DIAGNOSIS
☐ 724.2	Pain: Lower Back
☐ 727.6	Rupture of Achilles Tendon
☐ 780.1	Hallucinations
☐ 780.3	Convulsions
☐ 780.5	Sleep Disturbances
☐ 783.0	Anorexia
☐ 783.1	Abnormal Weight Gain
☐ 783.2	Abnormal Weight Loss
☐ 830.6	Dislocated Hip
☐ 830.9	Dislocated Shoulder
☐ 841.2	Sprained Wrist
☐ 842.5	Sprained Ankle
☐ 891.2	Fractured Tibia
☐ 892.0	Fractured Fibula
☐ 919.5	Insect Bite, Nonvenomous
☐ 921.1	Contus Eyelid/Perioc Area
☐ v16.3	Fam. Hist of Breast Cancer
☐ v17.4	Fam. Hist of Cardiovasc Dis
☐ v20.2	Well Child
☐ v22.0	Pregnancy - First Normal
☐ v22.1	Pregnancy - Normal

Previous Balance	Today's Charges	Total Due	Amount Paid	New Balance

Follow Up

PRN _____ Weeks _____   Months _____ Units _____

Next Appointment Date: Time:

I hereby authorize release of any information acquired in the course of
examination or treatment and allow a photocopy of my signature to be used.

TIP: Before you start each exercise, circle the patient number, doctor number, procedure, and diagnosis codes on the form. This will improve your accuracy.

RETRIEVING AN ACCOUNT

The Patient Retrieval screen allows rapid account location.

The prompt for Patient Retrieval appears in numerous places throughout **The Medical Manager** system and is shown in Figure 3-2. The Patient Retrieval screen allows you to retrieve a patient account by entering a name, account number, Social Security number, or ID #. A question mark ('?') plus all or part of one of these four items can be entered to display a related help window OR using the mouse, click on the Help button ('?') on the top toolbar to get a related help window.

Figure 3-2 Procedure Entry Patient Retrieval Prompt with Help Window

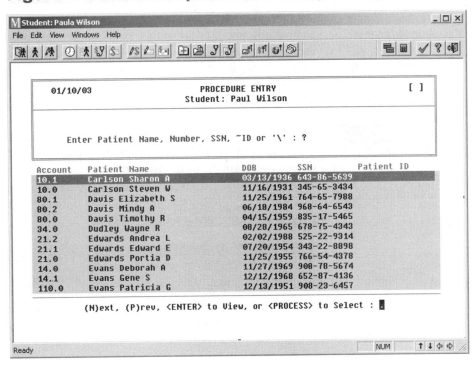

Although there are several methods for retrieving an account, you should use one of the simple methods described below.

1. *Enter the patient name.* Enter one of more letters of the patient's last name. If the complete last name is entered, type a comma (,) or a semicolon (;) and then all or part of the first name. Press **ENTER** and the screen will display the Patient Retrieval screen, discussed below.

2. *Enter the account number.* If you know the full patient number, you can enter it. For example, for the guarantor of account 10, you would key '10.0' and press **ENTER**. For the first dependent you would key '10.1' and press **ENTER**. If the full patient number is entered, **The Medical Manager** software assumes you know which patient is needed and will proceed directly to the screen being accessed for that specific patient. If the account number is entered without a decimal extension, the system will display the Patient Retrieval screen discussed below.

3. *Enter the Social Security number.* Key in the full Social Security number (with or without hyphens) and press **ENTER**. The system will bypass the Patient Retrieval screen and go directly to the specific patient being accessed.

4. *Enter a '\'.* The number of the most recently accessed patient appears in brackets in the upper right corner of the screen. Type a backward slash ('\') to display the retrieval screen for the patient last accessed in **The Medical Manager** system.

Press ENTER to retrieve this default patient number and bypass the Patient Retrieval screen.

Use the highlight bar or the mouse to select the appropriate patient and press **ENTER** to view the Retrieval screen. You can also press F1 or click on the PROCESS button ('√') to process and bypass the Retrieval screen.

POSTING AN ACCOUNT

Posting refers to entering charges, payments, and adjustments.

Data for posting accounts usually comes from an encounter form similar to the one shown in Figure 3-1. Encounter forms, sometimes called *superbills*, enable the physician to inform the front desk of a patient's diagnosis and the procedures that were performed during the examination. The doctor indicates the procedure(s) performed and diagnosis by a checkmark or "X" through the appropriate box on the encounter form. You will use information from Figure 3-1 to complete the practice exercise below.

STEP 1

Select option **2**, PROCEDURE Entry, at the Main Menu (Menu 1) and press **ENTER** OR using the mouse, double-click on option **2**. (Figure 3-3.) The Patient Retrieval prompt will appear on your screen. Follow the instructions below for posting patient accounts. Review Mr. Carlson's encounter form step by step as you enter the data.

Figure 3-3 Patient Retrieval Screen

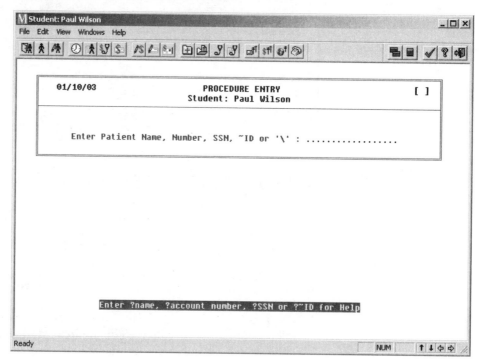

Enter the patient's name or number: '**Carlson,Steven**' or '**10**'

Do not key a space before the first name. The Patient Retrieval screen will display. Verify that this is the correct account and press **ENTER**. Review the encounter form shown in Figure 3-1 for an understanding of the services performed. Mr. Carlson is being charged for an extended office visit to treat a spastic colon. Enter the following data from his encounter form.

◆   a. Primary Insurance #: **2**

Select from the displayed list the insurance plan primarily responsible for payment and to which the bill is to be sent. Highlight the desired plan and press **ENTER** OR using the mouse, double-click on plan **2**.

Note: The highlight bar should default to the primary plan (plan 2), based on the coverage priority originally set for this patient.

Processing with an insurance plan number in this field will set this item to be billed to the selected insurance company. If the patient has no insurance coverage, these fields will not be displayed and the cursor will move directly to the Voucher # field. If this procedure is not being billed to insurance, then you would enter '0' in this field.

◆   b. Assign: (**Y**)es

This field is used to designate assignment or to create insurance estimates. Keying 'E' in this field would post the item as an estimate instead of a charge. Valid responses for this field are (Y)es, (N)o, or (E)stimate. You may press ENTER to default to 'Y'.

◆   c. Secondary Insurance #: **5**

Select the insurance plan secondarily responsible for payment of the procedure. If this procedure should not be billed to a secondary company, then you would enter '0' in this field.

◆   d. EMC Billable: (the cursor will not stop at this field)

This field is used to note whether or not this procedure should be billed electronically. Valid responses for this field are (Y)es and (N)o. The response is determined from the procedure code information and will be entered automatically by **The Medical Manager** software.

◆   e. Voucher #: **1050**

This field is used to store the encounter form number. The encounter form numbers are used to reconcile patients seen, procedures performed, and monies collected for each day of business. These numbers may also be used to track patients as they move throughout an office or other medical facility (e.g., hospital).

◆   f. Doctor #: **3**

This number changes depending on which doctor performs the service. Refer to the top right of the encounter form for the doctor's number. You may press ENTER to default to the primary care physician originally named on this patient's account. Usually, the primary care physician performs the treatment, although another doctor may substitute if the primary care physician is unavailable.

◆   g. Supervisor: **0**

Some medical services are performed by a physician assistant or other provider working under the supervision of a medical doctor. When this occurs, the supervising doctor is recorded in this field. The Student Edition does not have any exercises where this occurs. You may press ENTER to default to '0' for this field.

◆   h. Dept: **0**

Some medical practices credit procedures to certain departments, such as a laboratory or each individual physician's office. When departments are not credited, the default option, '0', may be used.

◆   i.   Location: (Press **ENTER** to leave this field blank)
> **TIP:** The default for this field is for it to remain blank

If procedures are posted by location, this field can be used.

◆   j.   Dates: (Press **ENTER** to default to current system date)

From Date/To Date can be entered for repetitive procedures, such as allergy shots given weekly or on an ongoing basis over time. This is accomplished by typing the first date and pressing ENTER for the From Date and then keying the second date and pressing ENTER for the To Date. You will use only the From Date in this exercise. You may press ENTER to default to the current system date of January 10, 2003, and press ENTER again to bypass the second date.

◆   k.   Place of Service (P.O.S.) Code: **3**

This field contains the number representing the place where the service was performed. For this exercise, you may press ENTER to use the default Place of Service code of '3'. For the purposes of these exercises, the P.O.S. of '3' will be used unless otherwise specified.

The Medical Manager software has an internal, one-digit code that corresponds to different coding systems used by different insurance companies and agencies. **The Medical Manager** system user, in this case the student, only needs to enter the default code in the P.O.S. and T.O.S. fields (see Type of Service Code below). When P.O.S. or T.O.S. codes are provided to an insurance company on an insurance form, they will automatically be cross-referenced to the correct code for that company.

◆   l.   Procedure Code: **99214**

Enter the first procedure code marked on the encounter form. The description of the procedure code and its charge will display on the screen. If an improper code is entered, the following message will appear:

"**PROCEDURE CODE NOT FOUND**"

> **TIP:** A help window is available at the Procedure Code field to assist you in determining the code for a procedure not listed on the encounter form. Key a question mark '?' at the field and press ENTER OR using the mouse, click on the Help button ('?') on the top toolbar to view a help window for this field.

Note: Descriptions of both diagnosis and procedure codes may differ slightly from encounter form to encounter form, and from practice to practice. Although the wording of these descriptions varies, you will notice that the actual meaning does not.

◆   m.   Modifier Code: (Press **ENTER** to bypass this field)

The modifier code refers to codes for special procedures performed during a primary procedure. You will press ENTER to bypass this field.

◆   n.   Diagnosis 1–4: **564.1**

Four fields are provided for the physician's diagnoses. The primary diagnosis for field 1 is required, and the other three diagnoses are optional. The other diagnoses will be skipped in these exercises, so you may press ENTER to advance the cursor to the Units field OR using the mouse, simply click in the Units field to relocate the cursor to this point. If an improper diagnosis code is entered, the following message will appear:

"**DIAGNOSIS CODE NOT FOUND**"

Once a patient has been seen, a default of the patient's last diagnosis is available. This can be useful when a patient is seen repeatedly for the same condition. A description of the diagnosis code will be displayed on the screen.

A help window is available at the Diagnosis Code field to help you locate the code for a diagnosis not preprinted (i.e., generally handwritten by the physician) on the encounter form. To view a help window at the field, enter a question mark '?' and press ENTER OR click on the Help button ('?') on the top toolbar.

◆ o. Units: **1.0**

Units refers to the number of times the procedure was repeated during the date or dates of service. The procedure must have been performed by the same doctor on the same patient. You may press ENTER to default to '1', because this is usually the number of times a procedure is performed.

◆ p. Charges: (Press **ENTER** to accept default amount)

The procedure charge, less discount percent, plus tax, times the number of units, is automatically entered into this field. This fee can also be determined by which doctor performed the service or which insurance company is being billed. Press ENTER to accept this amount, or key in a new amount and press ENTER. The amount displayed in this field is the total amount that the patient will be charged for the services performed.

◆ q. Type of Service (T.O.S.) Code: **1**

This field refers to the type of service rendered to the patient. The standard T.O.S. codes accepted by insurance companies are available in a help window. You may press ENTER to use the default, '1', for this field.

◆ r. Comment: (Press **ENTER** to leave blank)

Key any comment to be communicated to the insurance company about the procedure. This comment can appear on insurance forms or patient statements and bills. Unless otherwise specified, the comment field will be skipped in these exercises.

STEP 2 Review and edit the screen. If any fields have not been entered, you will be returned to these fields for proper entry. When you are sure your screen is complete, press **F1** OR click on the PROCESS button ('√') on the top toolbar to process. Your screen should be similar to Figure 3-4.

You will now be asked about ailment detail. Answer '**0**' for 'None' to not add an ailment and press **ENTER**. This topic will be covered later in Unit 3 after you have had an opportunity to post additional exercises.

As each entry is processed, the charge will be displayed as a summary line in the lower part of the screen. The summary line will include the service date, insurance company, doctor number, procedure code, diagnosis code, units, charge, and a running total.

Figure 3-4 Posted Account

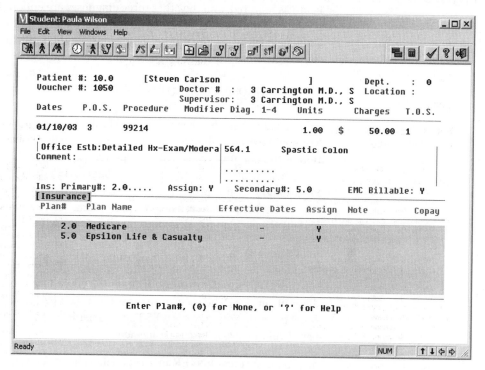

After you have completed Mr. Carlson's procedure entry, keyed '0' for ailment, and pressed ENTER then ESCAPE, a warning message will appear that will allow you to allocate payment to the account. This payment option will be covered in Unit 6. Press **ESCAPE** to exit so that a procedure may be posted for a different patient. The Patient Retrieval screen will display so that you can access the next patient's account.

APPLYING YOUR KNOWLEDGE

Encounter forms for five patients are provided below. Complete the exercises by referring to the encounter form for each patient. Refer to the practice exercise when you have questions about the content of any field.

All information must be completed correctly for an encounter. If you exit Procedure Entry and re-enter the modules, you may not be able to get your screen to match the figures in the text unless you first go to Edit Activity Records, delete the partially posted charges, and begin the exercise again. Similarly, you should carefully check each screen before pressing 'F1' or clicking the PROCESS ('√') button because you cannot go back to a screen once you leave it. If you process a screen with errors, you will correct the error in Edit Activity. Edit Activity will be covered in Unit 4. Ask your instructor before proceeding to Unit 4 out of sequence to correct errors.

EXERCISE 1: Sharon A. Carlson

Posting Procedures to a Dependent

Before attempting data entry, study the encounter form shown in Figure 3-5 and answer the following questions:

1. Who is the guarantor on the patient account?

2. Who is the patient listed on the encounter form?

3. Is the guarantor the patient who received services indicated on the encounter form?

Figure 3-5 Sharon Carlson's Encounter Form—Voucher 1051

Sydney Carrington & Associates P.A.
34 Sycamore Street   Suite 300
Madison, CA 95653

Date: 01/10/2003

Voucher No.: 1051

Time: 11:30

Patient: Sharon Carlson
Guarantor: Steven W. Carlson

Patient No: 10.1
Doctor: 3 - S. Carrington

CPT	DESCRIPTION	FEE
OFFICE/HOSPITAL CONSULTS		
☐ 99201	Office New:Focused Hx-Exam	
☐ 99202	Office New:Expanded Hx-Exam	
☐ 99211	Office Estb:Min/None Hx-Exa	
☐ 99212	Office Estb:Focused Hx-Exam	
☒ 99213	Office Estb:Expanded Hx-Exa	$40.00
☐ 99214	Office Estb:Detailed Hx-Exa	
☐ 99215	Office Estb:Comprhn Hx-Exam	
☐ 99221	Hosp. Initial:Comprh Hx-	
☐ 99223	Hosp.Ini:Comprh Hx-Exam/Hi	
☐ 99231	Hosp. Subsequent: S-Fwd	
☐ 99232	Hosp. Subsequent: Comprhn Hx	
☐ 99233	Hosp. Subsequent: Ex/Hi	
☐ 99238	Hospital Visit Discharge Ex	
☐ 99371	Telephone Consult - Simple	
☐ 99372	Telephone Consult - Intermed	
☐ 99373	Telephone Consult - Complex	
☐ 90843	Counseling - 25 minutes	
☐ 90844	Counseling - 50 minutes	
☐ 90865	Counseling - Special Interview	
IMMUNIZATIONS/INJECTIONS		
☐ 90585	BCG Vaccine	
☐ 90659	Influenza Virus Vaccine	
☐ 90701	Immunization-DTP	
☐ 90702	DT Vaccine	
☐ 90703	Tetanus Toxoids	
☐ 90732	Pneumococcal Vaccine	
☐ 90746	Hepatitis B Vaccine	
☐ 90749	Immunization; Unlisted	

CPT	DESCRIPTION	FEE
LABORATORY/RADIOLOGY		
☐ 81000	Urinalysis	
☐ 81002	Urinalysis; Pregnancy Test	
☐ 82951	Glucose Tolerance Test	
☐ 84478	Triglycerides	
☐ 84550	Uric Acid: Blood Chemistry	
☐ 84830	Ovulation Test	
☐ 85014	Hematocrit	
☐ 85031	Hemogram, Complete Blood Wk	
☐ 86403	Particle Agglutination Test	
☐ 86485	Skin Test; Candida	
☐ 86580	TB Intradermal Test	
☐ 86585	TB Tine Test	
☐ 87070	Culture	
☐ 70190	X-Ray; Optic Foramina	
☐ 70210	X-Ray Sinuses Complete	
☐ 71010	Radiological Exam Ent Spine	
☐ 71020	X-Ray Chest Pa & Lat	
☐ 72050	X-Ray Spine, Cerv (4 views)	
☐ 72090	X-Ray Spine; Scoliosis Ex	
☐ 72110	Spine, lumbosacral; a/p & Lat	
☐ 73030	Shoulder-Comp, min w/ 2vws	
☐ 73070	Elbow, anteropost & later vws	
☐ 73120	X-Ray; Hand, 2 views	
☐ 73560	X-Ray, Knee, 1 or 2 views	
☐ 74022	X-Ray; Abdomen, Complete	
☐ 75552	Cardiac Magnetic Res Img	
☐ 76020	X-Ray; Bone Age Studies	
☐ 76088	Mammary Ductogram Complete	
☐ 78465	Myocardial Perfusion Img	

CPT	DESCRIPTION	FEE
PROCEDURES/TESTS		
☐ 00452	Anesthesia for Rad Surgery	
☐ 11100	Skin Biopsy	
☐ 15852	Dressing Change	
☐ 29075	Cast Appl. - Lower Arm	
☐ 29530	Strapping of Knee	
☐ 29705	Removal/Revis of Cast w/Exa	
☐ 53670	Catheterization Incl. Suppl	
☐ 57452	Colposcopy	
☐ 57505	ECC	
☐ 69420	Myringotomy	
☐ 92081	Visual Field Examination	
☐ 92100	Serial Tonometry Exam	
☐ 92120	Tonography	
☐ 92552	Pure Tone Audiometry	
☐ 92567	Tympanometry	
☐ 93000	Electrocardiogram	
☐ 93015	Exercise Stress Test (ETT)	
☐ 93017	ETT Tracing Only	
☐ 93040	Electrocardiogram - Rhythm	
☐ 96100	Psychological Testing	
☐ 99000	Specimen Handling	
☐ 99058	Office Emergency Care	
☐ 99070	Surgical Tray - Misc.	
☐ 99080	Special Reports of Med Rec	
☐ 99195	Phlebotomy	
☐		
☐		
☐		

ICD-9	CODE DIAGNOSIS
☐ 009.0	Ill-defined Intestinal Infect
☐ 133.2	Establish Baseline
☐ 174.9	Breast Cancer
☐ 185.0	Prostate Cancer
☐ 250	Diabetes Mellitus
☐ 272.4	Hyperlipidemia
☐ 282.5	Anemia - Sickle Trait
☐ 282.60	Anemia - Sickle Cell
☐ 285.9	Anemia, Unspecified
☐ 300.4	Neurotic Depression
☐ 340	Multiple Sclerosis
☐ 342.9	Hemiplegia - Unspecified
☐ 346.9	Migraine Headache
☐ 352.9	Cranial Neuralgia
☐ 354.0	Carpal Tunnel Syndrome
☐ 355.0	Sciatic Nerve Root Lesion
☐ 366.9	Cataract
☐ 386.0	Vertigo
☐ 401.1	Essential Hypertension
☐ 414.9	Ischemic Hearth Disease
☐ 428.0	Congestive Heart Failure

ICD-9	CODE DIAGNOSIS
☐ 435.0	Basilar Artery Syndrome
☐ 440.0	Atherosclerosis
☐ 442.81	Carotid Artery
☐ 460.0	Common Cold
☒ 461.9	Acute Sinusitis
☐ 474.0	Tonsillitis
☐ 477.9	Hay Fever
☐ 487.0	Flu
☐ 496	Chronic Airway Obstruction
☐ 522	Low Red Blood Count
☐ 524.6	Temporo-Mandibular Jnt Synd
☐ 538.8	Stomach Pain
☐ 553.3	Hiatal Hernia
☐ 564.1	Spastic Colon
☐ 571.4	Chronic Hepatitis
☐ 571.5	Cirrhosis of Liver
☐ 573.3	Hepatitis
☐ 575.2	Obstruction of Gallbladder
☐ 648.2	Anemia - Compl. Pregnancy
☐ 715.90	Osteoarthritis - Unspec
☐ 721.3	Lumbar Osteo/Spondylarthrit

ICD-9	CODE DIAGNOSIS
☐ 724.2	Pain: Lower Back
☐ 727.6	Rupture of Achilles Tendon
☐ 780.1	Hallucinations
☐ 780.3	Convulsions
☐ 780.5	Sleep Disturbances
☐ 783.0	Anorexia
☐ 783.1	Abnormal Weight Gain
☐ 783.2	Abnormal Weight Loss
☐ 830.6	Dislocated Hip
☐ 830.9	Dislocated Shoulder
☐ 841.2	Sprained Wrist
☐ 842.5	Sprained Ankle
☐ 891.2	Fractured Tibia
☐ 892.0	Fractured Fibula
☐ 919.5	Insect Bite, Nonvenomous
☐ 921.1	Contus Eyelid/Perioc Area
☐ v16.3	Fam. Hist of Breast Cancer
☐ v17.4	Fam. Hist of Cardiovasc Dis
☐ v20.2	Well Child
☐ v22.0	Pregnancy - First Normal
☐ v22.1	Pregnancy - Normal

Previous Balance	Today's Charges	Total Due	Amount Paid	New Balance

Follow Up

PRN _____ Weeks _____ Months _____ Units _____

Next Appointment Date: _____   Time: _____

I hereby authorize release of any information acquired in the course of examination or treatment and allow a photocopy of my signature to be used.

4. Who is the doctor who performed the services for the patient?

5. What procedure did the doctor perform for the patient?

6. What was the doctor's diagnosis of the patient's condition?

You should already be at the Procedure Entry Patient Retrieval screen. If not, return to the Main Menu (Menu 1) and choose option **2**, PROCEDURE Entry, and press **ENTER**. In this exercise, the patient to be treated is Steven Carlson's wife, Sharon. Refer to Mrs. Carlson's encounter form, shown in Figure 3-5, for the necessary patient information.

STEP 1

Key in Mrs. Carlson's patient number, '**10.1**', and press **ENTER** to begin the exercise. Note that the Patient Retrieval screen will be bypassed because the complete account number was entered.

STEP 2

Only one insurance plan displays, Pan American. This is due to the patient coverage list you set up for the patient in Unit 2. Press **ENTER** to select and bill Pan American as Mrs. Carlson's primary coverage. Press **ENTER** again at both the Assignment and Secondary Insurance fields to accept the default responses.

STEP 3

Key '**1051**' in the Voucher number field and press **ENTER**. The cursor will move to the Dr # field. Press **ENTER** to accept the default doctor # and supervisor for this patient, Dr. Sydney Carrington. Press **ENTER** twice to bypass the Department and Location fields.

STEP 4

Press **ENTER** to accept the current system date (01/10/03) as the date of the visit, and press **ENTER** to leave the second date field blank. Press **ENTER** at the Place of Service field to default to code '3' (for Doctor's Office).

STEP 5

Key the procedure code listed on Mrs. Carlson's Encounter Form, '**99213**', and press **ENTER**. Then, press **ENTER** to bypass the Modifier field. Key the diagnosis code shown at the bottom of the encounter form, '**461.9**', and press **ENTER**.

STEP 6

After you post all information shown on Mrs. Carlson's encounter form, carefully review to make sure you have entered the correct voucher number and that the proper doctor's number appears when you use the default. Compare your screen with Figure 3-6, then press **F1** or click the PROCESS button ('√') on the top toolbar to

Figure 3-6 Sharon Carlson's Completed Procedure Entry Screen

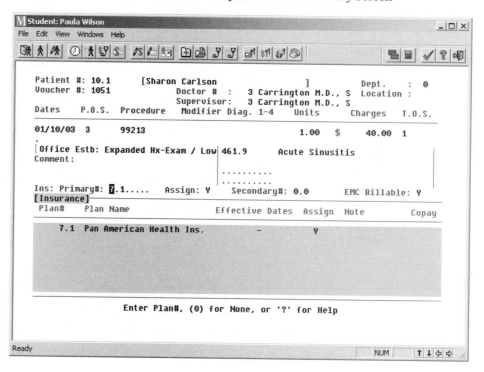

process. Respond '**0**' at the Ailment Detail screen, as you did in the exercise for Mr. Carlson and press **ENTER**.

Press **ESCAPE** twice or click twice on the EXIT button on the top toolbar to return to the Patient Retrieval screen for the next patient.

EXERCISE 2: Alice J. Spivey

Posting Multiple Procedures to a Patient with a Different Last Name Than Guarantor

Before attempting data entry, study the encounter form shown in Figure 3-7 and answer the following questions:

1. Does the encounter form indicate that Terry Williams was seen by the doctor on January 10, 2003?

2. According to the encounter form, who was seen by the doctor?

3. According to the encounter form, who is responsible for the account?

4. What is the name of the physician who saw Alice Spivey?

5. How many procedures and diagnosis codes were checked by the physician?

The next two patients are the daughters of Ms. Terry Williams (remember that these children do not share her last name). Starting from the Main Menu (Menu 1), choose option **2**, PROCEDURE Entry. Retrieve Ms. Williams's account as guarantor by entering the patient's last name 'Spivey' into the Patient Retrieval screen.

Once you access the account with 'Alice Spivey', highlight Alice's name and press ENTER OR using the mouse, double-click on Alice's name to highlight and select her account. If you access the account by keying the full account number, '120.2', and pressing ENTER, the correct patient will be immediately selected and the Patient Retrieval screen will be bypassed.

You could have also accessed the account by entering the guarantor's last name 'Williams'. If you access the account with the name 'Terry Williams', highlight Alice's name on the list and press **ENTER** OR using the mouse, double-click on Alice's name to highlight and select her.

STEP 1
Alice is covered under two insurance plans: her mother's HMO plan and a policy through her father. Using the keyboard or mouse, indicate the HMO plan as primary coverage and the Epsilon Life and Casualty as secondary insurance. Key voucher #'**1052**', Doctor #'**1**', and press **ENTER** at both the Department and Location fields. Press **ENTER** again at both date fields and at the P.O.S. field.

STEP 2
Alice is being seen for a General Check-Up and a routine immunization booster shot. (See Figure 3-7.) Enter procedure code, '**99211**', and her diagnosis code, '**V20.2**'. This is a special diagnosis code used to indicate that the procedures being performed are part of a regular Well-Child visit and that Alice is in good health.

STEP 3
Press **F1** to process or click on the PROCESS button ('√') on the top toolbar. Then, key '**0**' for 'None' for Ailment Detail and press **ENTER** and the cursor returns to the procedure code field. The bottom of the screen will display the first procedure you just posted. Now you can enter Alice's second procedure code, '**90701**'. Press **F1** or click on the PROCESS button ('√') on the top toolbar to process, and answer '**0**' for 'None' to Ailment Detail again and press **ENTER**.

Figure 3-7 Alice Spivey's Encounter Form—Voucher 1052

Sydney Carrington & Associates P.A.
34 Sycamore Street   Suite 300
Madison, CA 95653

Date: 01/10/2003

Time: 10:00

Voucher No.:   1052

Patient: Alice Spivey
Guarantor: Terry L. Williams

Patient No: 120.2
Doctor: 1 - J. Monroe

☐ CPT	DESCRIPTION	FEE
OFFICE/HOSPITAL CONSULTS		
☐ 99201	Office New:Focused Hx-Exam	
☐ 99202	Office New:Expanded Hx-Exam	
☒ 99211	Office Estb:Min/None Hx-Exa	$25.00
☐ 99212	Office Estb:Focused Hx-Exam	
☐ 99213	Office Estb:Expanded Hx-Exa	
☐ 99214	Office Estb:Detailed Hx-Exa	
☐ 99215	Office Estb:Comprhn Hx-Exam	
☐ 99221	Hosp. Initial:Comprh Hx-	
☐ 99223	Hosp.Ini:Comprh Hx-Exam/Hi	
☐ 99231	Hosp. Subsequent: S-Fwd	
☐ 99232	Hosp. Subsequent: Comprhn Hx	
☐ 99233	Hosp. Subsequent: Ex/Hi	
☐ 99238	Hospital Visit Discharge Ex	
☐ 99371	Telephone Consult - Simple	
☐ 99372	Telephone Consult - Intermed	
☐ 99373	Telephone Consult - Complex	
☐ 90843	Counseling - 25 minutes	
☐ 90844	Counseling - 50 minutes	
☐ 90865	Counseling - Special Interview	
IMMUNIZATIONS/INJECTIONS		
☐ 90585	BCG Vaccine	
☐ 90659	Influenza Virus Vaccine	
☒ 90701	Immunization-DTP	$14.00
☐ 90702	DT Vaccine	
☐ 90703	Tetanus Toxoids	
☐ 90732	Pneumococcal Vaccine	
☐ 90746	Hepatitis B Vaccine	
☐ 90749	Immunization; Unlisted	

☐ CPT	DESCRIPTION	FEE
LABORATORY/RADIOLOGY		
☐ 81000	Urinalysis	
☐ 81002	Urinalysis; Pregnancy Test	
☐ 82951	Glucose Tolerance Test	
☐ 84478	Triglycerides	
☐ 84550	Uric Acid: Blood Chemistry	
☐ 84830	Ovulation Test	
☐ 85014	Hematocrit	
☐ 85031	Hemogram, Complete Blood Wk	
☐ 86403	Particle Agglutination Test	
☐ 86485	Skin Test; Candida	
☐ 86580	TB Intradermal Test	
☐ 86585	TB Tine Test	
☐ 87070	Culture	
☐ 70190	X-Ray; Optic Foramina	
☐ 70210	X-Ray Sinuses Complete	
☐ 71010	Radiological Exam Ent Spine	
☐ 71020	X-Ray Chest Pa & Lat	
☐ 72050	X-Ray Spine, Cerv (4 views)	
☐ 72090	X-Ray Spine; Scoliosis Ex	
☐ 72110	Spine, lumbosacral; a/p & Lat	
☐ 73030	Shoulder-Comp, min w/ 2vws	
☐ 73070	Elbow, anteropost & later vws	
☐ 73120	X-Ray; Hand, 2 views	
☐ 73560	X-Ray, Knee, 1 or 2 views	
☐ 74022	X-Ray; Abdomen, Complete	
☐ 75552	Cardiac Magnetic Res Img	
☐ 76020	X-Ray; Bone Age Studies	
☐ 76088	Mammary Ductogram Complete	
☐ 78465	Myocardial Perfusion Img	

☐ CPT	DESCRIPTION	FEE
PROCEDURES/TESTS		
☐ 00452	Anesthesia for Rad Surgery	
☐ 11100	Skin Biopsy	
☐ 15852	Dressing Change	
☐ 29075	Cast Appl. - Lower Arm	
☐ 29530	Strapping of Knee	
☐ 29705	Removal/Revis of Cast w/Exa	
☐ 53670	Catheterization Incl. Suppl	
☐ 57452	Colposcopy	
☐ 57505	ECC	
☐ 69420	Myringotomy	
☐ 92081	Visual Field Examination	
☐ 92100	Serial Tonometry Exam	
☐ 92120	Tonography	
☐ 92552	Pure Tone Audiometry	
☐ 92567	Tympanometry	
☐ 93000	Electrocardiogram	
☐ 93015	Exercise Stress Test (ETT)	
☐ 93017	ETT Tracing Only	
☐ 93040	Electrocardiogram - Rhythm	
☐ 96100	Psychological Testing	
☐ 99000	Specimen Handling	
☐ 99058	Office Emergency Care	
☐ 99070	Surgical Tray - Misc.	
☐ 99080	Special Reports of Med Rec	
☐ 99195	Phlebotomy	
☐ ___	_____	
☐ ___	_____	
☐ ___	_____	

☐ ICD-9	CODE DIAGNOSIS
☐ 009.0	Ill-defined Intestinal Infect
☐ 133.2	Establish Baseline
☐ 174.9	Breast Cancer
☐ 185.0	Prostate Cancer
☐ 250	Diabetes Mellitus
☐ 272.4	Hyperlipidemia
☐ 282.5	Anemia - Sickle Trait
☐ 282.60	Anemia - Sickle Cell
☐ 285.9	Anemia, Unspecified
☐ 300.4	Neurotic Depression
☐ 340	Multiple Sclerosis
☐ 342.9	Hemiplegia - Unspecified
☐ 346.9	Migraine Headache
☐ 352.9	Cranial Neuralgia
☐ 354.0	Carpal Tunnel Syndrome
☐ 355.0	Sciatic Nerve Root Lesion
☐ 366.9	Cataract
☐ 386.0	Vertigo
☐ 401.1	Essential Hypertension
☐ 414.9	Ischemic Hearth Disease
☐ 428.0	Congestive Heart Failure

☐ ICD-9	CODE DIAGNOSIS
☐ 435.0	Basilar Artery Syndrome
☐ 440.0	Atherosclerosis
☐ 442.81	Carotid Artery
☐ 460.0	Common Cold
☐ 461.9	Acute Sinusitis
☐ 474.0	Tonsillitis
☐ 477.9	Hay Fever
☐ 487.0	Flu
☐ 496	Chronic Airway Obstruction
☐ 522	Low Red Blood Count
☐ 524.6	Temporo-Mandibular Jnt Synd
☐ 538.8	Stomach Pain
☐ 553.3	Hiatal Hernia
☐ 564.1	Spastic Colon
☐ 571.4	Chronic Hepatitis
☐ 571.5	Cirrhosis of Liver
☐ 573.3	Hepatitis
☐ 575.2	Obstruction of Gallbladder
☐ 648.2	Anemia - Compl. Pregnancy
☐ 715.90	Osteoarthritis - Unspec
☐ 721.3	Lumbar Osteo/Spondylarthrit

☐ ICD-9	CODE DIAGNOSIS
☐ 724.2	Pain: Lower Back
☐ 727.6	Rupture of Achilles Tendon
☐ 780.1	Hallucinations
☐ 780.3	Convulsions
☐ 780.5	Sleep Disturbances
☐ 783.0	Anorexia
☐ 783.1	Abnormal Weight Gain
☐ 783.2	Abnormal Weight Loss
☐ 830.6	Dislocated Hip
☐ 830.9	Dislocated Shoulder
☐ 841.2	Sprained Wrist
☐ 842.5	Sprained Ankle
☐ 891.2	Fractured Tibia
☐ 892.0	Fractured Fibula
☐ 919.5	Insect Bite, Nonvenomous
☐ 921.1	Contus Eyelid/Perioc Area
☐ v16.3	Fam. Hist of Breast Cancer
☐ v17.4	Fam. Hist of Cardiovasc Dis
☒ v20.2	Well Child
☐ v22.0	Pregnancy - First Normal
☐ v22.1	Pregnancy - Normal

Previous Balance	Today's Charges	Total Due	Amount Paid	New Balance
_____	_____	_____	_____	_____

Follow Up

PRN _____ Weeks _____ Months _____ Units _____

Next Appointment Date: _____   Time: _____

I hereby authorize release of any information acquired in the course of examination or treatment and allow a photocopy of my signature to be used.

_____

You have completed posting for this patient. Compare your screen with Figure 3-8. Two charges should appear on the screen to match the two charges shown on her encounter form. The charge amount showing in the posting window should equal the amount shown on the encounter form. Press **F1** or click on the PROCESS button ('√') on the top toolbar to process. Press **ESCAPE** twice or click twice on the EXIT button on the top toolbar to return to the Patient Retrieval screen and select the next patient.

Figure 3-8 Alice Spivey's Procedure Entry Screen

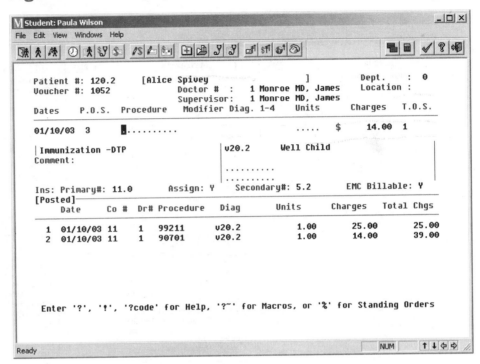

EXERCISE 3: Laura S. Simmons

Posting a Procedure for a Work-In Patient

Ms. Williams brought Laura along for a General Check-Up because she already had an appointment for her other daughter, Alice. Since Laura didn't have an appointment, she does not have a preprinted encounter form. For that reason a "Work-In" form is used (Figure 3-9). A "Work-In" form is simply a blank encounter form that is completed by hand and attached to the patient's chart.

STEP 1 At the Procedure Entry Patient Retrieval screen, key '**120.1**' and press **ENTER** to retrieve Laura's account. Verify that Laura's name is at the top of the Procedure Entry screen. Using the keyboard or mouse, enter only one insurance plan, '**11**', for the primary insurance number, since Laura is not covered on the other plan. Type **WorkIn** for the voucher number since "Work-In" is too large for this field. Key '**1**' at the Doctor # field and press **ENTER** at both the Department and Location fields. Press **ENTER** again at both of the dates fields and at the P.O.S. field.

STEP 2 Enter the procedure code shown for Laura, **99211**, press **ENTER** to bypass the Modifier field, and key '**V20.2**' in the Diagnosis field. Press **F1** or click on the PROCESS button ('√') on the top toolbar to process, then answer '**0**' for 'None' to Ailment Detail

Figure 3-9 Laura Simmon's Encounter Form—Voucher Work-In

Sydney Carrington & Associates P.A.

34 Sycamore Street   Suite 300
Madison, CA 95653

Date: 01/10/2003

Time: 10:05

Patient: Laura Simmons
Guarantor: Terry L. Williams

Voucher No.: Work-In

Patient No: 120.1
Doctor: 1 - J. Monroe

	CPT	DESCRIPTION	FEE
		OFFICE/HOSPITAL CONSULTS	
☐	99201	Office New:Focused Hx-Exam	
☐	99202	Office New:Expanded Hx-Exam	
☒	99211	Office Estb:Min/None Hx-Exa	$25.00
☐	99212	Office Estb:Focused Hx-Exam	
☐	99213	Office Estb:Expanded Hx-Exa	
☐	99214	Office Estb:Detailed Hx-Exa	
☐	99215	Office Estb:Comprhn Hx-Exam	
☐	99221	Hosp. Initial:Comprh Hx-	
☐	99223	Hosp.Ini:Comprh Hx-Exam/Hi	
☐	99231	Hosp. Subsequent: S-Fwd	
☐	99232	Hosp. Subsequent: Comprhn Hx	
☐	99233	Hosp. Subsequent: Ex/Hi	
☐	99238	Hospital Visit Discharge Ex	
☐	99371	Telephone Consult - Simple	
☐	99372	Telephone Consult - Intermed	
☐	99373	Telephone Consult - Complex	
☐	90843	Counseling - 25 minutes	
☐	90844	Counseling - 50 minutes	
☐	90865	Counseling - Special Interview	
		IMMUNIZATIONS/INJECTIONS	
☐	90585	BCG Vaccine	
☐	90659	Influenza Virus Vaccine	
☐	90701	Immunization-DTP	
☐	90702	DT Vaccine	
☐	90703	Tetanus Toxoids	
☐	90732	Pneumococcal Vaccine	
☐	90746	Hepatitis B Vaccine	
☐	90749	Immunization; Unlisted	

	CPT	DESCRIPTION	FEE
		LABORATORY/RADIOLOGY	
☐	81000	Urinalysis	
☐	81002	Urinalysis; Pregnancy Test	
☐	82951	Glucose Tolerance Test	
☐	84478	Triglycerides	
☐	84550	Uric Acid: Blood Chemistry	
☐	84830	Ovulation Test	
☐	85014	Hematocrit	
☐	85031	Hemogram, Complete Blood Wk	
☐	86403	Particle Agglutination Test	
☐	86485	Skin Test; Candida	
☐	86580	TB Intradermal Test	
☐	86585	TB Tine Test	
☐	87070	Culture	
☐	70190	X-Ray; Optic Foramina	
☐	70210	X-Ray Sinuses Complete	
☐	71010	Radiological Exam Ent Spine	
☐	71020	X-Ray Chest Pa & Lat	
☐	72050	X-Ray Spine, Cerv (4 views)	
☐	72090	X-Ray Spine; Scoliosis Ex	
☐	72110	Spine, lumbosacral; a/p & Lat	
☐	73030	Shoulder-Comp, min w/ 2vws	
☐	73070	Elbow, anteropost & later vws	
☐	73120	X-Ray; Hand, 2 views	
☐	73560	X-Ray, Knee, 1 or 2 views	
☐	74022	X-Ray; Abdomen, Complete	
☐	75552	Cardiac Magnetic Res Img	
☐	76020	X-Ray; Bone Age Studies	
☐	76088	Mammary Ductogram Complete	
☐	78465	Myocardial Perfusion Img	

	CPT	DESCRIPTION	FEE
		PROCEDURES/TESTS	
☐	00452	Anesthesia for Rad Surgery	
☐	11100	Skin Biopsy	
☐	15852	Dressing Change	
☐	29075	Cast Appl. - Lower Arm	
☐	29530	Strapping of Knee	
☐	29705	Removal/Revis of Cast w/Exa	
☐	53670	Catheterization Incl. Suppl	
☐	57452	Colposcopy	
☐	57505	ECC	
☐	69420	Myringotomy	
☐	92081	Visual Field Examination	
☐	92100	Serial Tonometry Exam	
☐	92120	Tonography	
☐	92552	Pure Tone Audiometry	
☐	92567	Tympanometry	
☐	93000	Electrocardiogram	
☐	93015	Exercise Stress Test (ETT)	
☐	93017	ETT Tracing Only	
☐	93040	Electrocardiogram - Rhythm	
☐	96100	Psychological Testing	
☐	99000	Specimen Handling	
☐	99058	Office Emergency Care	
☐	99070	Surgical Tray - Misc.	
☐	99080	Special Reports of Med Rec	
☐	99195	Phlebotomy	
☐			
☐			
☐			

	ICD-9	CODE DIAGNOSIS
☐	009.0	Ill-defined Intestinal Infect
☐	133.2	Establish Baseline
☐	174.9	Breast Cancer
☐	185.0	Prostate Cancer
☐	250	Diabetes Mellitus
☐	272.4	Hyperlipidemia
☐	282.5	Anemia - Sickle Trait
☐	282.60	Anemia - Sickle Cell
☐	285.9	Anemia, Unspecified
☐	300.4	Neurotic Depression
☐	340	Multiple Sclerosis
☐	342.9	Hemiplegia - Unspecified
☐	346.9	Migraine Headache
☐	352.9	Cranial Neuralgia
☐	354.0	Carpal Tunnel Syndrome
☐	355.0	Sciatic Nerve Root Lesion
☐	366.9	Cataract
☐	386.0	Vertigo
☐	401.1	Essential Hypertension
☐	414.9	Ischemic Hearth Disease
☐	428.0	Congestive Heart Failure

	ICD-9	CODE DIAGNOSIS
☐	435.0	Basilar Artery Syndrome
☐	440.0	Atherosclerosis
☐	442.81	Carotid Artery
☐	460.0	Common Cold
☐	461.9	Acute Sinusitis
☐	474.0	Tonsillitis
☐	477.9	Hay Fever
☐	487.0	Flu
☐	496	Chronic Airway Obstruction
☐	522	Low Red Blood Count
☐	524.6	Temporo-Mandibular Jnt Synd
☐	538.8	Stomach Pain
☐	553.3	Hiatal Hernia
☐	564.1	Spastic Colon
☐	571.4	Chronic Hepatitis
☐	571.5	Cirrhosis of Liver
☐	573.3	Hepatitis
☐	575.2	Obstruction of Gallbladder
☐	648.2	Anemia - Compl. Pregnancy
☐	715.90	Osteoarthritis - Unspec
☐	721.3	Lumbar Osteo/Spondylarthrit

	ICD-9	CODE DIAGNOSIS
☐	724.2	Pain: Lower Back
☐	727.6	Rupture of Achilles Tendon
☐	780.1	Hallucinations
☐	780.3	Convulsions
☐	780.5	Sleep Disturbances
☐	783.0	Anorexia
☐	783.1	Abnormal Weight Gain
☐	783.2	Abnormal Weight Loss
☐	830.6	Dislocated Hip
☐	830.9	Dislocated Shoulder
☐	841.2	Sprained Wrist
☐	842.5	Sprained Ankle
☐	891.2	Fractured Tibia
☐	892.0	Fractured Fibula
☐	919.5	Insect Bite, Nonvenomous
☐	921.1	Contus Eyelid/Perioc Area
☐	v16.3	Fam. Hist of Breast Cancer
☐	v17.4	Fam. Hist of Cardiovasc Dis
☒	v20.2	Well Child
☐	v22.0	Pregnancy - First Normal
☐	v22.1	Pregnancy - Normal

Previous Balance	Today's Charges	Total Due	Amount Paid	New Balance

Follow Up

PRN _____ Weeks _____   Months _____ Units _____

Next Appointment Date: Time:

I hereby authorize release of any information acquired in the course of
examination or treatment and allow a photocopy of my signature to be used.

_____

and press **ENTER**. The cursor returns to the Procedure Code field and the bottom of the screen displays the procedure you just posted.

You have completed posting for this patient. Compare the completed screen with Figure 3-10. One charge should appear on the screen to match the charge shown on the encounter form. The total amount showing in the posting window should equal the total shown on the encounter form. Press **ESCAPE** twice or click twice on the EXIT button on the top toolbar to return to the Patient Retrieval screen and select the next patient.

Figure 3-10 Posted Window for Laura Simmons

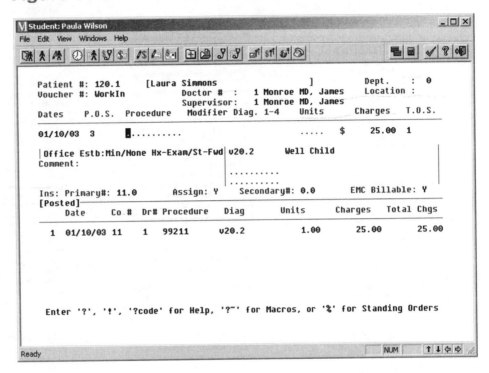

EXERCISE 4: Wayne R. Dudley

Posting Four Charges

Mr. Wayne Dudley has a full examination with multiple tests (Figure 3-11). Using the keyboard or mouse, follow the steps below to post each procedure code and diagnosis information until you have completed all the marked items on his encounter form.

STEP 1   At the Procedure Entry Patient Retrieval screen, key Mr. Dudley's account number, '**34.0**', and press **ENTER** to retrieve his account. Press **ENTER** to select Cross and Shield Insurance Plan as Mr. Dudley's primary coverage. Press **ENTER** again at both the Assignment and Secondary insurance fields to accept the default responses.

STEP 2   Key '**1053**' in the Voucher number field and press **ENTER**. The cursor will move to the Dr. # field. Press **ENTER** to accept the default doctor and supervisor for this patient, Dr. Sydney Carrington. Press **ENTER** twice to bypass the Department and Location fields.

STEP 3   Press **ENTER** to accept the current system date (01/10/03) as the date of the visit, and press **ENTER** to leave the second date field blank. Press **ENTER** at the Place of Service field to default to code 3 (for Doctor's Office).

Figure 3-11 Wayne Dudley's Encounter Form—Voucher 1053

Sydney Carrington & Associates P.A.
34 Sycamore Street   Suite 300
Madison, CA 95653

Date: 01/10/2003

Time: 11:00

Patient: Wayne Dudley
Guarantor: Wayne R. Dudley

Voucher No.: 1053

Patient No: 34.0
Doctor: 3 - S. Carrington

CPT	DESCRIPTION	FEE
OFFICE/HOSPITAL CONSULTS		
☐ 99201	Office New:Focused Hx-Exam	
☐ 99202	Office New:Expanded Hx-Exam	
☐ 99211	Office Estb:Min/None Hx-Exa	
☐ 99212	Office Estb:Focused Hx-Exam	
☐ 99213	Office Estb:Expanded Hx-Exa	
☐ 99214	Office Estb:Detailed Hx-Exa	
☒ 99215	Office Estb:Comprhn Hx-Exam	$85.00
☐ 99221	Hosp. Initial:Comprh Hx	
☐ 99223	Hosp.Ini:Comprh Hx-Exam/Hi	
☐ 99231	Hosp. Subsequent: S-Fwd	
☐ 99232	Hosp. Subsequent: Comprhn Hx	
☐ 99233	Hosp. Subsequent: Ex/Hi	
☐ 99238	Hospital Visit Discharge Ex	
☐ 99371	Telephone Consult - Simple	
☐ 99372	Telephone Consult - Intermed	
☐ 99373	Telephone Consult - Complex	
☐ 90843	Counseling - 25 minutes	
☐ 90844	Counseling - 50 minutes	
☐ 90865	Counseling - Special Interview	
IMMUNIZATIONS/INJECTIONS		
☐ 90585	BCG Vaccine	
☐ 90659	Influenza Virus Vaccine	
☐ 90701	Immunization-DTP	
☐ 90702	DT Vaccine	
☐ 90703	Tetanus Toxoids	
☐ 90732	Pneumococcal Vaccine	
☐ 90746	Hepatitis B Vaccine	
☐ 90749	Immunization; Unlisted	

CPT	DESCRIPTION	FEE
LABORATORY/RADIOLOGY		
☒ 81000	Urinalysis	$8.00
☐ 81002	Urinalysis; Pregnancy Test	
☐ 82951	Glucose Tolerance Test	
☐ 84478	Triglycerides	
☐ 84550	Uric Acid: Blood Chemistry	
☐ 84830	Ovulation Test	
☐ 85014	Hematocrit	
☐ 85031	Hemogram, Complete Blood Wk	
☐ 86403	Particle Agglutination Test	
☐ 86485	Skin Test; Candida	
☐ 86580	TB Intradermal Test	
☐ 86585	TB Tine Test	
☐ 87070	Culture	
☐ 70190	X-Ray; Optic Foramina	
☐ 70210	X-Ray Sinuses Complete	
☐ 71010	Radiological Exam Ent Spine	
☐ 71020	X-Ray Chest Pa & Lat	
☒ 72050	X-Ray Spine, Cerv (4 views)	$150.00
☐ 72090	X-Ray Spine; Scoliosis Ex	
☐ 72110	Spine, lumbosacral; a/p & Lat	
☐ 73030	Shoulder-Comp, min w/ 2vws	
☐ 73070	Elbow, anteropost & later vws	
☐ 73120	X-Ray; Hand, 2 views	
☐ 73560	X-Ray, Knee, 1 or 2 views	
☐ 74022	X-Ray; Abdomen, Complete	
☐ 75552	Cardiac Magnetic Res Img	
☐ 76020	X-Ray; Bone Age Studies	
☐ 76088	Mammary Ductogram Complete	
☐ 78465	Myocardial Perfusion Img	

CPT	DESCRIPTION	FEE
PROCEDURES/TESTS		
☐ 00452	Anesthesia for Rad Surgery	
☐ 11100	Skin Biopsy	
☐ 15852	Dressing Change	
☐ 29075	Cast Appl. - Lower Arm	
☐ 29530	Strapping of Knee	
☐ 29705	Removal/Revis of Cast w/Exa	
☐ 53670	Catheterization Incl. Suppl	
☐ 57452	Colposcopy	
☐ 57505	ECC	
☐ 69420	Myringotomy	
☐ 92081	Visual Field Examination	
☐ 92100	Serial Tonometry Exam	
☐ 92120	Tonography	
☐ 92552	Pure Tone Audiometry	
☐ 92567	Tympanometry	
☒ 93000	Electrocardiogram	$57.00
☐ 93015	Exercise Stress Test (ETT)	
☐ 93017	ETT Tracing Only	
☐ 93040	Electrocardiogram - Rhythm	
☐ 96100	Psychological Testing	
☐ 99000	Specimen Handling	
☐ 99058	Office Emergency Care	
☐ 99070	Surgical Tray - Misc.	
☐ 99080	Special Reports of Med Rec	
☐ 99195	Phlebotomy	
☐		
☐		
☐		

ICD-9	CODE DIAGNOSIS
☐ 009.0	Ill-defined Intestinal Infect
☐ 133.2	Establish Baseline
☐ 174.9	Breast Cancer
☐ 185.0	Prostate Cancer
☐ 250	Diabetes Mellitus
☐ 272.4	Hyperlipidemia
☐ 282.5	Anemia - Sickle Trait
☐ 282.60	Anemia - Sickle Cell
☐ 285.9	Anemia, Unspecified
☐ 300.4	Neurotic Depression
☐ 340	Multiple Sclerosis
☐ 342.9	Hemiplegia - Unspecified
☒ 346.9	Migraine Headache
☐ 352.9	Cranial Neuralgia
☐ 354.0	Carpal Tunnel Syndrome
☐ 355.0	Sciatic Nerve Root Lesion
☐ 366.9	Cataract
☐ 386.0	Vertigo
☐ 401.1	Essential Hypertension
☐ 414.9	Ischemic Hearth Disease
☐ 428.0	Congestive Heart Failure

ICD-9	CODE DIAGNOSIS
☐ 435.0	Basilar Artery Syndrome
☐ 440.0	Atherosclerosis
☐ 442.81	Carotid Artery
☐ 460.0	Common Cold
☐ 461.9	Acute Sinusitis
☐ 474.0	Tonsillitis
☐ 477.9	Hay Fever
☐ 487.0	Flu
☐ 496	Chronic Airway Obstruction
☐ 522	Low Red Blood Count
☐ 524.6	Temporo-Mandibular Jnt Synd
☐ 538.8	Stomach Pain
☐ 553.3	Hiatal Hernia
☐ 564.1	Spastic Colon
☐ 571.4	Chronic Hepatitis
☐ 571.5	Cirrhosis of Liver
☐ 573.3	Hepatitis
☐ 575.2	Obstruction of Gallbladder
☐ 648.2	Anemia - Compl. Pregnancy
☐ 715.90	Osteoarthritis - Unspec
☐ 721.3	Lumbar Osteo/Spondylarthrit

ICD-9	CODE DIAGNOSIS
☐ 724.2	Pain: Lower Back
☐ 727.6	Rupture of Achilles Tendon
☐ 780.1	Hallucinations
☐ 780.3	Convulsions
☐ 780.5	Sleep Disturbances
☐ 783.0	Anorexia
☐ 783.1	Abnormal Weight Gain
☐ 783.2	Abnormal Weight Loss
☐ 830.6	Dislocated Hip
☐ 830.9	Dislocated Shoulder
☐ 841.2	Sprained Wrist
☐ 842.5	Sprained Ankle
☐ 891.2	Fractured Tibia
☐ 892.0	Fractured Fibula
☐ 919.5	Insect Bite, Nonvenomous
☐ 921.1	Contus Eyelid/Perioc Area
☐ v16.3	Fam. Hist of Breast Cancer
☐ v17.4	Fam. Hist of Cardiovasc Dis
☐ v20.2	Well Child
☐ v22.0	Pregnancy - First Normal
☐ v22.1	Pregnancy - Normal

Previous Balance	Today's Charges	Total Due	Amount Paid	New Balance

Follow Up

PRN _____ Weeks _____   Months _____ Units _____

Next Appointment Date: _____   Time: _____

I hereby authorize release of any information acquired in the course of examination or treatment and allow a photocopy of my signature to be used.

STEP 4   Enter the first procedure code shown on Mr. Dudley's encounter form, '**99215**', and press **ENTER**. Then, press **ENTER** to bypass the Modifier field. Enter the diagnosis code shown at the bottom of the encounter form, '**346.9**', and press **ENTER**. Press **F1**

or click the PROCESS button ('√') on the top toolbar to process. Respond '**0**' at the Ailment Detail prompt as you did in previous exercises and press **ENTER**.

STEP 5
Enter the second through fourth procedure codes shown on Mr. Dudley's encounter form. Press **F1** or click the PROCESS button ('√') to process after each code is entered. This will also match each subsequently entered procedure code with the original diagnosis code (**346.9**). Remember that you will need to respond '**0**' at the Ailment Detail prompt for each additional procedure code entered.

After you post all information shown on Mr. Dudley's encounter form, carefully review to make sure you have entered the correct voucher number and that the proper doctor's number appears when you use the default. Compare your screen with Figure 3-12, then press **F1** or click the PROCESS button ('√') on the top toolbar to process.

Press **ESCAPE** twice or click twice on the EXIT button on the top toolbar to return to the Patient Retrieval screen and post charges for the next patient.

Figure 3-12 Posted Window for Wayne Dudley

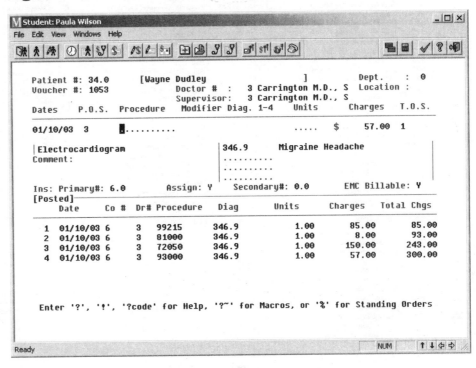

EXERCISE 5: Claire E. League

Posting Multiple Procedures with Different Diagnoses

In addition to multiple procedures, Ms. Claire League has multiple diagnoses (Figure 3-13). Key '**30.0**' at the Procedure Entry Patient Retrieval screen and press **ENTER** to retrieve Ms. League's account.

STEP 1
Use the keyboard or mouse to select the highlighted plan '**2.0**', Medicare, as Ms. League's primary insurance plan. Press **ENTER** to accept the default response at the Assignment field. Using the keyboard or mouse, choose plan '**10.0**', Medicare Plus, as her secondary coverage. Key '**1054**' in the Voucher Number field and press **ENTER**. Press **ENTER** to accept the default doctor and supervisor for this patient, Dr. James Monroe. Press **ENTER** again at the Department Location, both Dates fields, and the P.O.S. field.

Figure 3-13 Claire League's Encounter Form—Voucher 1054

Sydney Carrington & Associates P.A.
34 Sycamore Street Suite 300
Madison, CA 95653

Date: 01/10/2003

Time: 01:00

Patient: Claire League
Guarantor: Claire E. League

Voucher No.: 1054

Patient No: 30.0
Doctor: 1 - J. Monroe

CPT	DESCRIPTION	FEE
OFFICE/HOSPITAL CONSULTS		
☐ 99201	Office New:Focused Hx-Exam	____
☐ 99202	Office New:Expanded Hx-Exam	____
☐ 99211	Office Estb:Min/None Hx-Exa	____
☐ 99212	Office Estb:Focused Hx-Exam	____
☒ 99213	Office Estb:Expanded Hx-Exa	$40.00
☐ 99214	Office Estb:Detailed Hx-Exa	____
☐ 99215	Office Estb:Comprhn Hx-Exam	____
☐ 99221	Hosp. Initial:Comprh Hx-	____
☐ 99223	Hosp.Ini:Comprh Hx-Exam/Hi	____
☐ 99231	Hosp. Subsequent: S-Fwd	____
☐ 99232	Hosp. Subsequent: Comprhn Hx	____
☐ 99233	Hosp. Subsequent: Ex/Hi	____
☐ 99238	Hospital Visit Discharge Ex	____
☐ 99371	Telephone Consult - Simple	____
☐ 99372	Telephone Consult - Intermed	____
☐ 99373	Telephone Consult - Complex	____
☐ 90843	Counseling - 25 minutes	____
☐ 90844	Counseling - 50 minutes	____
☐ 90865	Counseling - Special Interview	____
IMMUNIZATIONS/INJECTIONS		
☐ 90585	BCG Vaccine	____
☐ 90659	Influenza Virus Vaccine	____
☐ 90701	Immunization-DTP	____
☐ 90702	DT Vaccine	____
☐ 90703	Tetanus Toxoids	____
☐ 90732	Pneumococcal Vaccine	____
☐ 90746	Hepatitis B Vaccine	____
☐ 90749	Immunization; Unlisted	____

CPT	DESCRIPTION	FEE
LABORATORY/RADIOLOGY		
☐ 81000	Urinalysis	____
☐ 81002	Urinalysis; Pregnancy Test	____
☐ 82951	Glucose Tolerance Test	____
☐ 84478	Triglycerides	____
☐ 84550	Uric Acid: Blood Chemistry	____
☐ 84830	Ovulation Test	____
☒ 85014	Hematocrit	$18.00
☐ 85031	Hemogram, Complete Blood Wk	____
☐ 86403	Particle Agglutination Test	____
☐ 86485	Skin Test; Candida	____
☐ 86580	TB Intradermal Test	____
☐ 86585	TB Tine Test	____
☐ 87070	Culture	____
☐ 70190	X-Ray; Optic Foramina	____
☐ 70210	X-Ray Sinuses Complete	____
☐ 71010	Radiological Exam Ent Spine	____
☐ 71020	X-Ray Chest Pa & Lat	____
☐ 72050	X-Ray Spine, Cerv (4 views)	____
☐ 72090	X-Ray Spine; Scoliosis Ex	____
☐ 72110	Spine, lumbosacral; a/p & Lat	____
☐ 73030	Shoulder-Comp, min w/ 2vws	____
☐ 73070	Elbow, anteropost & later vws	____
☐ 73120	X-Ray; Hand, 2 views	____
☐ 73560	X-Ray, Knee, 1 or 2 views	____
☐ 74022	X-Ray; Abdomen, Complete	____
☐ 75552	Cardiac Magnetic Res Img	____
☐ 76020	X-Ray; Bone Age Studies	____
☐ 76088	Mammary Ductogram Complete	____
☐ 78465	Myocardial Perfusion Img	____

CPT	DESCRIPTION	FEE
PROCEDURES/TESTS		
☐ 00452	Anesthesia for Rad Surgery	____
☐ 11100	Skin Biopsy	____
☐ 15852	Dressing Change	____
☐ 29075	Cast Appl. - Lower Arm	____
☐ 29530	Strapping of Knee	____
☐ 29705	Removal/Revis of Cast w/Exa	____
☐ 53670	Catheterization Incl. Suppl	____
☐ 57452	Colposcopy	____
☐ 57505	ECC	____
☐ 69420	Myringotomy	____
☐ 92081	Visual Field Examination	____
☐ 92100	Serial Tonometry Exam	____
☐ 92120	Tonography	____
☐ 92552	Pure Tone Audiometry	____
☐ 92567	Tympanometry	____
☐ 93000	Electrocardiogram	____
☐ 93015	Exercise Stress Test (ETT)	____
☐ 93017	ETT Tracing Only	____
☐ 93040	Electrocardiogram - Rhythm	____
☐ 96100	Psychological Testing	____
☐ 99000	Specimen Handling	____
☐ 99058	Office Emergency Care	____
☐ 99070	Surgical Tray - Misc.	____
☐ 99080	Special Reports of Med Rec	____
☐ 99195	Phlebotomy	____
☐	_____	____
☐	_____	____
☐	_____	____
☐	_____	____

ICD-9	CODE DIAGNOSIS
☐ 009.0	Ill-defined Intestinal Infect
☐ 133.2	Establish Baseline
☐ 174.9	Breast Cancer
☐ 185.0	Prostate Cancer
☐ 250	Diabetes Mellitus
☐ 272.4	Hyperlipidemia
☐ 282.5	Anemia - Sickle Trait
☐ 282.60	Anemia - Sickle Cell
☒ 285.9	Anemia, Unspecified
☐ 300.4	Neurotic Depression
☐ 340	Multiple Sclerosis
☐ 342.9	Hemiplegia - Unspecified
☐ 346.9	Migraine Headache
☐ 352.9	Cranial Neuralgia
☐ 354.0	Carpal Tunnel Syndrome
☐ 355.0	Sciatic Nerve Root Lesion
☐ 366.0	Cataract
☐ 386.0	Vertigo
☐ 401.1	Essential Hypertension
☐ 414.9	Ischemic Hearth Disease
☐ 428.0	Congestive Heart Failure

ICD-9	CODE DIAGNOSIS
☐ 435.0	Basilar Artery Syndrome
☐ 440.0	Atherosclerosis
☐ 442.81	Carotid Artery
☐ 460.0	Common Cold
☐ 461.9	Acute Sinusitis
☐ 474.0	Tonsillitis
☐ 477.9	Hay Fever
☐ 487.0	Flu
☐ 496	Chronic Airway Obstruction
☐ 522	Low Red Blood Count
☐ 524.6	Temporo-Mandibular Jnt Synd
☐ 538.8	Stomach Pain
☐ 553.3	Hiatal Hernia
☐ 564.1	Spastic Colon
☐ 571.4	Chronic Hepatitis
☒ 571.5	Cirrhosis of Liver
☐ 573.3	Hepatitis
☐ 575.2	Obstruction of Gallbladder
☐ 648.2	Anemia - Compl. Pregnancy
☐ 715.90	Osteoarthritis - Unspec
☐ 721.3	Lumbar Osteo/Spondylarthrit

ICD-9	CODE DIAGNOSIS
☐ 724.2	Pain: Lower Back
☐ 727.6	Rupture of Achilles Tendon
☐ 780.1	Hallucinations
☐ 780.3	Convulsions
☐ 780.5	Sleep Disturbances
☐ 783.0	Anorexia
☐ 783.1	Abnormal Weight Gain
☐ 783.2	Abnormal Weight Loss
☐ 830.6	Dislocated Hip
☐ 830.9	Dislocated Shoulder
☐ 841.2	Sprained Wrist
☐ 842.5	Sprained Ankle
☐ 891.2	Fractured Tibia
☐ 892.0	Fractured Fibula
☐ 919.5	Insect Bite, Nonvenomous
☐ 921.1	Contus Eyelid/Perioc Area
☐ v16.3	Fam. Hist of Breast Cancer
☐ v17.4	Fam. Hist of Cardiovasc Dis
☐ v20.2	Well Child
☐ v22.0	Pregnancy - First Normal
☐ v22.1	Pregnancy - Normal

Previous Balance	Today's Charges	Total Due	Amount Paid	New Balance
_____	_____	_____	_____	_____

Follow Up

PRN _____ Weeks _____ Months _____ Units _____

Next Appointment Date: _____   Time: _____

I hereby authorize release of any information acquired in the course of examination or treatment and allow a photocopy of my signature to be used.

_____

_____

STEP 2   Post the first procedure code, '**99213**', and match it with the diagnosis code, '**285.9**', by pressing **F1** or clicking on the PROCESS button ('√') on the top toolbar. Respond '**0**' at the Ailment Detail prompt as you did previous exercises.

STEP 3

Key the second procedure code, '**85014**'; then press **ENTER** or use the down arrow until the cursor is over the diagnosis code. Using the mouse, you may also move the mouse pointer to the diagnosis code field and click to move the cursor. Because **The Medical Manager** software is in typeover mode, key in '**571.5**' over the first diagnosis code, and press **ENTER**. This diagnosis code will automatically match with the second procedure code you entered.

Compare your screen with Figure 3-14, then press **F1** or click on the PROCESS button ('√') on the top toolbar to process. Respond '**0**' again at the Ailment Detail prompt as you did when you posted the first procedure code and press **ENTER**.

> **TIP:** Do not proceed further in this unit until you understand how to locate procedure and diagnosis codes marked by the doctor and to post them correctly in the proper sequence. If you need help ask your instructor.

Figure 3-14 Posted Window for Claire League

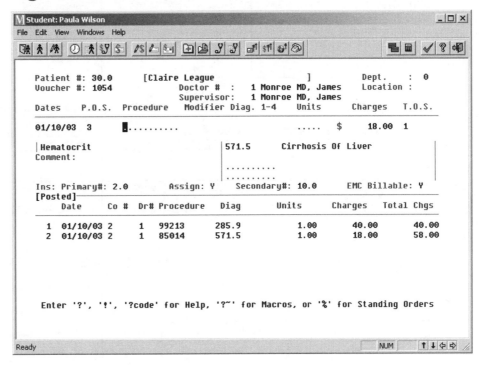

POSTING AILMENT DETAILS

Ailment Detail gives information about an illness.

Insurance claim forms are very detailed because insurance carriers must have enough information to make sound decisions about whether to pay claims and, if so, what fees to pay. Although much of the information needed for patient claim forms is entered at the time the patient is added to the system, additional information may be required depending on the reason for the visit.

Ailment Detail

A function called *Ailment Detail* allows you to complete the more detailed sections of a claim form. Ailment Detail is the basic information about an incident, illness, or accident. For a better understanding of how Ailment Detail will be used, compare the questions on the Ailment Detail screen (shown later in Figure 3-18) with the middle portion of the CMS-1500 insurance claim form shown in Figure 3-15. You will notice

Figure 3-15 Health Insurance Claim Form Showing Ailment Detail Fields

PLEASE
DO NOT
STAPLE
IN THIS
AREA

CARRIER

| | PICA | | **HEALTH INSURANCE CLAIM FORM** | PICA | |

1. MEDICARE   MEDICAID   CHAMPUS   CHAMPVA   GROUP HEALTH PLAN   FECA BLK LUNG   OTHER
(Medicare #) (Medicaid #) (Sponsor's SSN) (VA File #) (SSN or ID) (SSN) (ID)

1a. INSURED'S I.D. NUMBER   (FOR PROGRAM IN ITEM 1)

2. PATIENT'S NAME (Last Name, First Name, Middle Initial)

3. PATIENT'S BIRTH DATE   MM   DD   YY   SEX   M   F

4. INSURED'S NAME (Last Name, First Name, Middle Initial)

5. PATIENT'S ADDRESS (No., Street)

6. PATIENT RELATIONSHIP TO INSURED   Self   Spouse   Child   Other

7. INSURED'S ADDRESS (No., Street)

CITY   STATE

8. PATIENT STATUS   Single   Married   Other
Employed   Full-Time Student   Part-Time Student

CITY   STATE

ZIP CODE   TELEPHONE (Include Area Code)   (   )

ZIP CODE   TELEPHONE (INCLUDE AREA CODE)   (   )

9. OTHER INSURED'S NAME (Last Name, First Name, Middle Initial)

10. IS PATIENT'S CONDITION RELATED TO:

11. INSURED'S POLICY GROUP OR FECA NUMBER

a. OTHER INSURED'S POLICY OR GROUP NUMBER

a. EMPLOYMENT? (CURRENT OR PREVIOUS)   YES   NO

a. INSURED'S DATE OF BIRTH   MM   DD   YY   SEX   M   F

b. OTHER INSURED'S DATE OF BIRTH   MM   DD   YY   SEX   M   F

b. AUTO ACCIDENT?   PLACE (State)   YES   NO

b. EMPLOYER'S NAME OR SCHOOL NAME

c. EMPLOYER'S NAME OR SCHOOL NAME

c. OTHER ACCIDENT?   YES   NO

c. INSURANCE PLAN NAME OR PROGRAM NAME

d. INSURANCE PLAN NAME OR PROGRAM NAME

10d. RESERVED FOR LOCAL USE

d. IS THERE ANOTHER HEALTH BENEFIT PLAN?   YES   NO   If yes, return to and complete item 9 a-d.

READ BACK OF FORM BEFORE COMPLETING & SIGNING THIS FORM.
12. PATIENT'S OR AUTHORIZED PERSON'S SIGNATURE I authorize the release of any medical or other information necessary to process this claim. I also request payment of government benefits either to myself or to the party who accepts assignment below.

SIGNED _____   DATE _____

13. INSURED'S OR AUTHORIZED PERSON'S SIGNATURE I authorize payment of medical benefits to the undersigned physician or supplier for services described below.

SIGNED _____

14. DATE OF CURRENT: MM   DD   YY   ILLNESS (First symptom) OR INJURY (Accident) OR PREGNANCY(LMP)

15. IF PATIENT HAS HAD SAME OR SIMILAR ILLNESS. GIVE FIRST DATE   MM   DD   YY

16. DATES PATIENT UNABLE TO WORK IN CURRENT OCCUPATION   FROM   MM   DD   YY   TO   MM   DD   YY

17. NAME OF REFERRING PHYSICIAN OR OTHER SOURCE

17a. I.D. NUMBER OF REFERRING PHYSICIAN

18. HOSPITALIZATION DATES RELATED TO CURRENT SERVICES   FROM   MM   DD   YY   TO   MM   DD   YY

19. RESERVED FOR LOCAL USE

20. OUTSIDE LAB?   YES   NO $ CHARGES

21. DIAGNOSIS OR NATURE OF ILLNESS OR INJURY. (RELATE ITEMS 1,2,3 OR 4 TO ITEM 24E BY LINE)

1. L___ . ___   3. L___ . ___
2. L___ . ___   4. L___ . ___

22. MEDICAID RESUBMISSION CODE   ORIGINAL REF. NO.

23. PRIOR AUTHORIZATION NUMBER

24. A DATE(S) OF SERVICE From MM DD YY To MM DD YY	B Place of Service	C Type of Service	D PROCEDURES, SERVICES, OR SUPPLIES (Explain Unusual Circumstances) CPT/HCPCS MODIFIER	E DIAGNOSIS CODE	F $ CHARGES	G DAYS OR UNITS	H EPSDT Family Plan	I EMG	J COB	K RESERVED FOR LOCAL USE
1										
2										
3										
4										
5										
6										

25. FEDERAL TAX I.D. NUMBER   SSN   EIN

26. PATIENT'S ACCOUNT NO.

27. ACCEPT ASSIGNMENT? (For govt. claims, see back)   YES   NO

28. TOTAL CHARGE $

29. AMOUNT PAID $

30. BALANCE DUE $

31. SIGNATURE OF PHYSICIAN OR SUPPLIER INCLUDING DEGREES OR CREDENTIALS (I certify that the statements on the reverse apply to this bill and are made a part thereof.)

SIGNED _____   DATE _____

32. NAME AND ADDRESS OF FACILITY WHERE SERVICES WERE RENDERED (If other than home or office)

33. PHYSICIAN'S, SUPPLIER'S BILLING NAME, ADDRESS, ZIP CODE & PHONE #

PIN#   GRP#

(APPROVED BY AMA COUNCIL ON MEDICAL SERVICE 8/88)   **PLEASE PRINT OR TYPE**   APPROVED OMB-0938-0008 FORM HCFA-1500 (12-90),   FORM RRB-1500,
APPROVED OMB-1215-0055 FORM OWCP-1500,   APPROVED OMB-0720-0001 (CHAMPUS)

PATIENT AND INSURED INFORMATION

PHYSICIAN OR SUPPLIER INFORMATION

that the information requested in boxes 10, 14, 15, 16, 17, 18, 19, 20, 22, and 23 is the same information gathered from the Ailment Detail screen. Some examples of this information include whether the patient's condition is related or not to the patient's employment, an accident, an auto accident, or other; specific details of the current illness; and so on.

Figure 3-16 Timothy Davis' Encounter Form—Voucher 1055

Sydney Carrington & Associates P.A.
34 Sycamore Street Suite 300
Madison, CA 95653

Date: 01/10/2003

Voucher No.: 1055

Time: 10:00

Patient: Timothy Davis
Guarantor: Timothy R. Davis

Patient No: 80.0
Doctor: 2 - F. Simpson

CPT	DESCRIPTION	FEE
OFFICE/HOSPITAL CONSULTS		
☐ 99201	Office New:Focused Hx-Exam	
☐ 99202	Office New:Expanded Hx-Exam	
☐ 99211	Office Estb:Min/None Hx-Exa	
☐ 99212	Office Estb:Focused Hx-Exam	
☒ 99213	Office Estb:Expanded Hx-Exa	$40.00
☐ 99214	Office Estb:Detailed Hx-Exa	
☐ 99215	Office Estb:Comprhn Hx-Exam	
☐ 99221	Hosp. Initial:Comprh Hx-	
☐ 99223	Hosp.Ini:Comprh Hx-Exam/Hi	
☐ 99231	Hosp. Subsequent: S-Fwd	
☐ 99232	Hosp. Subsequent: Comprhn Hx	
☐ 99233	Hosp. Subsequent: Ex/Hi	
☐ 99238	Hospital Visit Discharge Ex	
☐ 99371	Telephone Consult - Simple	
☐ 99372	Telephone Consult - Intermed	
☐ 99373	Telephone Consult - Complex	
☐ 90843	Counseling - 25 minutes	
☐ 90844	Counseling - 50 minutes	
☐ 90865	Counseling - Special Interview	
IMMUNIZATIONS/INJECTIONS		
☐ 90585	BCG Vaccine	
☐ 90659	Influenza Virus Vaccine	
☐ 90701	Immunization-DTP	
☐ 90702	DT Vaccine	
☐ 90703	Tetanus Toxoids	
☐ 90732	Pneumococcal Vaccine	
☐ 90746	Hepatitis B Vaccine	
☐ 90749	Immunization; Unlisted	

CPT	DESCRIPTION	FEE
LABORATORY/RADIOLOGY		
☐ 81000	Urinalysis	
☐ 81002	Urinalysis; Pregnancy Test	
☐ 82951	Glucose Tolerance Test	
☐ 84478	Triglycerides	
☐ 84550	Uric Acid: Blood Chemistry	
☐ 84830	Ovulation Test	
☐ 85014	Hematocrit	
☐ 85031	Hemogram, Complete Blood Wk	
☐ 86403	Particle Agglutination Test	
☐ 86485	Skin Test; Candida	
☐ 86580	TB Intradermal Test	
☐ 86585	TB Tine Test	
☐ 87070	Culture	
☐ 70190	X-Ray; Optic Foramina	
☐ 70210	X-Ray Sinuses Complete	
☐ 71010	Radiological Exam Ent Spine	
☐ 71020	X-Ray Chest Pa & Lat	
☐ 72050	X-Ray Spine, Cerv (4 views)	
☐ 72090	X-Ray Spine; Scoliosis Ex	
☐ 72110	Spine, lumbosacral; a/p & Lat	
☐ 73030	Shoulder-Comp, min w/ 2vws	
☐ 73070	Elbow, anteropost & later vws	
☐ 73120	X-Ray; Hand, 2 views	
☐ 73560	X-Ray, Knee, 1 or 2 views	
☐ 74022	X-Ray; Abdomen, Complete	
☐ 75552	Cardiac Magnetic Res Img	
☐ 76020	X-Ray; Bone Age Studies	
☐ 76088	Mammary Ductogram Complete	
☐ 78465	Myocardial Perfusion Img	

CPT	DESCRIPTION	FEE
PROCEDURES/TESTS		
☐ 00452	Anesthesia for Rad Surgery	
☐ 11100	Skin Biopsy	
☐ 15852	Dressing Change	
☒ 29075	Cast Appl. - Lower Arm	$48.00
☐ 29530	Strapping of Knee	
☐ 29705	Removal/Revis of Cast w/Exa	
☐ 53670	Catheterization Incl. Suppl	
☐ 57452	Colposcopy	
☐ 57505	ECC	
☐ 69420	Myringotomy	
☐ 92081	Visual Field Examination	
☐ 92100	Serial Tonometry Exam	
☐ 92120	Tonography	
☐ 92552	Pure Tone Audiometry	
☐ 92567	Tympanometry	
☐ 93000	Electrocardiogram	
☐ 93015	Exercise Stress Test (ETT)	
☐ 93017	ETT Tracing Only	
☐ 93040	Electrocardiogram - Rhythm	
☐ 96100	Psychological Testing	
☐ 99000	Specimen Handling	
☐ 99058	Office Emergency Care	
☐ 99070	Surgical Tray - Misc.	
☐ 99080	Special Reports of Med Rec	
☐ 99195	Phlebotomy	
☐		
☐		
☐		
☐		

ICD-9	CODE DIAGNOSIS
☐ 009.0	Ill-defined Intestinal Infect
☐ 133.2	Establish Baseline
☐ 174.9	Breast Cancer
☐ 185.0	Prostate Cancer
☐ 250	Diabetes Mellitus
☐ 272.4	Hyperlipidemia
☐ 282.5	Anemia - Sickle Trait
☐ 282.60	Anemia - Sickle Cell
☐ 285.9	Anemia, Unspecified
☐ 300.4	Neurotic Depression
☐ 340	Multiple Sclerosis
☐ 342.9	Hemiplegia - Unspecified
☐ 346.9	Migraine Headache
☐ 352.9	Cranial Neuralgia
☐ 354.0	Carpal Tunnel Syndrome
☐ 355.5	Sciatic Nerve Root Lesion
☐ 366.9	Cataract
☐ 386.0	Vertigo
☐ 401.1	Essential Hypertension
☐ 414.9	Ischemic Hearth Disease
☐ 428.0	Congestive Heart Failure

ICD-9	CODE DIAGNOSIS
☐ 435.0	Basilar Artery Syndrome
☐ 440.0	Atherosclerosis
☐ 442.81	Carotid Artery
☐ 460.0	Common Cold
☐ 461.9	Acute Sinusitis
☐ 474.0	Tonsillitis
☐ 477.9	Hay Fever
☐ 487.0	Flu
☐ 496	Chronic Airway Obstruction
☐ 522	Low Red Blood Count
☐ 524.6	Temporo-Mandibular Jnt Synd
☐ 538.8	Stomach Pain
☐ 553.3	Hiatal Hernia
☐ 564.1	Spastic Colon
☐ 571.4	Chronic Hepatitis
☐ 571.5	Cirrhosis of Liver
☐ 573.3	Hepatitis
☐ 575.2	Obstruction of Gallbladder
☐ 648.2	Anemia - Compl. Pregnancy
☐ 715.90	Osteoarthritis - Unspec
☐ 721.3	Lumbar Osteo/Spondylarthrit

ICD-9	CODE DIAGNOSIS
☐ 724.2	Pain: Lower Back
☐ 727.6	Rupture of Achilles Tendon
☐ 780.1	Hallucinations
☐ 780.3	Convulsions
☐ 780.5	Sleep Disturbances
☐ 783.0	Anorexia
☐ 783.1	Abnormal Weight Gain
☐ 783.2	Abnormal Weight Loss
☐ 830.6	Dislocated Hip
☐ 830.9	Dislocated Shoulder
☒ 841.2	Sprained Wrist
☐ 842.5	Sprained Ankle
☐ 891.2	Fractured Tibia
☐ 892.0	Fractured Fibula
☐ 919.5	Insect Bite, Nonvenomous
☐ 921.1	Contus Eyelid/Perioc Area
☐ v16.3	Fam. Hist of Breast Cancer
☐ v17.4	Fam. Hist of Cardiovasc Dis
☐ v20.2	Well Child
☐ v22.0	Pregnancy - First Normal
☐ v22.1	Pregnancy - Normal

Previous Balance	Today's Charges	Total Due	Amount Paid	New Balance

Follow Up

PRN _____ Weeks _____ Months _____ Units _____

Next Appointment Date: _____ Time: _____

I hereby authorize release of any information acquired in the course of examination or treatment and allow a photocopy of my signature to be used.

How to Use Ailment Detail

If a patient is seen several times for different conditions, multiple ailment records can be created. Some of the reasons for creating a new Ailment Detail record are:

1. A new ailment condition for the patient.

2. A move to a different hospital or different hospital dates than shown on a previous Ailment Detail record.

3. Outside laboratory work done at a different laboratory.

4. Any condition in which the detail would require overwriting the detail held on a previous ailment record.

Ailment Detail is generally used for all insurance responsible charges and can be selected or created during Procedure Entry.

STEP 1

From the Main Menu (Menu 1), select option **2**, PROCEDURE Entry. Retrieve the account for Mr. Timothy Davis. Mr. Davis visited the doctor today for treatment of a sprained wrist he received at work. Because this was an on-the-job injury, he will file a claim with his company's Worker's Compensation insurer. Therefore, Ailment Detail is needed. Information for the Ailment Detail will be taken from his encounter form, shown in Figure 3-16.

Using the keyboard or mouse, post both the procedure code ('**99213**') and diagnosis code ('**841.2**') from the encounter form, then press **F1** or click on the PROCESS button ('√') on the top toolbar to process the information. Compare your screen with Figure 3-17.

STEP 2

When you are prompted for Ailment Detail, select option (**A**)dd to allow the system to create a new Ailment Detail for Mr. Davis. Then, press **ENTER** to accept the default of (**N**)ormal billing, and key in the following information. Press **ENTER** to bypass any other field not listed below. Note that the Ailment Detail screen is different from most of **The Medical Manager** system screens in that it may be processed at any time without completing all of the fields. Therefore, you need to enter only the relevant information before processing.

◆ a. Hold Claim: (**N**)o
   This field allows insurance billing to be held for all items associated with the ailment. In this case it is not desired to hold insurance billing. Press **ENTER** to default the field to '**N**'.

◆ b. Date First Consulted: (Press **ENTER** to accept default date of 01/10/03)
   Enter the date when the physician is first consulted by the patient regarding the particular condition for this ailment. Press **ENTER** to accept the default of today's date.

◆ c. Facility #: '**0**'
   If a procedure is performed at a facility other than the physician's office the information is recorded in Ailment by entering the service facility number. A Service Facility Help window is available. Press **ENTER** to default to "**0**" No, indicating that an outside facility was not used.

Figure 3-17 First Procedure, Add Ailment Screen

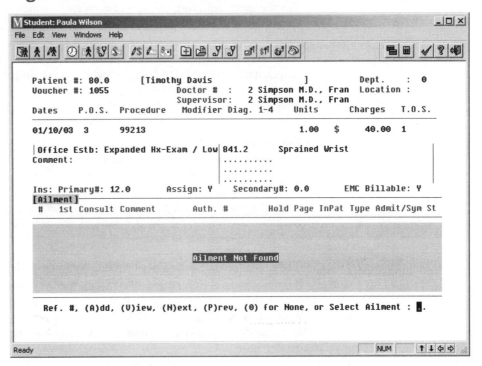

♦ d. Comment Field: **wc wrist**
   Key information useful to identifying this ailment. Formerly, this comment would not appear on insurance forms; it is generally used in the Ailment Help window to aid the user in associating procedures with the proper ailment. Press **ENTER**.

   Prior Authorization #: (Press **ENTER** to leave blank)

   If an insurance plan has issued a prior authorization or an authorized referral, a special authorization number is often assigned to it.

♦ e. Inpatient: (**N**)o
   If a service facility was indicated above and the patient was admitted to the above facility as an inpatient enter '**Yes**', otherwise press **ENTER** to default to 'No'.

♦ f. Specialty:
   This field is used to override the performing doctor's default specialty code. If a specialty is entered in this field, it will be reported on any claims associated with this ailment and in place of the performing doctor's specialty code. This field is not entered in the Student Edition.

♦ g. Ref. Doctor #: **4** (Jason Detrasnick)
   Key the number of the doctor who referred the patient or press **ENTER** to accept the patient's default referring doctor.

♦ h. Related to Employment: (**Y**)es
   If the condition is related to the patient's employment, key '**Y**' and press **ENTER**. If not, type '**N**' and press **ENTER**.

◆ i. Accident: (**W**)ork
Key the letter indicating the type of accident to which the condition is related. Valid entries are as follows: (**A**)uto, (**H**)ome, (**W**)ork, (**O**)ther, (**N**)one.

TIP: Ailment Help messages appear at the bottom of the screen and change as you move from field to field. In this case the Help message indicates that you may also enter (**W**)ork or (**H**)ome even though the accident field lists (**A**)uto, (**O**)ther and (**N**)one.

◆ j. Old Symptoms: (**N**)o
This contains a code describing the patient's symptoms. This field could contain a two-letter code describing the patient's symptoms and type of symptom. Valid entries for the first character are '**Y**' if it is an old symptom and '**N**' if it is a new symptom. Valid entries for the second character are (**I**)llness, (**P**)regnancy, (**A**)ccident. Example: If this were an old symptom related to a previous accident, the entry would be '**YA**'. If this is a new symptom due to an illness the entry would be '**NI**'.

TIP: Similar to the Accident field, additional instructions are provided in the help message which appears at the bottom of the screen.

◆ k. Emergency: **N**
If this was an emergency situation key '**Y**' and press **ENTER**. If not, key '**N**'.

◆ l. Date of First Symptom: **01102003**
The date the first symptoms were noted by the patient.

◆ m. Date Resumed Work: **01112003**
This is the date the patient resumed working regular employment.

◆ n. Special: (Press **ENTER** to leave blank)
Any special information that we require but which is unavailable from any other field.

◆ o. Date Disability (Partial)–From: **01102003** To: Press **ENTER** to leave blank

If the patient was partially disabled, type the beginning date of the patient's disability. If the patient has returned to regular work, type the ending date of the patient's disability. In this case type **01102003** in the From date and press **ENTER** to leave the "TO" date field blank.

◆ p. Date of Total Disability: (Press **ENTER** to leave blank in both fields)
If the patient was or is totally disabled, type the beginning and ending dates of total disability.

◆ q. Date of Similar Illness: (Press **ENTER** to leave blank)
If the patient was previously ill with a similar type ailment, type the beginning and ending dates of the similar illness.

◆ r. Dates of Hospitalization: (Press **ENTER** to leave blank in both fields)
If the patient was hospitalized type the beginning and ending dates of hospitalization.

TIP: If the dates of hospitalization are completed, the inpatient field should say 'yes' and the service facility should have a valid entry.

◆ s. Outside Laboratory: (Press **ENTER** to leave blank)
Outside laboratory refers to "purchase diagnostic tests". If the practice purchases diagnostic tests from an outside laboratory and then charges the patient for the test, this and

the following two fields must be completed. If the practice orders laboratory tests from an outside laboratory that directly bills the patient or the insurance, then these fields are not completed.

◆   t.   Laboratory Charges: (Press **ENTER** to leave blank)
If the practice purchased tests from an outside laboratory, it enters the actual cost to the practice for the laboratory tests.

◆   u.   Laboratory Facility #: (Press **ENTER** to leave blank)
If the practice purchased diagnostic tests from an outside laboratory enter the facility number of the laboratory.

◆   v.   ESPDT: (Press **ENTER** to leave blank)
ESPDT is early and periodic screen for diagnostics and treatment of children. If services on this visit were done under the auspices of the ESPDT Program enter **Yes**. Otherwise press **ENTER** to leave blank.

◆   w.   Family Planning: (Press **ENTER** to leave blank)
If family planning services are involved enter '**Yes**'. Otherwise press **ENTER** to leave blank.

The physician will inform Mr. Davis's employer that although he may be unable to perform his regular duties, he can do supervisory work. He may return to work the next day but should be considered partially disabled until his cast is removed. He can resume his regular duties after the cast is removed. Compare your screen with Figure 3-18, then press **F1** or click on the PROCESS button ('√') on the top toolbar.

Figure 3-18 Enter Ailment Detail Screen

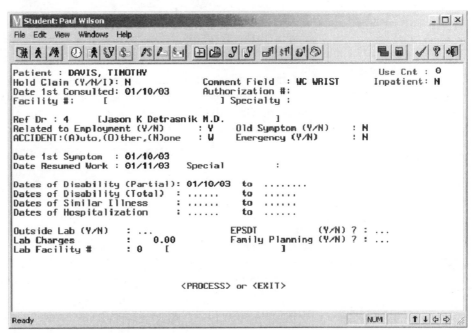

STEP 3   After the screen is processed, the Procedure Code field will clear and be ready for a new procedure code. Enter the second code for the application of a cast to hold the sprain in place. From the patient's encounter form, you will see that the procedure code for cast

Figure 3-19 Post Second Charge Screen

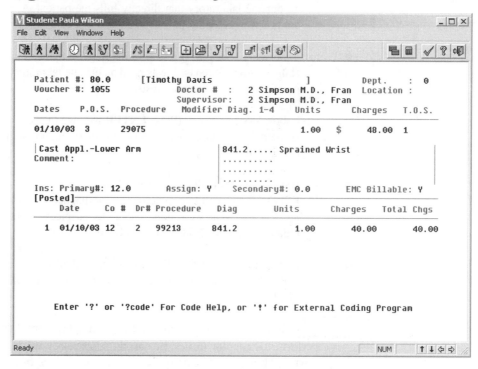

is '**29075**'. Compare your screen with Figure 3-19. After you process the data and are asked for Ailment Detail, you may select (**S**)ame to represent the same ailment as for the previous charge. This concludes Mr. Davis's record. Press **ESCAPE** twice or click twice on the EXIT button on the top toolbar.

APPLYING YOUR KNOWLEDGE

Encounter forms for three patients are provided on the following pages. Review each encounter form carefully; then post the Ailment Detail, when applicable, for each person as you did in the preceding example.

EXERCISE 6: Patricia G. Evans

Posting a Visit and an Ailment

Ms. Patricia Evans has a serious illness (breast cancer) that will likely require hospitalization; therefore, an Ailment Detail should be created at this time. Often, the first time a patient is seen is the best time to determine the date of the first symptom and the date of first consultation, both of which are part of the Ailment Detail. Referring to Ms. Evans's encounter form (Figure 3-20), post the charges for her visit and add Ailment Detail.

STEP 1 When you choose the PROCEDURE Entry option (option **2**) from the Main Menu (Menu 1) and are presented with the Patient Retrieval screen, you will enter the last name '**?Evans**'. Because more than one patient has the last name Evans, **The Medical Manager** software will present a list of names from which you can choose. Use the up/down arrow keys to select Patricia Evans, then press **ENTER**. Using the mouse, you may also double-click on Ms. Evans to highlight and select her account. You will then be presented with some demographic information about the patient and the patient's dependents. Using the keyboard or the mouse, choose the patient for whom you want to post charges.

Figure 3-20 Patricia Evans's Encounter Form—Voucher 1056

Sydney Carrington & Associates P.A.
34 Sycamore Street   Suite 300
Madison, CA 95653

Date: 01/10/2003   Voucher No.: 1056

Time: 02:00

Patient: Patricia Evans   Patient No: 110.0
Guarantor: Patricia G. Evans   Doctor: 3 - S. Carrington

CPT	DESCRIPTION	FEE
OFFICE/HOSPITAL CONSULTS		
☐ 99201	Office New:Focused Hx-Exam	
☐ 99202	Office New:Expanded Hx-Exam	
☐ 99211	Office Estb:Min/None Hx-Exa	
☐ 99212	Office Estb:Focused Hx-Exam	
☐ 99213	Office Estb:Expanded Hx-Exa	
☒ 99214	Office Estb:Detailed Hx-Exa	$50.00
☐ 99215	Office Estb:Comprhn Hx-Exam	
☐ 99221	Hosp. Initial:Comprh Hx-	
☐ 99223	Hosp.Ini:Comprh Hx-Exam/Hi	
☐ 99231	Hosp. Subsequent: S-Fwd	
☐ 99232	Hosp. Subsequent: Comprhn Hx	
☐ 99233	Hosp. Subsequent: Ex/Hi	
☐ 99238	Hospital Visit Discharge Ex	
☐ 99371	Telephone Consult - Simple	
☐ 99372	Telephone Consult - Intermed	
☐ 99373	Telephone Consult - Complex	
☐ 90843	Counseling - 25 minutes	
☐ 90844	Counseling - 50 minutes	
☐ 90865	Counseling - Special Interview	
IMMUNIZATIONS/INJECTIONS		
☐ 90585	BCG Vaccine	
☐ 90659	Influenza Virus Vaccine	
☐ 90701	Immunization-DTP	
☐ 90702	DT Vaccine	
☐ 90703	Tetanus Toxoids	
☐ 90732	Pneumococcal Vaccine	
☐ 90746	Hepatitis B Vaccine	
☐ 90749	Immunization; Unlisted	

CPT	DESCRIPTION	FEE
LABORATORY/RADIOLOGY		
☐ 81000	Urinalysis	
☐ 81002	Urinalysis; Pregnancy Test	
☐ 82951	Glucose Tolerance Test	
☐ 84478	Triglycerides	
☐ 84550	Uric Acid: Blood Chemistry	
☐ 84830	Ovulation Test	
☐ 85014	Hematocrit	
☐ 85031	Hemogram, Complete Blood Wk	
☐ 86403	Particle Agglutination Test	
☐ 86485	Skin Test; Candida	
☐ 86580	TB Intradermal Test	
☐ 86585	TB Tine Test	
☐ 87070	Culture	
☐ 70190	X-Ray; Optic Foramina	
☐ 70210	X-Ray Sinuses Complete	
☐ 71010	Radiological Exam Ent Spine	
☒ 71020	X-Ray Chest Pa & Lat	$58.00
☐ 72050	X-Ray Spine, Cerv (4 views)	
☐ 72090	X-Ray Spine; Scoliosis Ex	
☐ 72110	Spine, lumbosacral; a/p & Lat	
☐ 73030	Shoulder-Comp, min w/ 2vws	
☐ 73070	Elbow, anteropost & later vws	
☐ 73120	X-Ray; Hand, 2 views	
☐ 73560	X-Ray, Knee, 1 or 2 views	
☐ 74022	X-Ray; Abdomen, Complete	
☐ 75552	Cardiac Magnetic Res Img	
☐ 76020	X-Ray; Bone Age Studies	
☒ 76088	Mammary Ductogram Complete	$125.00
☐ 78465	Myocardial Perfusion Img	

CPT	DESCRIPTION	FEE
PROCEDURES/TESTS		
☐ 00452	Anesthesia for Rad Surgery	
☐ 11100	Skin Biopsy	
☐ 15852	Dressing Change	
☐ 29075	Cast Appl. - Lower Arm	
☐ 29530	Strapping of Knee	
☐ 29705	Removal/Revis of Cast w/Exa	
☐ 53670	Catheterization Incl. Suppl	
☐ 57452	Colposcopy	
☐ 57505	ECC	
☐ 69420	Myringotomy	
☐ 92081	Visual Field Examination	
☐ 92100	Serial Tonometry Exam	
☐ 92120	Tonography	
☐ 92552	Pure Tone Audiometry	
☐ 92567	Tympanometry	
☐ 93000	Electrocardiogram	
☐ 93015	Exercise Stress Test (ETT)	
☐ 93017	ETT Tracing Only	
☐ 93040	Electrocardiogram - Rhythm	
☐ 96100	Psychological Testing	
☐ 99000	Specimen Handling	
☐ 99058	Office Emergency Care	
☐ 99070	Surgical Tray - Misc.	
☐ 99080	Special Reports of Med Rec	
☐ 99195	Phlebotomy	
☐		
☐		
☐		

ICD-9	CODE DIAGNOSIS
☐ 009.0	Ill-defined Intestinal Infect
☐ 133.2	Establish Baseline
☒ 174.9	Breast Cancer
☐ 185.0	Prostate Cancer
☐ 250	Diabetes Mellitus
☐ 272.4	Hyperlipidemia
☐ 282.5	Anemia - Sickle Trait
☐ 282.60	Anemia - Sickle Cell
☐ 285.9	Anemia, Unspecified
☐ 300.4	Neurotic Depression
☐ 340	Multiple Sclerosis
☐ 342.9	Hemiplegia - Unspecified
☐ 346.9	Migraine Headache
☐ 352.9	Cranial Neuralgia
☐ 354.0	Carpal Tunnel Syndrome
☐ 355.0	Sciatic Nerve Root Lesion
☐ 366.9	Cataract
☐ 386.0	Vertigo
☐ 401.1	Essential Hypertension
☐ 414.9	Ischemic Hearth Disease
☐ 428.0	Congestive Heart Failure

ICD-9	CODE DIAGNOSIS
☐ 435.0	Basilar Artery Syndrome
☐ 440.0	Atherosclerosis
☐ 442.81	Carotid Artery
☐ 460.0	Common Cold
☐ 461.9	Acute Sinusitis
☐ 474.0	Tonsillitis
☐ 477.9	Hay Fever
☐ 487.0	Flu
☐ 496	Chronic Airway Obstruction
☐ 522	Low Red Blood Count
☐ 524.6	Temporo-Mandibular Jnt Synd
☐ 538.8	Stomach Pain
☐ 553.3	Hiatal Hernia
☐ 564.1	Spastic Colon
☐ 571.4	Chronic Hepatitis
☐ 571.5	Cirrhosis of Liver
☐ 573.3	Hepatitis
☐ 575.2	Obstruction of Gallbladder
☐ 648.2	Anemia - Compl. Pregnancy
☐ 715.90	Osteoarthritis - Unspec
☐ 721.3	Lumbar Osteo/Spondylarthrit

ICD-9	CODE DIAGNOSIS
☐ 724.2	Pain: Lower Back
☐ 727.6	Rupture of Achilles Tendon
☐ 780.1	Hallucinations
☐ 780.3	Convulsions
☐ 780.5	Sleep Disturbances
☐ 783.0	Anorexia
☐ 783.1	Abnormal Weight Gain
☐ 783.2	Abnormal Weight Loss
☐ 830.6	Dislocated Hip
☐ 830.9	Dislocated Shoulder
☐ 841.2	Sprained Wrist
☐ 842.5	Sprained Ankle
☐ 891.2	Fractured Tibia
☐ 892.0	Fractured Fibula
☐ 919.5	Insect Bite, Nonvenomous
☐ 921.1	Contus Eyelid/Perioc Area
☐ v16.3	Fam. Hist of Breast Cancer
☐ v17.4	Fam. Hist of Cardiovasc Dis
☐ v20.2	Well Child
☐ v22.0	Pregnancy - First Normal
☐ v22.1	Pregnancy - Normal

Previous Balance	Today's Charges	Total Due	Amount Paid	New Balance

Follow Up

PRN _____ Weeks _____ Months _____ Units _____

Next Appointment Date: _____   Time: _____

I hereby authorize release of any information acquired in the course of examination or treatment and allow a photocopy of my signature to be used.

STEP 2 Once you have located Ms. Evans's account, press **ENTER** to select Epsilon Life and Casualty as her primary insurance coverage. Press **ENTER** again at both the Assignment and Secondary Insurance fields to accept the default responses for each of these fields. Key '**1056**' in the Voucher Number field and press **ENTER**. The cursor will move to the

Doctor Number field. Press **ENTER** to accept the default doctor for this patient, Dr. Carrington. Press **ENTER** twice to bypass the Department and Location fields. Press **ENTER** at both of the Date fields to accept the default response for each. Press **ENTER** again at the Place of Service field to accept the default response of 3, Doctor's Office.

STEP 3

Post the charges for the first procedure, '**99214**', and press **ENTER**. Press **ENTER** again to bypass the Modifier field. Post the diagnosis shown on Ms. Evans's encounter form '**174.9**', and press **ENTER**. Press **F1** or click on the PROCESS button ('√') on the top toolbar and you will be prompted for Ailment Detail (Figure 3-21). Choose (**A**)dd to allow the system to create a new Ailment Detail for Ms. Evans and press ENTER. Because Ms. Evans has a serious, ongoing illness and it is likely that she will be hospitalized shortly, you will need Ailment Detail information for her hospitalization. It is more convenient to be able to record information such as the date of first symptom and the date of first consult at this time rather than having to pull the patient file later. Use the following information to complete the Ailment Detail screen:

Figure 3-21 First Procedure, Add Ailment Screen

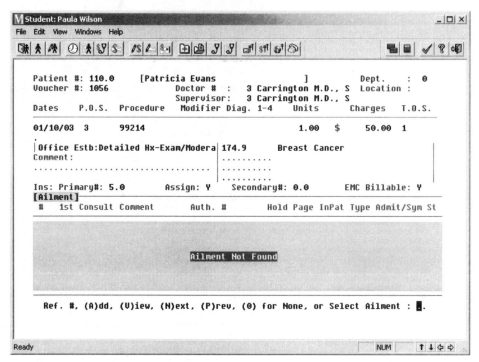

Hold Claim (Y/N): [Press **ENTER** to accept the default of (**N**)ormal billing]
Date First Consulted: **01102003**
Facility #: (Press **ENTER** to leave blank)
Comment Field: **Cancer**
Prior Authorization #: (Press **ENTER** to leave blank)
Inpatient (Y/N): (**N**)o
Ref. Doctor #: (Press **ENTER** to accept the default doctor 2, Leland W. Groves, M.D.)
Related To Employment (Y/N): (**N**)o
Accident (Y/N): (**N**)o
Old Symptom (Y/N): (**N**)o
Emergency (Y/N): (**N**)o
Date First Symptom: **12/30/2002** (Be careful that you *do not* accept the default date at this field.)

Compare your screen to Figure 3-22 and press **F1** or click on the PROCESS button ('√') on the top toolbar now to process this screen without completing the remaining fields at this time.

Figure 3-22 Ailment Detail Screen

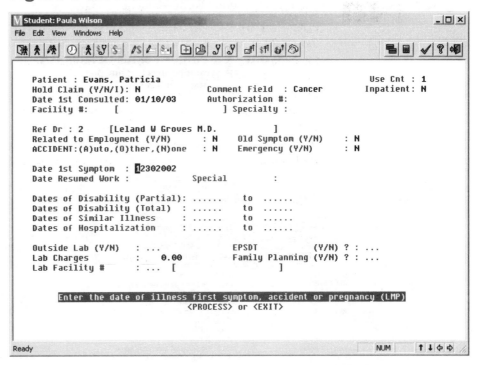

Complete this exercise by posting the other two procedures (**71020** and **76088**). *Remember to press* **F1** *or click on the PROCESS button ('√') to process each procedure you post.* When you post the second and third charges, enter '**S**' to indicate the (S)ame Ailment Detail is to be used. Press **ESCAPE** twice or click twice on the EXIT button on the top toolbar when you have completed posting the charges shown on Ms. Evans's encounter form.

EXERCISE 7: Andrea L. Edwards

Posting an Ailment with Three Charges

Mrs. Portia Edwards's daughter, Andrea, is being treated for anorexia nervosa, which may be a psychological condition. Her charges are to be billed to the family insurance plan. The insurance plan will want to know if Andrea's problem is a recurrence of an old condition, so an Ailment Detail will be necessary.

From the Procedure Entry Patient Retrieval screen, retrieve Andrea's account by keying '**21.2**' and pressing **ENTER**. Once you have located Andrea's account, press **ENTER** to select Epsilon Life and Casualty as her primary insurance coverage. Press **ENTER** again at both the Assignment and Secondary Insurance fields to accept the default responses for each of these fields. Key '**1057**' in the Voucher Number field and press **ENTER**. The cursor will move to the Doctor Number field. Press **ENTER** to accept the default doctor for this patient, Dr. Carrington. Press **ENTER** twice to bypass the Department and Location fields. Press **ENTER** at both of the Date fields to accept the default response for each. Press **ENTER** again at the Place of Service field to accept the default response of 3, Doctor's Office.

STEP 2   Referring to Figure 3-23, post the charges for the first procedure, '**99213**', and press **ENTER**. Press **ENTER** again to bypass the Modifier field. Post the diagnosis shown on Andrea's encounter form, '**783.0**', and press **ENTER**. Press **F1** or click on the PROCESS

Figure 3-23 Andrea Edwards's Encounter Form—Voucher 1057

Sydney Carrington & Associates P.A.
34 Sycamore Street   Suite 300
Madison, CA 95653

Date: 01/10/2003   Voucher No.: 1057

Time: 09:00

Patient: Andrea Edwards   Patient No: 21.2
Guarantor: Portia D. Edwards   Doctor: 3 - S. Carrington

CPT	DESCRIPTION	FEE		CPT	DESCRIPTION	FEE		CPT	DESCRIPTION	FEE
OFFICE/HOSPITAL CONSULTS				**LABORATORY/RADIOLOGY**				**PROCEDURES/TESTS**		
99201	Office New:Focused Hx-Exam		☒	81000	Urinalysis	$8.00		00452	Anesthesia for Rad Surgery	
99202	Office New:Expanded Hx-Exam			81002	Urinalysis; Pregnancy Test			11100	Skin Biopsy	
99211	Office Estb:Min/None Hx-Exa			82951	Glucose Tolerance Test			15852	Dressing Change	
99212	Office Estb:Focused Hx-Exam			84478	Triglycerides			29075	Cast Appl. - Lower Arm	
☒ 99213	Office Estb:Expanded Hx-Exa	$40.00		84550	Uric Acid: Blood Chemistry			29530	Strapping of Knee	
99214	Office Estb:Detailed Hx-Exa			84830	Ovulation Test			29705	Removal/Revis of Cast w/Exa	
99215	Office Estb:Comprhn Hx-Exam		☒	85014	Hematocrit	$18.00		53670	Catheterization Incl. Suppl	
99221	Hosp. Initial:Comprh Hx-			85031	Hemogram, Complete Blood Wk			57452	Colposcopy	
99223	Hosp.Ini:Comprh Hx-Exam/Hi			86403	Particle Agglutination Test			57505	ECC	
99231	Hosp. Subsequent: S-Fwd			86485	Skin Test; Candida			69420	Myringotomy	
99232	Hosp. Subsequent: Comprhn Hx			86580	TB Intradermal Test			92081	Visual Field Examination	
99233	Hosp. Subsequent: Ex/Hi			86585	TB Tine Test			92100	Serial Tonometry Exam	
99238	Hospital Visit Discharge Ex			87070	Culture			92120	Tonography	
99371	Telephone Consult - Simple			70190	X-Ray; Optic Foramina			92552	Pure Tone Audiometry	
99372	Telephone Consult - Intermed			70210	X-Ray Sinuses Complete			92567	Tympanometry	
99373	Telephone Consult - Complex			71010	Radiological Exam Ent Spine			93000	Electrocardiogram	
90843	Counseling - 25 minutes			71020	X-Ray Chest Pa & Lat			93015	Exercise Stress Test (ETT)	
90844	Counseling - 50 minutes			72050	X-Ray Spine, Cerv (4 views)			93017	ETT Tracing Only	
90865	Counseling - Special Interview			72090	X-Ray Spine; Scoliosis Ex			93040	Electrocardiogram - Rhythm	
				72110	Spine, lumbosacral; a/p & Lat			96100	Psychological Testing	
IMMUNIZATIONS/INJECTIONS				73030	Shoulder-Comp, min w/ 2vws			99000	Specimen Handling	
90585	BCG Vaccine			73070	Elbow, anteropost & later vws			99058	Office Emergency Care	
90659	Influenza Virus Vaccine			73120	X-Ray; Hand, 2 views			99070	Surgical Tray - Misc.	
90701	Immunization-DTP			73560	X-Ray, Knee, 1 or 2 views			99080	Special Reports of Med Rec	
90702	DT Vaccine			74022	X-Ray; Abdomen, Complete			99195	Phlebotomy	
90703	Tetanus Toxoids			75552	Cardiac Magnetic Res Img					
90732	Pneumococcal Vaccine			76020	X-Ray; Bone Age Studies					
90746	Hepatitis B Vaccine			76088	Mammary Ductogram Complete					
90749	Immunization; Unlisted			78465	Myocardial Perfusion Img					

ICD-9	CODE DIAGNOSIS		ICD-9	CODE DIAGNOSIS		ICD-9	CODE DIAGNOSIS
009.0	Ill-defined Intestinal Infect		435.0	Basilar Artery Syndrome		724.2	Pain: Lower Back
133.2	Establish Baseline		440.0	Atherosclerosis		727.6	Rupture of Achilles Tendon
174.9	Breast Cancer		442.81	Carotid Artery		780.1	Hallucinations
185.0	Prostate Cancer		460.0	Common Cold		780.3	Convulsions
250	Diabetes Mellitus		461.9	Acute Sinusitis		780.5	Sleep Disturbances
272.4	Hyperlipidemia		474.0	Tonsillitis	☒	783.0	Anorexia
282.5	Anemia - Sickle Trait		477.9	Hay Fever		783.1	Abnormal Weight Gain
282.60	Anemia - Sickle Cell		487.0	Flu		783.2	Abnormal Weight Loss
285.9	Anemia, Unspecified		496	Chronic Airway Obstruction		830.6	Dislocated Hip
300.4	Neurotic Depression		522	Low Red Blood Count		830.9	Dislocated Shoulder
340	Multiple Sclerosis		524.6	Temporo-Mandibular Jnt Synd		841.2	Sprained Wrist
342.9	Hemiplegia - Unspecified		538.8	Stomach Pain		842.5	Sprained Ankle
346.9	Migraine Headache		553.3	Hiatal Hernia		891.2	Fractured Tibia
352.9	Cranial Neuralgia		564.1	Spastic Colon		892.0	Fractured Fibula
354.0	Carpal Tunnel Syndrome		571.4	Chronic Hepatitis		919.5	Insect Bite, Nonvenomous
355.0	Sciatic Nerve Root Lesion		571.5	Cirrhosis of Liver		921.1	Contus Eyelid/Perioc Area
366.9	Cataract		573.3	Hepatitis		v16.3	Fam. Hist of Breast Cancer
386.0	Vertigo		575.2	Obstruction of Gallbladder		v17.4	Fam. Hist of Cardiovasc Dis
401.1	Essential Hypertension		648.2	Anemia - Compl. Pregnancy		v20.2	Well Child
414.9	Ischemic Hearth Disease		715.90	Osteoarthritis - Unspec		v22.0	Pregnancy - First Normal
428.0	Congestive Heart Failure		721.3	Lumbar Osteo/Spondylarthrit		v22.1	Pregnancy - Normal

Previous Balance	Today's Charges	Total Due	Amount Paid	New Balance		Follow Up
_____	_____	_____	_____	_____		PRN _____ Weeks _____ Months _____ Units _____
						Next Appointment Date: Time:

I hereby authorize release of any information acquired in the course of examination or treatment and allow a photocopy of my signature to be used.

---

button ('√') on the top toolbar and you will be prompted for Ailment Detail. Choose (**A**)dd to allow the system to create a new Ailment Detail for Andrea and press **ENTER**. Use the following information to complete the Ailment Detail screen:

Hold Claim (Y/N): [Press **ENTER** to accept the default of (**N**)ormal billing]

Date First Consulted: **01102003**

Facility #: (Press **ENTER** to leave blank)

Comment Field: **Weight Loss**

Prior Authorization #: (Press **ENTER** to leave blank)

Inpatient (Y/N): (**N**)o

Ref. Doctor #: (Press **ENTER** to accept the default doctor 2, Leland W. Groves, M.D.)

Related To Employment (Y/N): (**N**)o

Accident (Y/N): (**N**)o

Old Symptom (Y/N): (**N**)o

Emergency (Y/N): (**N**)o

Date First Symptom: **12/30/2002** (Be careful that you *do not* accept the default date at this field.)

Press **F1** or click on the PROCESS button ('√') on the top toolbar to process this screen without completing the remaining fields at this time.

STEP 3　Complete this exercise by posting the other two procedure codes. Remember to press the **F1** key or click on the PROCESS button ('√') to process each procedure you post. When you post the second and third charges (81000 and 85014), enter '**S**' to indicate the (S)ame Ailment Detail is to be used.

Compare your screens with Figures 3-24 through 3-27. Press **F1** or click on the PROCESS button ('√') to process the screen; then press **ESCAPE** twice or click twice on the EXIT button on the top toolbar.

Figure 3-24 Post First Charge Screen

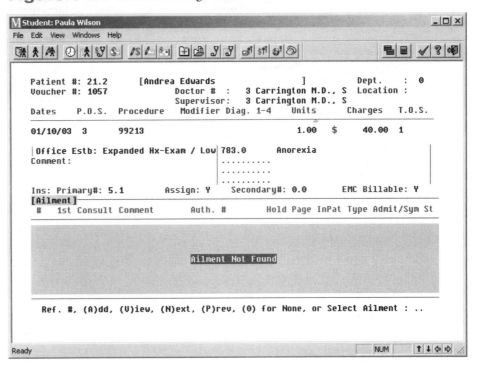

Figure 3-25 Ailment Detail Screen

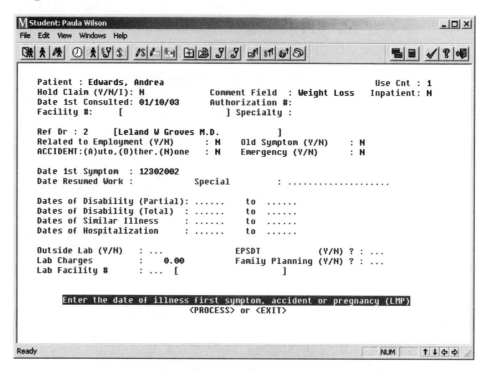

Figure 3-26 Second Charge Screen, Before Processing

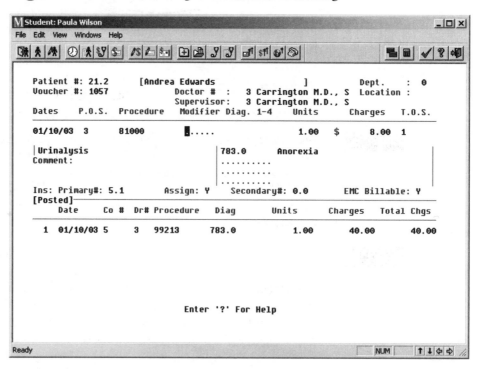

UNIT 3 Posting Your Entries

Figure 3-27 Third Charge Screen, Before Processing

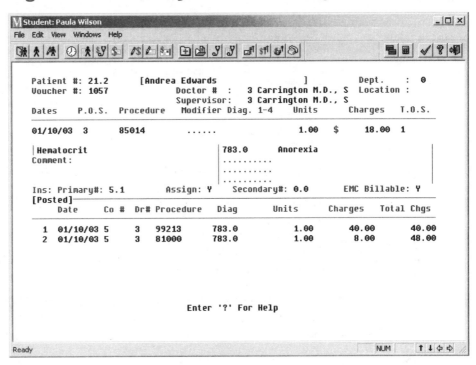

```
M Student: Paula Wilson                                                    _ | □ | X |
File  Edit  View  Windows  Help

 ╔═══════════════════════════════════════════════════════════════════════════╗

   Patient #: 21.2      [Andrea Edwards               ]       Dept.   :  0
   Voucher #: 1057                Doctor #  :   3 Carrington M.D., S  Location :
                                  Supervisor:   3 Carrington M.D., S
   Dates     P.O.S.  Procedure   Modifier Diag. 1-4   Units       Charges   T.O.S.

   01/10/03   3        85014        ......              1.00  $     18.00   1

   |Hematocrit                             |783.0      Anorexia
   Comment:                                |..........
                                           |..........
                                           |..........
   Ins: Primary#: 5.1         Assign: Y       Secondary#: 0.0      EMC Billable: Y
   [Posted]──────────────────────────────────────────────────────────────────
          Date     Co #  Dr# Procedure   Diag      Units     Charges   Total Chgs

      1  01/10/03 5      3   99213       783.0      1.00      40.00       40.00
      2  01/10/03 5      3   81000       783.0      1.00       8.00       48.00




                            Enter '?' For Help


 ╚═══════════════════════════════════════════════════════════════════════════╝
Ready                                                     NUM      ↑ ↓ ⇦ ⇨
```

EXERCISE 8: Mindy A. Davis

Posting a Procedure without Insurance

Mr. Timothy Davis brought his daughter, Mindy, with him to the doctor because she has a cold. Because Mr. Davis's insurance is for his Worker's Compensation coverage, it cannot be used for any other family member or for any other condition that Mr. Davis may incur. Mindy's coverage priority is set to no primary or secondary insurance. Therefore, no insurance plan information will display on this screen.

STEP 1 Using the keyboard or mouse, post the procedure and diagnosis code as usual, using the information on the encounter form shown in Figure 3-28. Note that since Mindy has no insurance coverage, the cursor will not go to the Insurance field. The field that you will complete next is Voucher #. However, the voucher number shown on Figure 3-28 will not fit in the designated space in the Procedure Entry screen. In this case enter '**WorkIn**' instead.

STEP 2 Post the procedure (**99213**) and diagnosis (**460.0**) codes shown on Mindy's encounter form. Then, compare your screen with Figure 3-29, and press **F1** or click on the PROCESS button ('√') on the top toolbar to process. Note that you will not be prompted for Ailment Detail because you did not indicate insurance responsibility. When you have completed posting the charge with no insurance, press **ESCAPE** twice or click twice on the EXIT button on the top toolbar.

Reminder: If an account has no insurance plans, the primary insurance field will automatically be set to '0.0'. If the procedure being performed is not to be billed to an insurance company, the ailment prompt will be skipped.

Figure 3-28 Mindy Davis's Encounter Form—Voucher Work-In

Sydney Carrington & Associates P.A.
34 Sycamore Street   Suite 300
Madison, CA 95653

Date: 01/10/2003

Time:

Patient: Mindy Davis
Guarantor: Timothy R. Davis

Voucher No.: Work-In

Patient No: 80.2
Doctor: 2 - F. Simpson

CPT	DESCRIPTION	FEE
OFFICE/HOSPITAL CONSULTS		
☐ 99201	Office New:Focused Hx-Exam	____
☐ 99202	Office New:Expanded Hx-Exam	____
☐ 99211	Office Estb:Min/None Hx-Exa	____
☐ 99212	Office Estb:Focused Hx-Exam	____
☒ 99213	Office Estb:Expanded Hx-Exa	$40.00
☐ 99214	Office Estb:Detailed Hx-Exa	____
☐ 99215	Office Estb:Comprhn Hx-Exam	____
☐ 99221	Hosp. Initial:Comprh Hx-	____
☐ 99223	Hosp.Ini:Comprh Hx-Exam/Hi	____
☐ 99231	Hosp. Subsequent: S-Fwd	____
☐ 99232	Hosp. Subsequent: Comprhn Hx	____
☐ 99233	Hosp. Subsequent: Ex/Hi	____
☐ 99238	Hospital Visit Discharge Ex	____
☐ 99371	Telephone Consult - Simple	____
☐ 99372	Telephone Consult - Intermed	____
☐ 99373	Telephone Consult - Complex	____
☐ 90843	Counseling - 25 minutes	____
☐ 90844	Counseling - 50 minutes	____
☐ 90865	Counseling - Special Interview	____
IMMUNIZATIONS/INJECTIONS		
☐ 90585	BCG Vaccine	____
☐ 90659	Influenza Virus Vaccine	____
☐ 90701	Immunization-DTP	____
☐ 90702	DT Vaccine	____
☐ 90703	Tetanus Toxoids	____
☐ 90732	Pneumococcal Vaccine	____
☐ 90746	Hepatitis B Vaccine	____
☐ 90749	Immunization; Unlisted	____

CPT	DESCRIPTION	FEE
LABORATORY/RADIOLOGY		
☐ 81000	Urinalysis	____
☐ 81002	Urinalysis; Pregnancy Test	____
☐ 82951	Glucose Tolerance Test	____
☐ 84478	Triglycerides	____
☐ 84550	Uric Acid: Blood Chemistry	____
☐ 84830	Ovulation Test	____
☐ 85014	Hematocrit	____
☐ 85031	Hemogram, Complete Blood Wk	____
☐ 86403	Particle Agglutination Test	____
☐ 86485	Skin Test; Candida	____
☐ 86580	TB Intradermal Test	____
☐ 86585	TB Tine Test	____
☐ 87070	Culture	____
☐ 70190	X-Ray; Optic Foramina	____
☐ 70210	X-Ray Sinuses Complete	____
☐ 71010	Radiological Exam Ent Spine	____
☐ 71020	X-Ray Chest Pa & Lat	____
☐ 72050	X-Ray Spine, Cerv (4 views)	____
☐ 72090	X-Ray Spine; Scoliosis Ex	____
☐ 72110	Spine, lumbosacral; a/p & Lat	____
☐ 73030	Shoulder-Comp, min w/ 2vws	____
☐ 73070	Elbow, anteropost & later vws	____
☐ 73120	X-Ray; Hand, 2 views	____
☐ 73560	X-Ray, Knee, 1 or 2 views	____
☐ 74022	X-Ray; Abdomen, Complete	____
☐ 75552	Cardiac Magnetic Res Img	____
☐ 76020	X-Ray; Bone Age Studies	____
☐ 76088	Mammary Ductogram Complete	____
☐ 78465	Myocardial Perfusion Img	____

CPT	DESCRIPTION	FEE
PROCEDURES/TESTS		
☐ 00452	Anesthesia for Rad Surgery	____
☐ 11100	Skin Biopsy	____
☐ 15852	Dressing Change	____
☐ 29075	Cast Appl. - Lower Arm	____
☐ 29530	Strapping of Knee	____
☐ 29705	Removal/Revis of Cast w/Exa	____
☐ 53670	Catheterization Incl. Suppl	____
☐ 57452	Colposcopy	____
☐ 57505	ECC	____
☐ 69420	Myringotomy	____
☐ 92081	Visual Field Examination	____
☐ 92100	Serial Tonometry Exam	____
☐ 92120	Tonography	____
☐ 92552	Pure Tone Audiometry	____
☐ 92567	Tympanometry	____
☐ 93000	Electrocardiogram	____
☐ 93015	Exercise Stress Test (ETT)	____
☐ 93017	ETT Tracing Only	____
☐ 93040	Electrocardiogram - Rhythm	____
☐ 96100	Psychological Testing	____
☐ 99000	Specimen Handling	____
☐ 99058	Office Emergency Care	____
☐ 99070	Surgical Tray - Misc.	____
☐ 99080	Special Reports of Med Rec	____
☐ 99195	Phlebotomy	____
☐ _____	_____	____
☐ _____	_____	____
☐ _____	_____	____

ICD-9	CODE DIAGNOSIS
☐ 009.0	Ill-defined Intestinal Infect
☐ 133.2	Establish Baseline
☐ 174.9	Breast Cancer
☐ 185.0	Prostate Cancer
☐ 250	Diabetes Mellitus
☐ 272.4	Hyperlipidemia
☐ 282.5	Anemia - Sickle Trait
☐ 282.60	Anemia - Sickle Cell
☐ 285.9	Anemia, Unspecified
☐ 300.4	Neurotic Depression
☐ 340	Multiple Sclerosis
☐ 342.9	Hemiplegia - Unspecified
☐ 346.9	Migraine Headache
☐ 352.9	Cranial Neuralgia
☐ 354.0	Carpal Tunnel Syndrome
☐ 355.0	Sciatic Nerve Root Lesion
☐ 366.9	Cataract
☐ 386.0	Vertigo
☐ 401.1	Essential Hypertension
☐ 414.9	Ischemic Hearth Disease
☐ 428.0	Congestive Heart Failure

ICD-9	CODE DIAGNOSIS
☐ 435.0	Basilar Artery Syndrome
☐ 440.0	Atherosclerosis
☐ 442.81	Carotid Artery
☒ 460.0	Common Cold
☐ 461.9	Acute Sinusitis
☐ 474.0	Tonsillitis
☐ 477.9	Hay Fever
☐ 487.0	Flu
☐ 496	Chronic Airway Obstruction
☐ 522	Low Red Blood Count
☐ 524.6	Temporo-Mandibular Jnt Synd
☐ 538.8	Stomach Pain
☐ 553.3	Hiatal Hernia
☐ 564.1	Spastic Colon
☐ 571.4	Chronic Hepatitis
☐ 571.5	Cirrhosis of Liver
☐ 573.3	Hepatitis
☐ 575.2	Obstruction of Gallbladder
☐ 648.2	Anemia - Compl. Pregnancy
☐ 715.90	Osteoarthritis - Unspec
☐ 721.3	Lumbar Osteo/Spondylarthrit

ICD-9	CODE DIAGNOSIS
☐ 724.2	Pain: Lower Back
☐ 727.6	Rupture of Achilles Tendon
☐ 780.1	Hallucinations
☐ 780.3	Convulsions
☐ 780.5	Sleep Disturbances
☐ 783.0	Anorexia
☐ 783.1	Abnormal Weight Gain
☐ 783.2	Abnormal Weight Loss
☐ 830.6	Dislocated Hip
☐ 830.9	Dislocated Shoulder
☐ 841.2	Sprained Wrist
☐ 842.5	Sprained Ankle
☐ 891.2	Fractured Tibia
☐ 892.0	Fractured Fibula
☐ 919.5	Insect Bite, Nonvenomous
☐ 921.1	Contus Eyelid/Perioc Area
☐ v16.3	Fam. Hist of Breast Cancer
☐ v17.4	Fam. Hist of Cardiovasc Dis
☐ v20.2	Well Child
☐ v22.0	Pregnancy - First Normal
☐ v22.1	Pregnancy - Normal

Previous Balance	Today's Charges	Total Due	Amount Paid	New Balance
_____	_____	_____	_____	_____

Follow Up

PRN _____ Weeks _____ Months _____ Units _____

Next Appointment Date: _____   Time: _____

I hereby authorize release of any information acquired in the course of examination or treatment and allow a photocopy of my signature to be used.

PRINTING DAILY REPORTS

The Daily Report provides a summary of the practice's activities.

The Daily Report or Daily Close refers to a list of the day's financial and patient activities. A Daily Report generates a report that includes full financial summaries by doctor for the

Figure 3-29 Post a Charge with No Insurance Screen

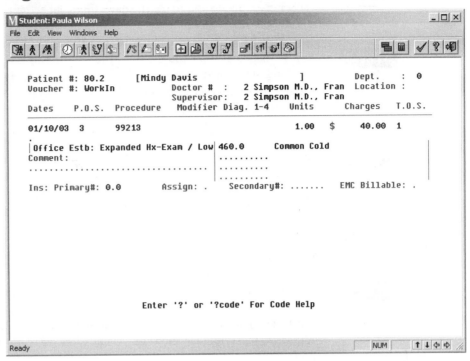

present day plus period-to-date and year-to-date financial activities. When you run a Daily Report, you may request a check register that prints changes in cash, the amount of the daily deposit, and a list of checks for the day. You may run a Trial Daily Report or a Final Daily Report. Follow the directions below for creating a Trial Daily Report.

STEP 1 Return to the Main Menu (Menu 1) and select option **5**, REPORT Generation. At the Reports Menu, select option **4**, DAILY Report. The screen in Figure 3-30 appears.

Figure 3-30 Daily Report Screen

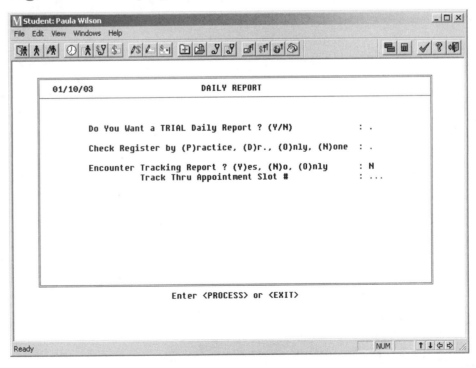

STEP 2   Key 'Y' to indicate that you desire a Trial Daily Report and press **ENTER**. The Trial Daily Report allows you to see the day's financial activities without the risk of closing the day's business prematurely.

STEP 3   Key 'P' to indicate that you desire a check register by practice and press **ENTER**. The check register provides a breakdown of the day's cash, checks, refunds, and other, and lists all checks received for the day. The breakdown of deposit amount per doctor is provided as part of each doctor's daily summary. The doctor's deposit amount will differ from daily receipts by the amount of daily refunds.

STEP 4   Because Encounter Form Tracking is turned off in the Student Edition of **The Medical Manager** software, the system will automatically default to 'N' to not provide an Encounter Tracking Report. Press **ENTER** to bypass the Selective Appointment Location field.

STEP 5   Key '**A**' for All to create a Daily Report for all doctors, operators, and locations and press **ENTER**.

STEP 6   Make sure your printer is on, has paper in it, and is online. Press **F1** or click on the PROCESS button ('√') on the top toolbar to process and then print the report. You may abort the report at any time by pressing **ESCAPE** or by clicking on the EXIT button. Although the reminder message "Daily Close NOT Performed" will appear, press **ENTER** to bypass it, as you will not run a Final Daily Report now. **Do not print a final report at this time**. Compare your reports to the Trial Daily Report shown in Figures 3-31 through 3-35. If there are any differences in the financial totals you may correct them by using Edit Activity as discussed in Unit 4. Ask your instructor if you should proceed to Unit 4 to familiarize yourself with Edit Activity. **Do not perform the final Daily Close if there are any financial errors**.

Note: You may run the Trial Daily Report and check it for accuracy as many times as you like. You may run the Final Daily Report only once.

Figure 3-31 Daily Report for 01/10/03—James Monroe, M.D

```
01/10/03                          DAILY REPORT FOR 01/10/03                          Page   1
                                    James T Monroe MD (1)

                                                          [to Vchr  Total  Ref Date]
Account   Patient Name    Dt Post  Type Dates of Service  Dept Voucher Proc Code  Units  Pri/Sec Ail Loc Exc   Amount
================================================================================================================
120.2    Spivey,Alice     01/10/03 CHG  01/10/03-          0    1052    99211     1.00    11/    5  N           25.00
120      Williams,Terry   01/10/03 A05  HMO Adj & Write-O  0           [1052      25.00          01/10/03]     -25.00
120.2    Spivey,Alice     01/10/03 CHG  01/10/03-          0    1052    90701     1.00    11/    5  N           14.00
120      Williams,Terry   01/10/03 A05  HMO Adj & Write-O  0           [1052      10.00          01/10/03]     -10.00
120.1    Simmons,Laura    01/10/03 CHG  01/10/03-          0    WorkIn  99211     1.00    11/    0  N           25.00
120      Williams,Terry   01/10/03 A05  HMO Adj & Write-O  0           [WorkIn    25.00          01/10/03]     -25.00
30.0     League,Claire    01/10/03 CHG  01/10/03-          0    1054    99213     1.00     2/   10  N           40.00
30.0     League,Claire    01/10/03 CHG  01/10/03-          0    1054    85014     1.00     2/   10  N           18.00

Exception Codes:
overrides: c= charge, p= profile, w= writedown, o= overpay, i= pmt not from resp. ins, e= item edited, x= rebuilt dlyfile.tmp used


                          Summary for : James T Monroe MD
         ---------------------------------------------------------------
            Item           Today       Period-to-Date        Year-to-Date
         Description      01/10/03    01/01/03 - 01/10/03   01/01/03 - 01/10/03
         ---------------------------------------------------------------
         Total Charges      122.00         122.00               122.00
         Total Receipts       0.00           0.00                 0.00
         Refunds              0.00           0.00                 0.00
         Cross-Alloc Unapplied 0.00          0.00                 0.00
         Total Adjustments   60.00          60.00                60.00
         Accounts Receivable 62.00          62.00                62.00
         Total # Procedures      5              5                    5
         Service Charges      0.00           0.00                 0.00
         Tax Charges          0.00           0.00                 0.00
         Copay Expected       0.00            ---                  ---
         Copay Paid           0.00            ---                  ---
         Deposit Amount       0.00            ---                  ---
              Checks     0.00
              Cash       0.00
              Other      0.00
         ---------------------------------------------------------------
```

Figure 3-32 Trial Daily Report for 01/10/03—Frances Simpson, M.D

```
01/10/03                          DAILY REPORT FOR 01/10/03                          Page   2
                                   Frances D Simpson M.D. (2)

                                                          [to Vchr  Total  Ref Date]
Account   Patient Name    Dt Post  Type Dates of Service  Dept Voucher Proc Code  Units  Pri/Sec Ail Loc Exc   Amount
================================================================================================================
80.0     Davis,Timothy    01/10/03 CHG  01/10/03-          0    1055    99213     1.00    12/    0  Y           40.00
80.0     Davis,Timothy    01/10/03 CHG  01/10/03-          0    1055    29075     1.00    12/    0  Y           48.00
80.2     Davis,Mindy      01/10/03 CHG  01/10/03-          0    WorkIn  99213     1.00     0/    0  N           40.00

Exception Codes:
overrides: c= charge, p= profile, w= writedown, o= overpay, i= pmt not from resp. ins, e= item edited, x= rebuilt dlyfile.tmp used


                          Summary for : Frances D Simpson M.D.
         ---------------------------------------------------------------
            Item           Today       Period-to-Date        Year-to-Date
         Description      01/10/03    01/01/03 - 01/10/03   01/01/03 - 01/10/03
         ---------------------------------------------------------------
         Total Charges      128.00         128.00               128.00
         Total Receipts       0.00           0.00                 0.00
         Refunds              0.00           0.00                 0.00
         Cross-Alloc Unapplied 0.00          0.00                 0.00
         Total Adjustments    0.00           0.00                 0.00
         Accounts Receivable 128.00        128.00               128.00
         Total # Procedures      3              3                    3
         Service Charges      0.00           0.00                 0.00
         Tax Charges          0.00           0.00                 0.00
         Copay Expected       0.00            ---                  ---
         Copay Paid           0.00            ---                  ---
         Deposit Amount       0.00            ---                  ---
              Checks     0.00
              Cash       0.00
              Other      0.00
         ---------------------------------------------------------------
```

Figure 3-33 Trial Daily Report for 01/10/03—Sydney Carrington, M.D.

```
01/10/03                              DAILY REPORT FOR 01/10/03                                    Page    3
                                     Sydney J Carrington M.D. (3)

                                                                     [to Vchr  Total  Ref Date]
Account    Patient Name      Dt Post   Type Dates of Service  Dept Voucher Proc Code  Units  Pri/Sec Ail  Loc  Exc  Amount
=========================================================================================================================
10.0       Carlson,Steven    01/10/03  CHG  01/10/03-           0   1050    99214     1.00    2/    5  N                 50.00
10.1       Carlson,Sharon    01/10/03  CHG  01/10/03-           0   1051    99213     1.00    7/    0  N                 40.00
34.0       Dudley,Wayne      01/10/03  CHG  01/10/03-           0   1053    99215     1.00    6/    0  N                 85.00
34.0       Dudley,Wayne      01/10/03  CHG  01/10/03-           0   1053    81000     1.00    6/    0  N                  8.00
34.0       Dudley,Wayne      01/10/03  CHG  01/10/03-           0   1053    72050     1.00    6/    0  N                150.00
34.0       Dudley,Wayne      01/10/03  CHG  01/10/03-           0   1053    93000     1.00    6/    0  N                 57.00
110.0      Evans,Patricia    01/10/03  CHG  01/10/03-           0   1056    99214     1.00    5/    0  Y                 50.00
110.0      Evans,Patricia    01/10/03  CHG  01/10/03-           0   1056    71020     1.00    5/    0  Y                 58.00
110.0      Evans,Patricia    01/10/03  CHG  01/10/03-           0   1056    76088     1.00    5/    0  Y                125.00
21.2       Edwards,Andrea    01/10/03  CHG  01/10/03-           0   1057    99213     1.00    5/    0  Y                 40.00
21.2       Edwards,Andrea    01/10/03  CHG  01/10/03-           0   1057    81000     1.00    5/    0  Y                  8.00
21.2       Edwards,Andrea    01/10/03  CHG  01/10/03-           0   1057    85014     1.00    5/    0  Y                 18.00

Exception Codes:
overrides: c= charge, p= profile, w= writedown, o= overpay, i= pmt not from resp. ins, e= item edited, x= rebuilt dlyfile.tmp used


                               Summary for : Sydney J Carrington M.D.
              ---------------------------------------------------------------------
                  Item            Today          Period-to-Date          Year-to-Date
                Description      01/10/03     01/01/03 - 01/10/03    01/01/03 - 01/10/03
              ---------------------------------------------------------------------
              Total Charges        689.00          689.00                  689.00
              Total Receipts         0.00            0.00                    0.00
              Refunds                0.00            0.00                    0.00
              Cross-Alloc Unapplied  0.00            0.00                    0.00
              Total Adjustments      0.00            0.00                    0.00
              Accounts Receivable  689.00          689.00                  689.00
              Total # Procedures      12              12                      12
              Service Charges        0.00            0.00                    0.00
              Tax Charges            0.00            0.00                    0.00
              Copay Expected         0.00            ---                     ---
              Copay Paid             0.00            ---                     ---
              Deposit Amount         0.00            ---                     ---
                     Checks    0.00
                     Cash      0.00
                     Other     0.00
              ---------------------------------------------------------------------
```

Figure 3-34 Cash Analysis Report for 01/10/03

```
01/10/03                              DAILY REPORT FOR 01/10/03                                    Page    4
                                        CASH ANALYSIS REPORT
                                        Student: Paul Wilson
=========================================================================================================================

          Change in Cash Position                              Daily Deposit
          -----------------------                              -------------

          CHECKS          0.00                       CHECKS          0.00
          CASH            0.00                       CASH            0.00
          OTHER           0.00                       OTHER           0.00
          REFUNDS         0.00
                       ==========                                 ==========
                            0.00                                       0.00

                                CHECK REGISTER FOR 01/10/03

          Ref #  Voucher    Dr.      Amount    Date Posted    Received From                Account
          ===============================================================================================
                                  ----------
                TOTAL CHECKS :           0.00
```

Figure 3-35 Trial Daily Report Totals for 01/10/03

==

TOTALS FOR 01/10/03

Doctor	Charges	Receipts	Adjustments	Net A/R	Total A/R	# Proc.	Serv Chg	Tax Chg
1. James T Monroe MD	122.00	0.00	60.00	62.00	62.00	5	0.00	0.00
2. Frances D Simpson M.D.	128.00	0.00	0.00	128.00	128.00	3	0.00	0.00
3. Sydney J Carrington M.D.	689.00	0.00	0.00	689.00	689.00	12	0.00	0.00
TOTAL	939.00	0.00	60.00	879.00	879.00	20	0.00	0.00

PERIOD-TO-DATE TOTALS FOR 01/01/03 - 01/10/03

Doctor	Charges	Receipts	Adjustments	Net A/R	Total A/R	# Proc.	Serv Chg	Tax Chg
1. James T Monroe MD	122.00	0.00	60.00	62.00	62.00	5	0.00	0.00
2. Frances D Simpson M.D.	128.00	0.00	0.00	128.00	128.00	3	0.00	0.00
3. Sydney J Carrington M.D.	689.00	0.00	0.00	689.00	689.00	12	0.00	0.00
TOTAL	939.00	0.00	60.00	879.00	879.00	20	0.00	0.00

YEAR-TO-DATE TOTALS FOR 01/01/03 - 01/10/03

Doctor	Charges	Receipts	Adjustments	Net A/R	Total A/R	# Proc.	Serv Chg	Tax Chg
1. James T Monroe MD	122.00	0.00	60.00	62.00	62.00	5	0.00	0.00
2. Frances D Simpson M.D.	128.00	0.00	0.00	128.00	128.00	3	0.00	0.00
3. Sydney J Carrington M.D.	689.00	0.00	0.00	689.00	689.00	12	0.00	0.00
TOTAL	939.00	0.00	60.00	879.00	879.00	20	0.00	0.00

********** Daily Close Has NOT Been Performed for 01/10/03 **********

APPLYING YOUR KNOWLEDGE

EXERCISE 9: Performing a Final Daily Close for January 10

Using the figures provided check the Trial Daily Report for accuracy and make necessary corrections. Refer to the section in this unit called *Editing Prior Entries* if you need to make corrections, then perform the Final Daily Report. *Remember to make a backup of your data BEFORE performing the Final Daily Close even if you are not at the end of a class session.*

STEP 1   Choose option **5**, REPORT Generation, at the Main Menu (Menu 1) and option **4**, DAILY Report, at the Reports Menu (Menu 7). Answer (**N**)o to indicate you do not want another Trial Daily Report, and answer '**P**' to ask for a check register for the practice. Enter '**0**' to indicate that you do not wish to purge appointments. Press **F1** or click on the PROCESS button ('√') on the top toolbar to process, and the report will be generated.

STEP 2   When the report is complete, accept the Final Daily Close by entering '**Y**' at the prompt "Do You Wish To Accept Daily Close? (Y/N)." Press **ENTER** at the prompt "Daily Close is Complete. Return to Log-On," so that you will be able to advance the date in the next exercise. Save all your pages from the final report and destroy all copies of the Trial Daily Report. Once you have run and accepted the Final Daily Close, you will not be able to make further corrections. Note that your Final Daily Close will contain more detail than your Trial Daily Report and will provide the additional pages as displayed in Figures 3-36 and 3-37. Hand in all pages of your Final Daily Close to your instructor.

Note: You must do a Final Daily Close, and it must be accurate, or information after today's date will be incorrect. You cannot change information once you have performed the Final Close.

Figure 3-36 GL Daily Distribution Report for 01/10/03

```
01/10/03                    GL DAILY DISTRIBUTION REPORT - FULL DETAIL                    Page    1
                                      Student: Paul Wilson
                                           01/10/03

   GL Account    Description     Dr     Pat #     Procedure    Date Post   Voucher      Debit           Credit
============================================================================================================
      15001.00
                 Accounts Rec     1     120.2                  01/10/03    1052          25.00
                 Accounts Rec     1     120.0                  01/10/03                                   25.00
                 Accounts Rec     1     120.2                  01/10/03    1052          14.00
                 Accounts Rec     1     120.0                  01/10/03                                   10.00
                 Accounts Rec     1     120.1                  01/10/03    WorkIn        25.00
                 Accounts Rec     1     120.0                  01/10/03                                   25.00
                 Accounts Rec     1      30.0                  01/10/03    1054          40.00
                 Accounts Rec     1      30.0                  01/10/03    1054          18.00
                                                                                       --------        --------
      15002.00                                 POST TO ACCOUNT    15001.00             122.00            60.00

                 Accounts Rec     2      80.0                  01/10/03    1055          40.00
                 Accounts Rec     2      80.0                  01/10/03    1055          48.00
                 Accounts Rec     2      80.2                  01/10/03    WorkIn        40.00
                                                                                       --------        --------
      15003.00                                 POST TO ACCOUNT    15002.00             128.00             0.00

                 Accounts Rec     3      10.0                  01/10/03    1050          50.00
                 Accounts Rec     3      10.1                  01/10/03    1051          40.00
                 Accounts Rec     3      34.0                  01/10/03    1053          85.00
                 Accounts Rec     3      34.0                  01/10/03    1053           8.00
                 Accounts Rec     3      34.0                  01/10/03    1053         150.00
                 Accounts Rec     3      34.0                  01/10/03    1053          57.00
                 Accounts Rec     3     110.0                  01/10/03    1056          50.00
                 Accounts Rec     3     110.0                  01/10/03    1056          58.00
                 Accounts Rec     3     110.0                  01/10/03    1056         125.00
                 Accounts Rec     3      21.2                  01/10/03    1057          40.00
                 Accounts Rec     3      21.2                  01/10/03    1057           8.00
                 Accounts Rec     3      21.2                  01/10/03    1057          18.00
                                                                                       --------        --------
      60001.00                                 POST TO ACCOUNT    15003.00             689.00             0.00

                 Revenue          1     120.2      99211       01/10/03    1052                          25.00
                 Revenue          1     120.2      90701       01/10/03    1052                          14.00
                 Revenue          1     120.1      99211       01/10/03    WorkIn                        25.00
                 Revenue          1      30.0      99213       01/10/03    1054                          40.00
                 Revenue          1      30.0      85014       01/10/03    1054                          18.00
                                                                                       --------        --------
      60002.00                                 POST TO ACCOUNT    60001.00               0.00           122.00

                 Revenue          2      80.0      99213       01/10/03    1055                          40.00
                 Revenue          2      80.0      29075       01/10/03    1055                          48.00
                 Revenue          2      80.2      99213       01/10/03    WorkIn                        40.00
                                                                                       --------        --------
      60003.00                                 POST TO ACCOUNT    60002.00               0.00           128.00

                 Revenue          3      10.0      99214       01/10/03    1050                          50.00
                 Revenue          3      10.1      99213       01/10/03    1051                          40.00
                 Revenue          3      34.0      99215       01/10/03    1053                          85.00
                 Revenue          3      34.0      81000       01/10/03    1053                           8.00
                 Revenue          3      34.0      72050       01/10/03    1053                         150.00
                 Revenue          3      34.0      93000       01/10/03    1053                          57.00
                 Revenue          3     110.0      99214       01/10/03    1056                          50.00
                 Revenue          3     110.0      71020       01/10/03    1056                          58.00
                 Revenue          3     110.0      76088       01/10/03    1056                         125.00
                 Revenue          3      21.2      99213       01/10/03    1057                          40.00
                 Revenue          3      21.2      81000       01/10/03    1057                           8.00
                 Revenue          3      21.2      85014       01/10/03    1057                          18.00
                                                                                       --------        --------
      60061.00                                 POST TO ACCOUNT    60003.00               0.00           689.00
```

EXERCISE 10: Advancing the Date to February 3

After you complete the Daily Close, the screen in Figure 3-38 appears to allow you to change the date.

Figure 3-37 Daily Close Status Report for 01/10/03

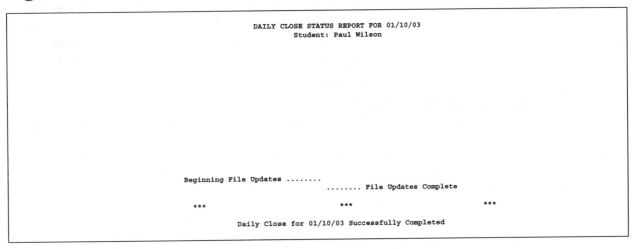

```
                      DAILY CLOSE STATUS REPORT FOR 01/10/03
                              Student: Paul Wilson




           Beginning File Updates ........
                                          ........ File Updates Complete

                  ***                  ***                  ***
                   Daily Close for 01/10/03 Successfully Completed
```

STEP 1 Key '**02032003**'. Check the date carefully. If you advance it incorrectly, you will have to restore your files from a backup. Press **ENTER** and you will receive the following warning message:

184: * WARNING * Skip > 7 Days: Continue (Y/N)

The system date is important. It is used throughout **The Medical Manager** system for financial purposes. Successful data entry will display **The Medical Manager** software's Main Menu (Menu 1). Do not change the date again until instructed to do so. In these lessons, you will usually just press **ENTER** at this screen to default to the system date.

STEP 2 Type '**Y**' and press **ENTER** to acknowledge that you are aware of the fact that you have chosen to advance the date more than seven days. You should never bypass a warning except when instructed to do so.

Figure 3-38 Advance Date

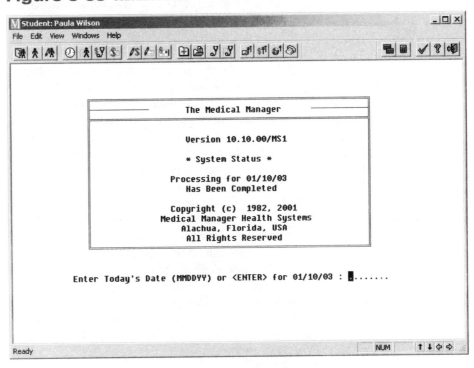

You will be prompted to reenter your password to verify the Date Advance. Key the student password, 'ICAN', and press **ENTER** to approve the date advance. Your system will return to the Main Menu (Menu 1) and the new date, 02/03/03, will appear in the upper left corner of your screen. If this date does not match your screen, notify your instructor immediately.

UNIT 3 SUMMARY

When a patient is examined or treated by a physician, charges for the procedures performed by the doctor are posted to the patient's account using a national standard coding system. Procedure or CPT Codes are used to record the procedure that was performed and Diagnosis or ICD-9 Codes are used to record the patient's disease, condition, or reason for the procedure.

Before a charge can be posted for a patient, you must retrieve the patient's account. The Patient Retrieval screen uses a common interface in all modules of **The Medical Manager**, allowing you to retrieve or find a patient by entering the last name, account number, Social Security number, an ID defined by the medical practice, or the full patient number. You may also enter a '?' plus all or part of the account number, Social Security number or patient last name to display a help window starting at a designated point in the patient file.

A patient number is the account number, a decimal point, and the patient's dependent number. For example, account 10 has two patients, 10. 0 Steven and 10. 1 Sharon. If you enter the full patient number, (e.g., 10.0) the system will directly invoke the selected module. If you retrieve a patient using any of the other methods discussed above, an intermediate patient screen will display the guarantor's name, address, and account balance information, as well as the patients or dependents on the account. Each patient's preferred physician, consent status, and type of primary insurance plan will display as you position the light bar on the dependent's name.

Charges are typically posted in the system based on information that the doctor has checked on the encounter form. When posting a charge, you will enter the doctor, date of service, procedure code, up to four diagnosis codes and the amount of the charge. Many of the charge entry fields, including insurance coverage, will default automatically, indicating which of the patient's policies are to be billed for these services. You can change the information on the screen in any of the fields even though they default.

When a practice bills the patient's insurance company for procedures that were performed, additional information is sometimes required. This information could include whether or not the charges are related to an accident or work injury; whether or not the patient was hospitalized, and so on. This additional information is stored in an Ailment Detail record. Patients can have more than one Ailment Detail record because they may be seen for different conditions at different times. Once an Ailment Detail record is created, it can be used on subsequent visits of the patient as long as the charges pertain to the same illness or injury as listed in the Ailment Detail record. New Ailment Detail records can be created or existing ailments can be selected during Procedure Entry.

At the end of the day, a Daily Close Report is run in trial mode. This will allow you to verify that the procedures you have posted in the system match those that were indicated by the doctor on the encounter form. You may edit incorrect entries or delete duplicate entries prior to daily close using the Edit Activity module discussed in Unit 4. Once you are satisfied that all charges and payment information is correct, you may run a Final Daily Close. A Final Daily Close seals the information so that the financial and doctor fields cannot be edited further.

Because certain charge and payment information cannot be edited once a Daily Close is performed, it is very important to back up your data before performing each Daily Close even if this occurs at a time in your class session where you would not normally perform a backup.

HW. p. 121

New accounts are entered by info. on the

1) Enter the last name field.

2) Look up that 1,

3) Extended · do not call
 * Through family & themselves. Yes.

4) Its imp. b/c it can affect mailing & get misinterpreted.
   UK phone #.

5) Its imp. b/c for emergencies.

6) A window to answer ques of specific fields. Click on the ? mark icon. They're imp b/c they can help us get through the Med. Manager.

1, 2, 3, 5

Unit 3:   the.

Ques 1-7

~~*~~

6) 3 components of the Daily Report   → show errors.
trial report 2 correct mistakes
verification- verify the procedures + make correct
final = ~~when all~~ to close out the tions.
DAY.

~~Hospital dates~~

7). Inal is to correct ~~mistakes~~ (where the
errors are shown. Final report - fix
errors & closes out the files.

4) Purpose of ailment Detail is to allow
us to complete the more detailed sections
of a claim form.

1) 2 methods of retrieving an account are:
type?. Last name
enter account #

2) helps you w/ anything u need.
press [?] icon.

3) They're posted as you ~~must~~.
what dr. checks on encounter
form.

5) · For the pt. + any cond. in which detail would
require overwriting the detail held on a previous Ahort

TESTING YOUR KNOWLEDGE

1. Describe any two methods of retrieving an account.

2. What is the purpose of a help window? How is this function accessed in **The Medical Manager** system?

3. Describe how procedure and diagnosis codes are posted in **The Medical Manager** software.

4. Describe the purpose of Ailment Detail.

(continues)

5. Name two reasons why you would create a new Ailment Detail.

6. Name three components of the Daily Report and their purposes.

7. Explain the difference between a Trial Daily Report and a Final Daily Report.

U N I T 4

Editing
Prior Entries

LEARNING OUTCOMES

After completing this unit, you should be able to:

◆ Retrieve a patient account.
◆ Modify or correct account or patient information.
◆ Retrieve and modify a referring doctor.
◆ Retrieve a previously posted charge.
◆ Modify or correct a previously posted charge.
◆ Retrieve and modify an ailment.

Refer to this chapter any time you need to correct or modify changes to your work. If you have made an error in a prior unit, your instructor may have asked you to read this chapter out of sequence. In this case, you may not be able to complete all of the exercises in this chapter. However, you will be able to learn from the instructions and apply them to your own situation. Once you thoroughly understand the process of making a correction, ask your instructor for assistance in applying it to the particular patient you are working on.

Most of the information in **The Medical Manager** is tied directly to a patient. If you have successfully completed Unit 3, you already know how to retrieve a patient account. You may skip the following section and proceed through the remainder of the Unit 4 exercises. Otherwise, make sure you understand how to retrieve a patient's account before continuing in this unit.

RETRIEVING A PATIENT'S ACCOUNT

The prompt for Patient Retrieval appears in numerous places throughout **The Medical Manager** and is shown in Figure 4-1. The Patient Retrieval screen allows you to retrieve a patient account by entering a name, account number, Social Security number, or ID #. *A questions mark ('?') plus all or part of one of these four items can be entered to display a related Help window OR using the mouse, click on the Help button ('?') on the top toolbar to get a Help window of patients as shown in Figure 4-2.*

Although there are several methods for retrieving an account, you should use one of the following simple methods:

1. *Enter the patient's name.* Enter one or more letters of the patient's last name. If the complete last name is entered, type a comma (,) or a semicolon (;) and then all or part of the first name. Press **ENTER** and the screen will display the Patient Retrieval screen, which is discussed below.

2. *Enter the account number.* If you know the full patient number, you can enter it. For example, for the guarantor of account 10, you would key 10.0 and press

Figure 4-1 Patient Retrieval Prompt

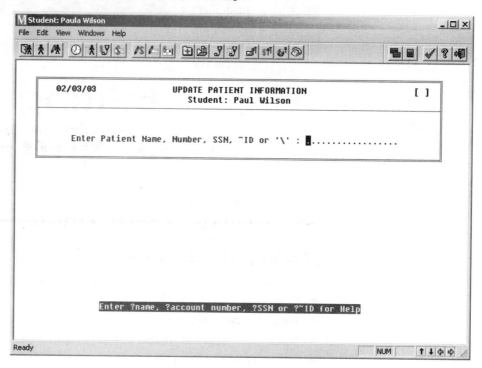

Figure 4-2 Patient Retrieval Prompt with Help Window

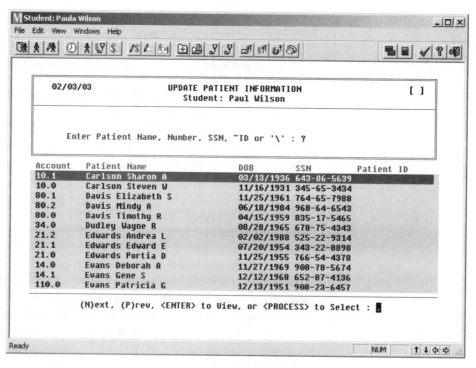

ENTER. For the first dependent you would key 10.1 and press **ENTER.** If the full patient number is entered, **The Medical Manager** assumes you know which patient is needed and will proceed directly to the screen being accessed for that specific patient. If the account number is entered without a decimal extension, the system will display the Patient Retrieval screen discussed below.

3. *Enter the Social Security number.* Key in the full Social Security number (with or without hyphens) and press **ENTER**. The system will bypass the Patient Retrieval screen and go directly to the specific patient being accessed.

4. *Enter a '\'.* The number of the most recently accessed patient appears in brackets in the upper right corner of the screen. Type a backward slash ('\') to display the retrieval screen for the patient last accessed in **The Medical Manager**. Press **ENTER** to retrieve this default patient number and bypass the Patient Retrieval screen.

Use the highlight bar or the mouse to select the appropriate patient and press **ENTER** to view the Patient Retrieval screen (Figure 4-3). You can also press **F1** or click on the PROCESS button ('√') to process and bypass the Patient Retrieval screen.

Figure 4-3 Patient Retrieval Screen

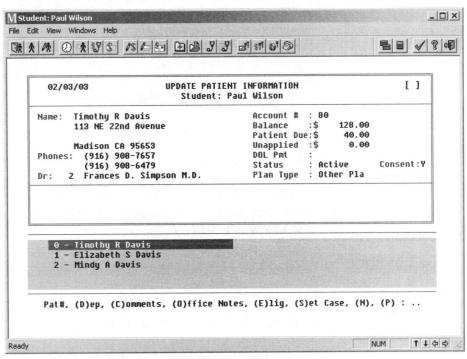

The Patient Retrieval screen displays demographic information about the guarantor of the account as well as financial information and a list of members on the account. Use the highlight bar or the mouse cursor to select the appropriate patient and press **ENTER**.

Changes to patient accounts occur frequently. For example, patients may move to a new address; change marital status, employers, or insurance companies; or add new dependents. Another example of the need for editing prior entries is when the procedure or diagnosis codes have been entered incorrectly. When an account requires editing, modifying, or deleting, this work is done through the File Maintenance Menu (Menu 2).

MODIFYING AN ACCOUNT

You may revise data you previously entered in **The Medical Manager** system by using the File Maintenance Menu (Menu 2). You can add, modify, or delete data in patient records, financial activity records, support files, payment records, procedure histories, and all related files. In most cases, the edit screens are nearly identical to the add screens, and updates within related files are performed automatically within **The Medical Manager** software.

EDITING PATIENT RECORDS

In the next section, you will learn how to edit as you work with a few examples. Because editing circumstances are virtually unlimited, use these examples to help you with similar editing situations in later units.

STEP 1

You should already be at the Main Menu (Menu 1). If not, return to the Main Menu (Menu 1) by keying '/**m1**' and pressing **ENTER**. Using the keyboard or mouse, select option **7**, FILE Maintenance. At the File Maintenance Menu (Menu 2), select option **1**, EDIT Patient Records.

Mr. Davis is currently being treated under his Worker's Compensation policy; therefore, billing statements should not be mailed to him. In order to modify Mr. Davis's account, you must first retrieve his account. If you are not familiar with this process, review the previous section on retrieving the patient's account.

When you added new patient information, you filled out a series of screens for each account. These included the guarantor information, any dependent information, and any insurance information or extended information. Screens were presented sequentially and automatically to allow you to quickly enter the account and dependent information. However when editing an account, you must first tell the computer which screen you want to go to to make changes. Once you have retrieved your patient's information, the first screen that is displayed is the Guarantor Information screen, which contains guarantor and account information. To change something on this screen, you will choose (**M**)odify. If you wish to change information on the insurance screen you will choose (**I**)nsurance. If you want to change the dependent information, you will choose (**D**)ependents. If you want to change the extended information, you will choose (**E**)xtended. When Mr. Davis's information is displayed on the screen, choose (**M**)odify account information. In the field called Bill Type, key '**10**', which marks the account to not receive a statement.

STEP 2

Compare your screen with Figure 4-4. Press **F1** or click on the PROCESS button ('√') and then press **ESCAPE** or click on the EXIT button to exit the screen.

Figure 4-4 Modify Guarantor Information Screen

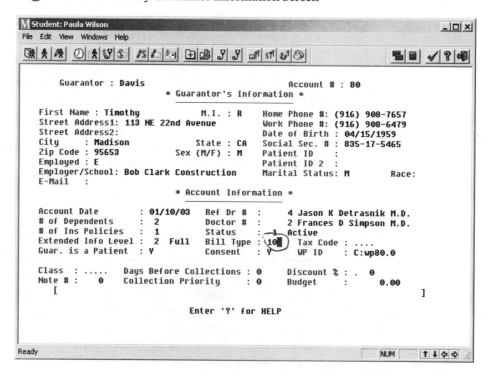

Exercise 1: Changing a Patient's Last Name

Mrs. Patricia Evans calls and says she has changed her marital status and is going back to her maiden name, which is Green.

STEP 1 From the File Maintenance menu select option **1** EDIT Patient Records and retrieve her account. Key (**M**)odify and press **ENTER**. The cursor will be located in the guarantor last name field. Press **F10** to clear the field and enter her maiden name "Green". Using the down arrow key or the mouse move your cursor to the marital status field and change her marital status by keying (**S**)ingle in the field .

STEP 2 Compare your screen with Figure 4-5. Press **F1** or click the PROCESS button ('√').

Note: Patricia Evans did not have any dependents. If she had any dependents, changing the guarantor's name would not automatically change the name of any dependents. Therefore, if it were desirable to change all of the members of the family's last name. you would go to each family member and change the dependent's last name, repeating the process for each member of the family.

Figure 4-5 Changing a Patient's Last Name

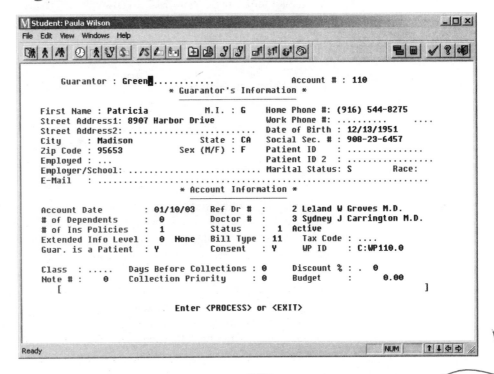

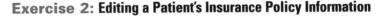

Exercise 2: Editing a Patient's Insurance Policy Information

Timothy Davis's employer calls your office and says that their Worker's Compensation carrier requires that you put the name of the division that Mr. Davis works for in the group name or number field.

STEP 1 From the File Maintenance menu select Option **1** EDIT Patient Records and retrieve Mr. Davis's account. Select (**I**)nsurance, and when the list of plans is displayed, choose Plan

12 Fringe Benefit Center by positioning the lightbar on Plan 12 Fringe Benefit Center and using your mouse or pressing **ENTER** to select the particular policy. Choose (**M**)odify and move your cursor to the group name or number field. Move the cursor to the end of the text Bob Clark Construction and add the text "**Div. 3**". Be sure you are at the end of the line so that you do not type over the name Bob Clark Construction. If you make an error, simply retype the entire text of the line.

STEP 2

When you have completed the entry, compare your screen with Figure 4-6. Press **F1** or click the PROCESS button ('√') to save your changes.

Figure 4-6 Timothy Davis's Worker's Compensation Policy

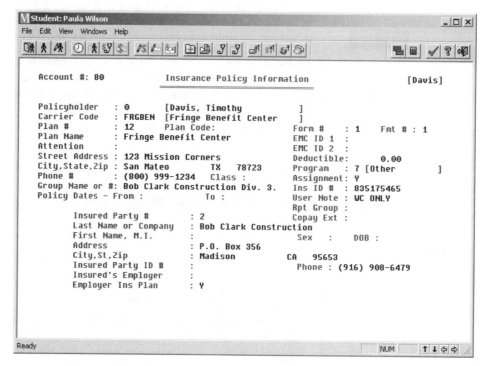

Notice that when you were editing Mr. Davis's insurance policy information, the cursor did not move to the name and address of the insurance plan. Only insurance policy fields were available, and these include the assignment, group name, policy dates, insurance ID, user note, report group, copay, and insured party information. Information about the plan, such as the plan address and telephone numbers, are edited from Support File Maintenance, Insurance Plan File. This is because plan information is shared across many patients within your practice. Similarly, if you needed to make a change to the Insured Party Information, you would change it through Support File Maintenance, Insured Party File Maintenance.

MODIFYING SUPPORT FILE ENTRIES

Similar to modifying entries in patient records, support files within **The Medical Manager** may also be changed. When information is changed in a support file, however, it affects all patients who are using that particular piece of data. Support File Maintenance programs allow you to retrieve items to be edited either by directly entering the desired code or number of the person, company, or item to be modified or by entering "?" for help in the first field of the screen. This will display a Help window of that particular type of support file information and will allow you to search that support file information by either code, description, name, or number according to the type of information you are looking for.

Exercise 3: Modifying a Referring Doctor

Dr. Summerfield's office called to report that there is a mistake in the address and that the address is simply **3434 Alafaya Trail**.

STEP 1 From the Main Menu select FILE MAINTENANCE (Menu 2), and from File Maintenance, select Option **3**, SUPPORT FILE MAINTENANCE. On the Support File Maintenance menu select Option **7**, REFERRING DOCTOR FILE. Once the Referring Doctor Maintenance screen is displayed, you may directly enter the number of the referring doctor if you know it or enter "**?**" for Help. In this exercise, enter "**?**" for help and locate referring doctor **Justine Summerfield**. Position the lightbar or mouse cursor on Dr. Summerfield and press **ENTER**. Choose (**M**)odify then move the cursor to the first line of the address field. Move the cursor to the end of the address field and using your backspace key, delete the abbreviation for "**Blvd**".

STEP 2 When you have completed this exercise, compare your work with Figure 4-7. Press **F1** or click the PROCESS ('√') button to save your work and EXIT back to the menu.

Editing of any other type of support file information is very similar to this process.

Figure 4-7 Editing the Referring Doctor

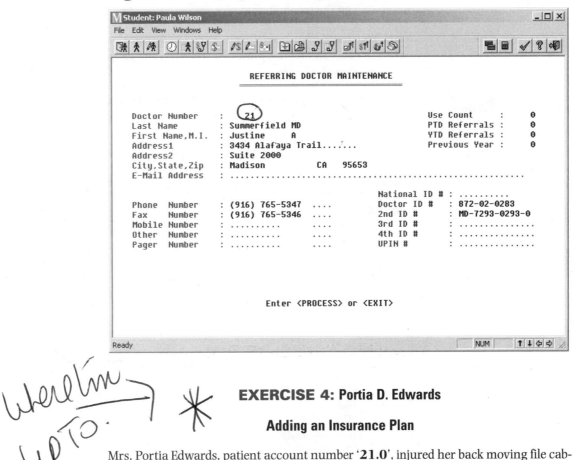

EXERCISE 4: Portia D. Edwards

Adding an Insurance Plan

Mrs. Portia Edwards, patient account number '**21.0**', injured her back moving file cabinets at work. She will be treated under her business insurance plan (a Worker's Compensation policy). Because information about this insurance plan is not on file, it must be added as an additional insurance plan before charges relating to her injury can be posted.

STEP 1

From the File Maintenance Menu (Menu 2), select option **1**, EDIT Patient Records, retrieve her account, select **(I)**nsurance, and when the existing plan is displayed, choose the **(A)**dd option. Enter the following information:

Policyholder: **0**
Carrier Code: **BENIND**
Plan #: **9** (Beneficial Industrial Co.)
Assignment (Y/N): **Y**
Group Name: **Portia Property Mgmt**.
(Since no Policy Dates are provided, press **ENTER** to bypass these fields)
Insurance ID #: **807152**
User Note: **WC only** (this means Worker's Compensation only)
(Press **ENTER** to bypass the Rpt Group and Copay Ext. fields, since no information is provided)
Insured Party #: 'Press **ENTER**, then select **(N)**ew. **The Medical Manager** system will provide the number'
Company Name: **Portia Property Mgmt**.
(Press **ENTER** to bypass the Sex and DOB fields, which do not apply since a company name is given)
Company Address: **487 James Road**
City, State, Zip: **Madison CA 95653**

Press **ENTER** to bypass each of the next three fields. Answer **(Y)**es to Employer Ins Plan. Compare your screen with Figure 4-8, then press **F1** or click on the PROCESS button ('√') on the top toolbar to process.

Note: You may also modify or delete insurance information or display the patient's other insurance plans by selecting the proper command at the prompt at the bottom of the screen.

STEP 2

Next, coverage priority needs to be set. Press **ESCAPE** or click on the EXIT button on the top toolbar; then choose **(S)**et Coverage Priority from the bottom of the Insurance

Figure 4-8 Insurance Plan with Insured Party Information Screen

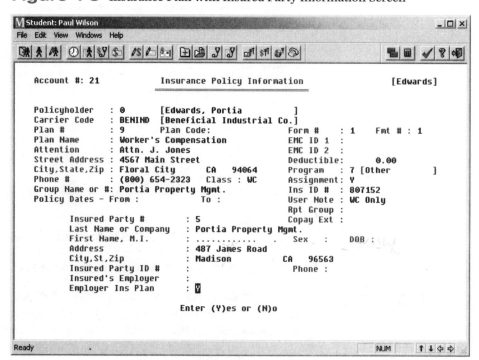

Policies Maintenance screen. Mrs. Edwards's name will be highlighted. Press **ENTER** or double-click on Mrs. Edwards's account to edit her coverage priority. Choose '**M**' to maintain her list. Press **ENTER** to bypass the fields in her primary insurance and add Insurance Plan # **9.0** as her secondary insurance. Enter '**O**' for (O)ther in the Relation to IPR field and press **ENTER**. The User Note will be used when posting to ensure the correct plan is being billed. Press **F1** or click on the PROCESS button ('√') to process and save this information.

STEP 3

Once you have processed the information, press **ESCAPE** or click on the EXIT button on the top toolbar to return to the Coverage Priority By Dependent screen. Notice that the two dependent insurance priorities read "Use Guarantor List." This was appropriate until we added the Worker's Compensation policy to the Guarantor (Portia) List. However, because the Worker's Compensation policy does not cover the dependents, it is now necessary to remove it from the dependents' Insurance Coverage Priority list.

Use the down arrow key to highlight the name of Mrs. Edwards's first dependent, Edward Edwards, and press **ENTER** or using the mouse, double-click on Edward Edwards to highlight and select his account. When Mr. Edwards's Insurance Coverage Priority screen appears, choose '**M**', then use the ENTER key or the mouse pointer to move the cursor to the Secondary Insurance Plan field. Press **F10** to clear this field. Press **ENTER** again and you will see that the Worker's Compensation policy has been removed from his coverage list. Then, press **F1** or click on the PROCESS button ('√') to process the screen. Repeat the same procedure for Mrs. Edwards's other dependent (Andrea Edwards). You have now created an updated Coverage Priority List for each dependent.

At this point, if you plan to proceed to Exercise 5, press **ESCAPE** *or click on the EXIT button on the top toolbar until you see the Update Patient Information screen.*

APPLYING YOUR KNOWLEDGE

EXERCISE 5: Changing a Patient's Last Name

Patricia Green (formerly Evans) called back and says she has decided not to revert to her maiden name. She wishes you to change the last name on her account back from Green to Evans.

Using what you learned in previous exercises, find the Edit Patient Records option and retrieve the account belonging to Patricia Green. Choose (**M**)odify and change her last name back to Evans. Save your changes by pressing **F1** or clicking the PROCESS button ('√').

EXERCISE 6: Terry L. Williams

Adding Dependents to an Existing Account

Today, Ms. Terry Williams will bring in her other two children, who must be added to her account before charges can be posted for them.

STEP 1

At the Update Patient Information screen, key '**Williams,Terry**' and press **ENTER** to retrieve Ms. Williams's account. Note that you will see the highlight bar covering Terry Williams's name. Press **ENTER** or double-click on Ms. Williams's name to retrieve more detailed information about the account and note the options shown at the bottom of the screen. Select (**D**)ependents to bring up Dependent Information. You will see then the Dependent Information Maintenance screen that allows you to change information about the dependents already listed, or to add new dependents.

Because your task is to add new dependents, select (**A**)dd. A new Dependent Information screen will be displayed. Using the information provided on the patient registration form shown in Figure 4-9, complete the screen for Thomas Williams. Note that information about the dependent's school is considered Extended Information.

Figure 4-9 Thomas Williams—Patient Registration Form

Patient Registration Form

Sydney Carrington & Associates
34 Sycamore Street • Madison, CA 95653

TODAY'S DATE: _02/03/2003_

PATIENT INFORMATION

Williams	_Thomas_	_C._
PATIENT LAST NAME	FIRST NAME	MI

Son
RELATIONSHIP TO GUARANTOR

_M_	_02/11/1993_	_Single_	_566-11-8852_
SEX (M/F)	DATE OF BIRTH	MARITAL STATUS	SOC. SEC. #

Wallace Elementary
EMPLOYER OR SCHOOL NAME

ADDRESS OF EMPLOYER OR SCHOOL

Wallace	_CA_	
CITY	STATE	ZIP CODE

	Leland Groves, M.D.
EMPLOYER OR SCHOOL PHONE	REFERRED BY

E-MAIL

GUARANTOR INFORMATION

Williams	_Terry_	_L._	_F_
RESPONSIBLE PARTY LAST NAME	FIRST NAME	MI	SEX (M/F)

P.O. Box 609	_207 Chestnut Street_
MAILING ADDRESS	STREET ADDRESS (IF DIFFERENT)

Wallace	_CA_	_95039_
CITY	STATE	ZIP CODE

_(916) 875-3256_	_(916) 875-3963_
(AREA CODE) HOME PHONE	(AREA CODE) WORK PHONE

_01/04/1960_	_Single_	_972-65-8971_
DATE OF BIRTH	MARITAL STATUS	SOC. SEC. #

Comptech Research
EMPLOYER NAME

693 Industrial Park Road
EMPLOYER ADDRESS

Palo Alto	_CA_	_94033_
CITY	STATE	ZIP CODE

PRIMARY INSURANCE

Health Maintenance Organization
NAME OF PRIMARY INSURANCE COMPANY

6632 3rd Avenue
ADDRESS

New York	_NY_	_10017_
CITY	STATE	ZIP CODE

_2289669820_	_Comptech Research_
IDENTIFICATION #	GROUP NAME AND/OR #

Terry Williams
INSURED PERSON'S NAME (IF DIFFERENT FROM THE RESPONSIBLE PARTY)

P.O. Box 609	_207 Chestnut Street_
ADDRESS (IF DIFFERENT)	

Wallace	_CA_	_95039_
CITY	STATE	ZIP CODE

_(800) 999-1234_	_972-65-8971_
PRIMARY INSURANCE PHONE NUMBER	SOC. SEC. #

Self
WHAT IS THE RESPONSIBLE PARTY'S RELATIONSHIP TO THE INSURED?

SECONDARY INSURANCE

NAME OF SECONDARY INSURANCE COMPANY

ADDRESS

CITY	STATE	ZIP CODE

IDENTIFICATION #	GROUP NAME AND/OR #

INSURED PERSON'S NAME (IF DIFFERENT FROM THE RESPONSIBLE PARTY)

ADDRESS (IF DIFFERENT)

CITY	STATE	ZIP CODE

SECONDARY INSURANCE PHONE NUMBER	SOC. SEC. #

WHAT IS THE RESPONSIBLE PARTY'S RELATIONSHIP TO THE INSURED?

I hereby consent for Sydney Carrington & Associates, P.A. to use or disclose my health information to carry out treatment, payment, and health care operations. I authorize the use of this signature on all insurance submissions. I understand that I am financially responsible for all charges whether or not paid by the insurance. I acknowledge receipt of the practice's privacy policy.

Terry L. Williams (Mother)	_02/03/2003_
PATIENT SIGNATURE	DATE

STEP 2

Thomas will automatically be assigned patient number 120.3 (as dependent number 3 on account 120) when the screen is completed. Key the date of 02/02/03 at the Date Became a Patient field. Compare your screen with Figure 4-10, then press **F1** or click on the PROCESS button ('√') on the top toolbar to process. Complete the Extended Information screen and process. Press **ESCAPE** or click on the EXIT button to get back to the Dependent Maintenance screen.

Figure 4-10 Additional Dependent Screen

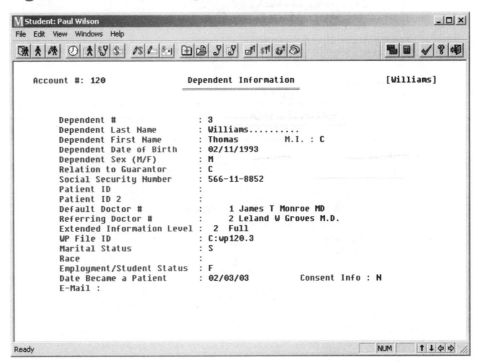

Select (**A**)dd to set up Janet, Terry Williams's final unlisted child. Complete the screen for Janet using the information provided in the patient registration form shown in Figure 4-11. Your screen should be similar to Figure 4-12. Press **F1** or click on the PROCESS button ('√') on the top toolbar to process the information about Janet.

Figure 4-11   Janet Williams—Patient Registration Form

Patient Registration Form

Sydney Carrington & Associates
34 Sycamore Street ● Madison, CA 95653

TODAY'S DATE: _02/03/2003_

FOR OFFICE USE ONLY	
ACCOUNT NO.:	**120**
DOCTOR:	**#1**
BILL TYPE:	**11**
EXTENDED INFO.:	**2**

PATIENT INFORMATION

Williams	_Janet_	_L._
PATIENT LAST NAME	FIRST NAME	MI

Daughter
RELATIONSHIP TO GUARANTOR

_F_	_10/02/1996_	_Single_	_563-18-4317_
SEX (M/F)	DATE OF BIRTH	MARITAL STATUS	SOC. SEC. #

Wallace Elementary
EMPLOYER OR SCHOOL NAME

ADDRESS OF EMPLOYER OR SCHOOL

Wallace	_CA_	
CITY	STATE	ZIP CODE

	Leland Groves, M.D.
EMPLOYER OR SCHOOL PHONE	REFERRED BY

E-MAIL

GUARANTOR INFORMATION

Williams	_Terry_	_L._	_F_
RESPONSIBLE PARTY LAST NAME	FIRST NAME	MI	SEX (M/F)

P.O. Box 609	_207 Chestnut Street_
MAILING ADDRESS	STREET ADDRESS (IF DIFFERENT)

Wallace	_CA_	_95039_
CITY	STATE	ZIP CODE

_(916) 875-3256_	_(916) 875-3963_
(AREA CODE) HOME PHONE	(AREA CODE) WORK PHONE

_01/04/1960_	_Single_	_972-65-8971_
DATE OF BIRTH	MARITAL STATUS	SOC. SEC. #

Comptech Research
EMPLOYER NAME

693 Industrial Park Road
EMPLOYER ADDRESS

Palo Alto	_CA_	_94033_
CITY	STATE	ZIP CODE

PRIMARY INSURANCE

Health Maintenance Organization
NAME OF PRIMARY INSURANCE COMPANY

6632 3rd Avenue
ADDRESS

New York	_NY_	_10017_
CITY	STATE	ZIP CODE

_2289669820_	_Comptech Research_
IDENTIFICATION #	GROUP NAME AND/OR #

Terry Williams
INSURED PERSON'S NAME (IF DIFFERENT FROM THE RESPONSIBLE PARTY)

P.O. Box 609	_207 Chestnut Street_
ADDRESS (IF DIFFERENT)	

Wallace	_CA_	_95039_
CITY	STATE	ZIP CODE

_(800) 999-1234_	_972-65-8971_
PRIMARY INSURANCE PHONE NUMBER	SOC. SEC. #

Self
WHAT IS THE RESPONSIBLE PARTY'S RELATIONSHIP TO THE INSURED?

SECONDARY INSURANCE

NAME OF SECONDARY INSURANCE COMPANY

ADDRESS

CITY	STATE	ZIP CODE

IDENTIFICATION #	GROUP NAME AND/OR #

INSURED PERSON'S NAME (IF DIFFERENT FROM THE RESPONSIBLE PARTY)

ADDRESS (IF DIFFERENT)

CITY	STATE	ZIP CODE

SECONDARY INSURANCE PHONE NUMBER	SOC. SEC. #

WHAT IS THE RESPONSIBLE PARTY'S RELATIONSHIP TO THE INSURED?

I hereby consent for Sydney Carrington & Associates, P.A. to use or disclose my health information to carry out treatment, payment, and health care operations. I authorize the use of this signature on all insurance submissions. I understand that I am financially responsible for all charges whether or not paid by the insurance. I acknowledge receipt of the practice's privacy policy.

Terry L. Williams (Mother)	_02/03/2003_
PATIENT SIGNATURE	DATE

Figure 4-12 Additional Dependent Screen

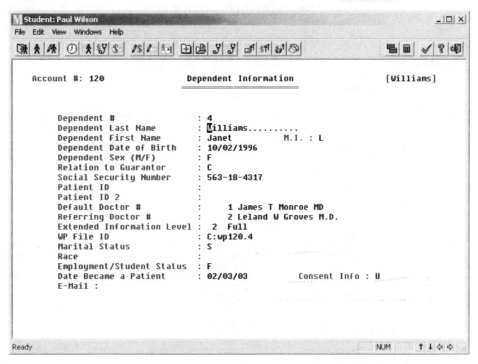

```
M Student: Paul Wilson                                              _ |□| X|
File  Edit  View  Windows  Help

[toolbar icons]


   Account #: 120                Dependent Information           [Williams]



          Dependent #                : 4
          Dependent Last Name        : Williams..........
          Dependent First Name       : Janet          M.I. : L
          Dependent Date of Birth    : 10/02/1996
          Dependent Sex (M/F)        : F
          Relation to Guarantor      : C
          Social Security Number     : 563-18-4317
          Patient ID                 :
          Patient ID 2               :
          Default Doctor #           :    1 James T Monroe MD
          Referring Doctor #         :    2 Leland W Groves M.D.
          Extended Information Level :  2  Full
          WP File ID                 : C:wp120.4
          Marital Status             : S
          Race                       :
          Employment/Student Status  : F
          Date Became a Patient      : 02/03/03        Consent Info : U
          E-Mail :




Ready                                              NUM      ↑ ↓ ⇦ ⇨
```

Press **ESCAPE** or click on the EXIT button until you are returned to the Main Menu (Menu 1).

EXERCISE 7: Janet S. Williams

Posting Charges for a New Patient

Charges must be posted for Janet and Thomas Williams from each of their encounter forms. From the Main Menu (Menu 1), use the mouse or keyboard to choose option **2**, PROCEDURE Entry. Key '**120.4**' and press **ENTER** to retrieve Janet Williams's account.

STEP 1 Janet is seen for the flu. Post the charges from her encounter form, Figure 4-13. Remember to press ENTER to bypass fields for which no information is provided.

Figure 4-13 Janet Williams's Encounter Form—Voucher 1058

Sydney Carrington & Associates P.A.
34 Sycamore Street   Suite 300
Madison, CA 95653

Date: 02/03/2003

Time: 09:45

Patient: Janet Williams
Guarantor: Terry L. Williams

Voucher No.: 1058

Patient No: 120.4

Doctor: 1 - J. Monroe

CPT	DESCRIPTION	FEE		CPT	DESCRIPTION	FEE		CPT	DESCRIPTION	FEE
OFFICE/HOSPITAL CONSULTS				**LABORATORY/RADIOLOGY**				**PROCEDURES/TESTS**		
☐ 99201	Office New:Focused Hx-Exam			☐ 81000	Urinalysis			☐ 00452	Anesthesia for Rad Surgery	
☐ 99202	Office New:Expanded Hx-Exam			☐ 81002	Urinalysis; Pregnancy Test			☐ 11100	Skin Biopsy	
☐ 99211	Office Estb:Min/None Hx-Exa			☐ 82951	Glucose Tolerance Test			☐ 15852	Dressing Change	
☒ 99212	Office Estb:Focused Hx-Exam	$30.00		☐ 84478	Triglycerides			☐ 29075	Cast Appl. - Lower Arm	
☐ 99213	Office Estb:Expanded Hx-Exa			☐ 84550	Uric Acid: Blood Chemistry			☐ 29530	Strapping of Knee	
☐ 99214	Office Estb:Detailed Hx-Exa			☐ 84830	Ovulation Test			☐ 29705	Removal/Revis of Cast w/Exa	
☐ 99215	Office Estb:Comprhn Hx-Exam			☐ 85014	Hematocrit			☐ 53670	Catheterization Incl. Suppl	
☐ 99221	Hosp. Initial:Comprh Hx-			☐ 85031	Hemogram, Complete Blood Wk			☐ 57452	Colposcopy	
☐ 99223	Hosp.Ini:Comprh Hx-Exam/Hi			☐ 86403	Particle Agglutination Test			☐ 57505	ECC	
☐ 99231	Hosp. Subsequent: S-Fwd			☐ 86485	Skin Test; Candida			☐ 69420	Myringotomy	
☐ 99232	Hosp. Subsequent: Comprhn Hx			☐ 86580	TB Intradermal Test			☐ 92081	Visual Field Examination	
☐ 99233	Hosp. Subsequent: Ex/Hi			☐ 86585	TB Tine Test			☐ 92100	Serial Tonometry Exam	
☐ 99238	Hospital Visit Discharge Ex			☐ 87070	Culture			☐ 92120	Tonography	
☐ 99371	Telephone Consult - Simple			☐ 70190	X-Ray; Optic Foramina			☐ 92552	Pure Tone Audiometry	
☐ 99372	Telephone Consult - Intermed			☐ 70210	X-Ray Sinuses Complete			☐ 92567	Tympanometry	
☐ 99373	Telephone Consult - Complex			☐ 71010	Radiological Exam Ent Spine			☐ 93000	Electrocardiogram	
☐ 90843	Counseling - 25 minutes			☐ 71020	X-Ray Chest Pa & Lat			☐ 93015	Exercise Stress Test (ETT)	
☐ 90844	Counseling - 50 minutes			☐ 72050	X-Ray Spine, Cerv (4 views)			☐ 93017	ETT Tracing Only	
☐ 90865	Counseling - Special Interview			☐ 72090	X-Ray Spine; Scoliosis Ex			☐ 93040	Electrocardiogram - Rhythm	
				☐ 72110	Spine, lumbosacral; a/p & Lat			☐ 96100	Psychological Testing	
IMMUNIZATIONS/INJECTIONS				☐ 73030	Shoulder-Comp, min w/ 2vws			☐ 99000	Specimen Handling	
☐ 90585	BCG Vaccine			☐ 73070	Elbow, anteropost & later vws			☐ 99058	Office Emergency Care	
☐ 90659	Influenza Virus Vaccine			☐ 73120	X-Ray; Hand, 2 views			☐ 99070	Surgical Tray - Misc.	
☐ 90701	Immunization-DTP			☐ 73560	X-Ray, Knee, 1 or 2 views			☐ 99080	Special Reports of Med Rec	
☐ 90702	DT Vaccine			☐ 74022	X-Ray; Abdomen, Complete			☐ 99195	Phlebotomy	
☐ 90703	Tetanus Toxoids			☐ 75552	Cardiac Magnetic Res Img			☐	_____	
☐ 90732	Pneumococcal Vaccine			☐ 76020	X-Ray; Bone Age Studies			☐	_____	
☐ 90746	Hepatitis B Vaccine			☐ 76088	Mammary Ductogram Complete			☐	_____	
☐ 90749	Immunization; Unlisted			☐ 78465	Myocardial Perfusion Img			☐	_____	

ICD-9	CODE DIAGNOSIS		ICD-9	CODE DIAGNOSIS		ICD-9	CODE DIAGNOSIS
☐ 009.0	Ill-defined Intestinal Infect		☐ 435.0	Basilar Artery Syndrome		☐ 724.2	Pain: Lower Back
☐ 133.2	Establish Baseline		☐ 440.0	Atherosclerosis		☐ 727.6	Rupture of Achilles Tendon
☐ 174.9	Breast Cancer		☐ 442.81	Carotid Artery		☐ 780.1	Hallucinations
☐ 185.0	Prostate Cancer		☐ 460.0	Common Cold		☐ 780.3	Convulsions
☐ 250	Diabetes Mellitus		☐ 461.9	Acute Sinusitis		☐ 780.5	Sleep Disturbances
☐ 272.4	Hyperlipidemia		☐ 474.0	Tonsillitis		☐ 783.0	Anorexia
☐ 282.5	Anemia - Sickle Trait		☐ 477.9	Hay Fever		☐ 783.1	Abnormal Weight Gain
☐ 282.60	Anemia - Sickle Cell		☒ 487.0	Flu		☐ 783.2	Abnormal Weight Loss
☐ 285.9	Anemia, Unspecified		☐ 496	Chronic Airway Obstruction		☐ 830.6	Dislocated Hip
☐ 300.4	Neurotic Depression		☐ 522	Low Red Blood Count		☐ 830.9	Dislocated Shoulder
☐ 340	Multiple Sclerosis		☐ 524.6	Temporo-Mandibular Jnt Synd		☐ 841.2	Sprained Wrist
☐ 342.9	Hemiplegia - Unspecified		☐ 538.8	Stomach Pain		☐ 842.5	Sprained Ankle
☐ 346.9	Migraine Headache		☐ 553.3	Hiatal Hernia		☐ 891.2	Fractured Tibia
☐ 352.9	Cranial Neuralgia		☐ 564.1	Spastic Colon		☐ 892.0	Fractured Fibula
☐ 354.0	Carpal Tunnel Syndrome		☐ 571.4	Chronic Hepatitis		☐ 919.5	Insect Bite, Nonvenomous
☐ 355.0	Sciatic Nerve Root Lesion		☐ 571.5	Cirrhosis of Liver		☐ 921.1	Contus Eyelid/Perioc Area
☐ 366.9	Cataract		☐ 573.3	Hepatitis		☐ v16.3	Fam. Hist of Breast Cancer
☐ 386.0	Vertigo		☐ 575.2	Obstruction of Gallbladder		☐ v17.4	Fam. Hist of Cardiovasc Dis
☐ 401.1	Essential Hypertension		☐ 648.2	Anemia - Compl. Pregnancy		☐ v20.2	Well Child
☐ 414.9	Ischemic Hearth Disease		☐ 715.90	Osteoarthritis - Unspec		☐ v22.0	Pregnancy - First Normal
☐ 428.0	Congestive Heart Failure		☐ 721.3	Lumbar Osteo/Spondylarthrit		☐ v22.1	Pregnancy - Normal

Previous Balance	Today's Charges	Total Due	Amount Paid	New Balance
_____	_____	_____	_____	_____

Follow Up

PRN _____ Weeks _____ Months _____ Units _____

Next Appointment Date: _____   Time: _____

I hereby authorize release of any information acquired in the course of examination or treatment and allow a photocopy of my signature to be used.

_____

STEP 2 Compare your screen with Figure 4-14. When you have made sure that all information has been entered correctly, press **F1** or click on the PROCESS button ('√') to process, then select '**O**' for no ailment and press **ENTER**. The screen will automatically be processed and when you check in the lower half of the screen you will see that the charge has been posted.

Figure 4-14 Janet Williams's Procedure Entry Screen

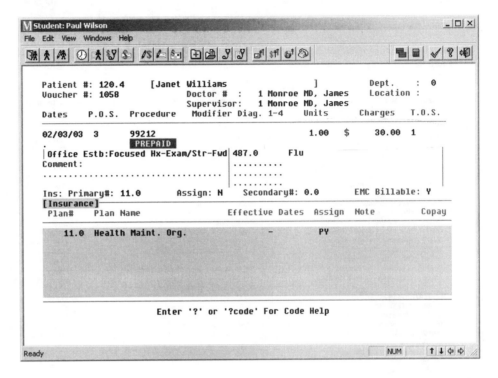

Because no other charges appear on Janet's encounter form, press **ESCAPE** twice or click twice on the EXIT button on the top toolbar to return to the Procedure Entry Patient Retrieval screen.

EXERCISE 8: Thomas C. Williams

Posting Charges for Another New Patient

Charges must now be posted for Thomas Williams. From the Procedure Entry Patient Retrieval screen, key '**120.3**' and press **ENTER** to retrieve Thomas's account.

STEP 1 Like his sister, Thomas is also seen for the flu. Use the information shown in Thomas's encounter form (Figure 4-15) to post his charges, as you did for his sister Janet. Remember to press ENTER to bypass each field for which you have no information.

STEP 2 Compare your screen with Figure 4-16. When you have made sure that all information has been entered correctly, press **F1** or click on the PROCESS button ('√') on the top toolbar to process, then select '**O**' for no ailment and press **ENTER**. The screen will automatically be processed and in the lower half of the screen you will see that the charge has been posted.

Because no other charges appear on Thomas's encounter form, press **ESCAPE** or click on the EXIT button to return to Procedure Entry. Press **ESCAPE** twice again or click twice on the EXIT button to return to the Main Menu (Menu 1) and begin Exercise 9.

Figure 4-15 Thomas Williams's Encounter Form—Voucher 1059

Sydney Carrington & Associates P.A.
34 Sycamore Street   Suite 300
Madison, CA 95653

Date: 02/03/2003

Voucher No.: 1059

Time: 10:00

Patient: Thomas Williams
Guarantor: Terry L. Williams

Patient No: 120.3
Doctor: 1 - J. Monroe

CPT	DESCRIPTION	FEE
OFFICE/HOSPITAL CONSULTS		
99201	Office New:Focused Hx-Exam	
99202	Office New:Expanded Hx-Exam	
99211	Office Estb:Min/None Hx-Exa	
☒ 99212	Office Estb:Focused Hx-Exam	$30.00
99213	Office Estb:Expanded Hx-Exa	
99214	Office Estb:Detailed Hx-Exa	
99215	Office Estb:Comprhn Hx-Exam	
99221	Hosp. Initial:Comprh Hx-	
99223	Hosp.Ini:Comprh Hx-Exam/Hi	
99231	Hosp. Subsequent: S-Fwd	
99232	Hosp. Subsequent: Comprhn Hx	
99233	Hosp. Subsequent: Ex/Hi	
99238	Hospital Visit Discharge Ex	
99371	Telephone Consult - Simple	
99372	Telephone Consult - Intermed	
99373	Telephone Consult - Complex	
90843	Counseling - 25 minutes	
90844	Counseling - 50 minutes	
90865	Counseling - Special Interview	
IMMUNIZATIONS/INJECTIONS		
90585	BCG Vaccine	
90659	Influenza Virus Vaccine	
90701	Immunization-DTP	
90702	DT Vaccine	
90703	Tetanus Toxoids	
90732	Pneumococcal Vaccine	
90746	Hepatitis B Vaccine	
90749	Immunization; Unlisted	

CPT	DESCRIPTION	FEE
LABORATORY/RADIOLOGY		
81000	Urinalysis	
81002	Urinalysis; Pregnancy Test	
82951	Glucose Tolerance Test	
84478	Triglycerides	
☒ 84550	Uric Acid: Blood Chemistry	
84830	Ovulation Test	
85014	Hematocrit	
85031	Hemogram, Complete Blood Wk	
86403	Particle Agglutination Test	
86485	Skin Test; Candida	
86580	TB Intradermal Test	
86585	TB Tine Test	
87070	Culture	
70190	X-Ray; Optic Foramina	
70210	X-Ray Sinuses Complete	
71010	Radiological Exam Ent Spine	
71020	X-Ray Chest Pa & Lat	
72050	X-Ray Spine, Cerv (4 views)	
72090	X-Ray Spine; Scoliosis Ex	
72110	Spine, lumbosacral; a/p & Lat	
73030	Shoulder-Comp, min w/ 2vws	
73070	Elbow, anteropost & later vws	
73120	X-Ray; Hand, 2 views	
73560	X-Ray, Knee, 1 or 2 views	
74022	X-Ray; Abdomen, Complete	
75552	Cardiac Magnetic Res Img	
76020	X-Ray; Bone Age Studies	
76088	Mammary Ductogram Complete	
78465	Myocardial Perfusion Img	

CPT	DESCRIPTION	FEE
PROCEDURES/TESTS		
00452	Anesthesia for Rad Surgery	
11100	Skin Biopsy	
15852	Dressing Change	
29075	Cast Appl. - Lower Arm	
29530	Strapping of Knee	
29705	Removal/Revis of Cast w/Exa	
53670	Catheterization Incl. Suppl	
57452	Colposcopy	
57505	ECC	
69420	Myringotomy	
92081	Visual Field Examination	
92100	Serial Tonometry Exam	
92120	Tonography	
92552	Pure Tone Audiometry	
92567	Tympanometry	
93000	Electrocardiogram	
93015	Exercise Stress Test (ETT)	
93017	ETT Tracing Only	
93040	Electrocardiogram - Rhythm	
96100	Psychological Testing	
99000	Specimen Handling	
99058	Office Emergency Care	
99070	Surgical Tray - Misc.	
99080	Special Reports of Med Rec	
99195	Phlebotomy	

ICD-9 CODE DIAGNOSIS		
009.0	Ill-defined Intestinal Infect	
133.2	Establish Baseline	
174.9	Breast Cancer	
185.0	Prostate Cancer	
250	Diabetes Mellitus	
272.4	Hyperlipidemia	
282.5	Anemia - Sickle Trait	
282.60	Anemia - Sickle Cell	
285.9	Anemia, Unspecified	
300.4	Neurotic Depression	
340	Multiple Sclerosis	
342.9	Hemiplegia - Unspecified	
346.9	Migraine Headache	
352.9	Cranial Neuralgia	
354.0	Carpal Tunnel Syndrome	
355.0	Sciatic Nerve Root Lesion	
366.9	Cataract	
386.0	Vertigo	
401.1	Essential Hypertension	
414.9	Ischemic Hearth Disease	
428.0	Congestive Heart Failure	

ICD-9 CODE DIAGNOSIS		
435.0	Basilar Artery Syndrome	
440.0	Atherosclerosis	
442.81	Carotid Artery	
460.0	Common Cold	
461.9	Acute Sinusitis	
474.0	Tonsillitis	
477.9	Hay Fever	
☒ 487.0	Flu	
496	Chronic Airway Obstruction	
522	Low Red Blood Count	
524.6	Temporo-Mandibular Jnt Synd	
538.8	Stomach Pain	
553.3	Hiatal Hernia	
564.1	Spastic Colon	
571.4	Chronic Hepatitis	
571.5	Cirrhosis of Liver	
573.3	Hepatitis	
575.2	Obstruction of Gallbladder	
648.2	Anemia - Compl. Pregnancy	
715.90	Osteoarthritis - Unspec	
721.3	Lumbar Osteo/Spondylarthrit	

ICD-9 CODE DIAGNOSIS		
724.2	Pain: Lower Back	
727.6	Rupture of Achilles Tendon	
780.1	Hallucinations	
780.3	Convulsions	
780.5	Sleep Disturbances	
783.0	Anorexia	
783.1	Abnormal Weight Gain	
783.2	Abnormal Weight Loss	
830.6	Dislocated Hip	
830.9	Dislocated Shoulder	
841.2	Sprained Wrist	
842.5	Sprained Ankle	
891.2	Fractured Tibia	
892.0	Fractured Fibula	
919.5	Insect Bite, Nonvenomous	
921.1	Contus Eyelid/Perioc Area	
v16.3	Fam. Hist of Breast Cancer	
v17.4	Fam. Hist of Cardiovasc Dis	
v20.2	Well Child	
v22.0	Pregnancy - First Normal	
v22.1	Pregnancy - Normal	

Previous Balance	Today's Charges	Total Due	Amount Paid	New Balance

Follow Up

PRN _____ Weeks _____   Months _____ Units _____

Next Appointment Date: _____   Time: _____

I hereby authorize release of any information acquired in the course of
examination or treatment and allow a photocopy of my signature to be used.

Figure 4-16 Thomas Williams's Procedure Entry Screen

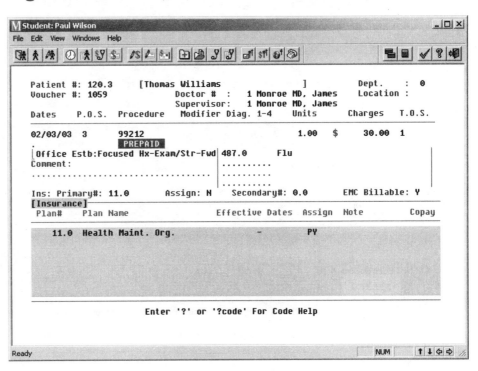

Note: You did not delete a patient record in these exercises; however, you may delete a record with the Edit Patient screen, so long as the patient has no outstanding charges. It is important to note that deleting or canceling a patient record is normally only done if an account has been added twice in error.

EXERCISE 9: Andrea L. Edwards

Editing Activity in a Patient Record

You receive a memo from the doctor, who indicates that the procedure code (99213) posted for Andrea Edwards was incorrect. Change the procedure code to 99214.

STEP 1
From the Main Menu (Menu 1), use the keyboard or mouse to choose option **7**, FILE Maintenance. Then, select option **2**, EDIT Activity Records and retrieve account number '**21.2**'.

The screen shown in Figure 4-17 will appear.

STEP 2
Use the keyboard or mouse to select the line (should be line 1) showing procedure code '**99213**'. (**M**)odify the item and change the procedure code to '**99214**'. Compare your screen with Figure 4-18, then press **F1** or click on the PROCESS button ('√') to process the change.

Press **ESCAPE** twice or click twice on the EXIT button when you have finished.

Note: Under certain conditions, procedure activities can be deleted via EDIT ACTIVITY and reentered in the PROCEDURE ENTRY module. Activity items may be deleted if the item does not have payments or adjustments, has not been daily closed, or insurance billed. Once an item has been daily closed, the doctor

Figure 4-17 Edit Account Activity Screen

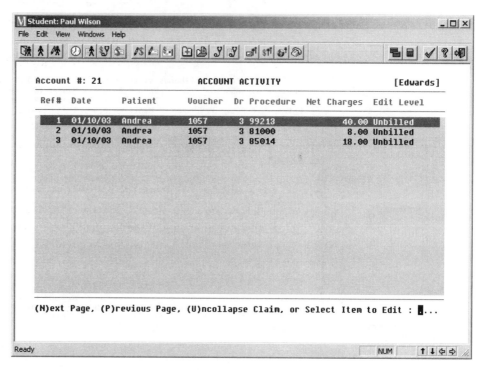

Figure 4-18 Edit Procedure Activity Screen

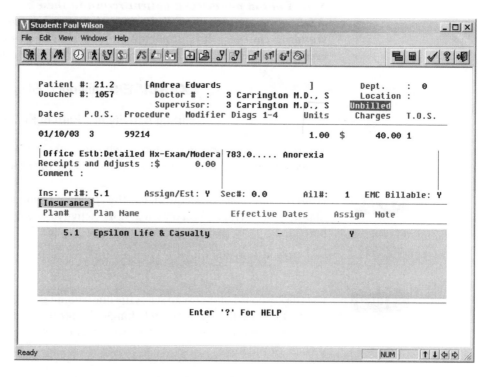

number, department number, charge, and units field may not be edited. Once the item has been billed to the patient's insurance, the doctor number, charge amount, units field, primary plan, and ailment number also may not be edited. This edit protection ensures accounting integrity and a proper audit trail for the office.

EXERCISE 10: Andrea L. Edwards

Editing a Patient's Procedure History

When procedures are posted and a Daily Close is done, this information is stored in a history file. If you must edit procedures after a Daily Close (which you just did at the end of Unit 3), you must also edit the history within **The Medical Manager** software. Now that Andrea's procedure code has been corrected in Edit Activity (see Exercise 9), a separate edit must be made to update the procedure history for the patient.

STEP 1
From the File Maintenance Menu (Menu 2), use the keyboard or mouse to select option **8**, EDIT Procedure History. At the Patient Retrieval screen, retrieve Andrea Edwards's account by keying '**21.2**' and pressing **ENTER**.

STEP 2
Choose to edit (**C**)harges and choose (**A**)ll to view all charges. Use the highlight bar or mouse to select line item of the office visit you wish to modify (**99213**) and press **ENTER**. Advance to the Procedure Code field and type over the field with the new procedure code '**99214**'.

Compare your screen with Figure 4-19, and then press **F1** or click on the PROCESS button ('√') on the top toolbar to process. Press **ESCAPE** twice or click twice on the EXIT button to return to the File Maintenance Menu (Menu 2).

Figure 4-19 Edit Procedure History Changes Screen

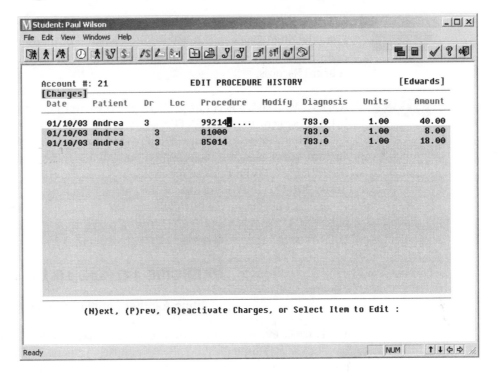

EXERCISE 11: Timothy R. Davis

Editing a Patient's Ailment

October 7.

The doctor wishes to take Mr. Timothy Davis off disability and to note this in his Ailment Detail before any billing occurs. Because Mr. Davis does not have a charge being posted, it is not possible to record this fact through the Procedure Entry screen. Edit Ailment will be used instead (Figure 4-20).

Figure 4-20 Edit Ailment Detail Screen

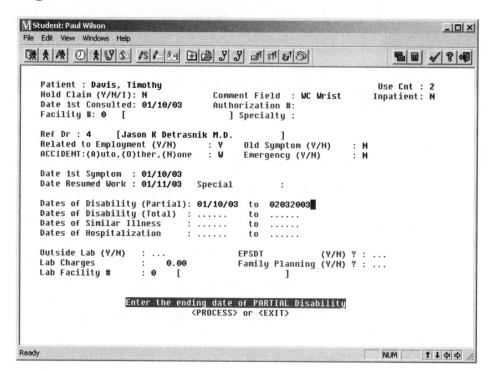

STEP 1 From the Main Menu (Menu 1), use the keyboard or mouse to choose option **7**, FILE Maintenance. Then, from the File Maintenance Menu (Menu 2), select option **9**, EDIT Ailment Records.

STEP 2 Retrieve Mr. Davis's account by keying '**80.0**' and pressing **ENTER** at the Patient Retrieval screen. Press the **ENTER** key again to choose the ailment shown. When the Ailment Detail appears, choose (**M**)odify, then use the ENTER key or mouse to move the cursor to the First Dates of Disability (Partial) field. The beginning date 01/10/03 is correct. Press **ENTER** or use the mouse to move the cursor to the next field and add '**02032003**' as the ending date of the Partial Disability.

Press **F1** or click on the PROCESS button ('√') on the top toolbar to process and then press **ESCAPE** or click on the EXIT button to return to the Patient Retrieval screen of EDIT Ailment. You are now ready to begin Exercise 12.

EXERCISE 12: Patricia G. Evans

Editing Another Patient's Ailment

Ms. Patricia Evans has recently been hospitalized for a serious medical condition, breast cancer. Hospitalization always requires Ailment Detail for date of hospitalization and name and address of the facility. Because some of the information was established when Ms. Evans was last seen in the office, Edit Ailment can now be used to complete the record.

STEP 1 If you attempt to retrieve Ms. Evans's account through the Patient Retrieval screen of Edit Ailments simply by keying '**Evans, Patricia**' and pressing **ENTER**, and you do not see her name listed, press (**N**)ext or click on the right arrow button ('→') on the bottom toolbar until her record is revealed. Then press **ENTER** to retrieve Ms. Evans's account and select the highlighted ailment OR using the mouse, simply double-click on Ms. Evans's account, then double-click on the highlighted ailment to select and modify it.

If you still cannot successfully retrieve her account, you may not have completed Exercise 5. Review that exercise to determine if she is still listed under her maiden name "Green".

STEP 2

The facility number needs to be added. Type '**4**' for Regional Hospital of Madison and press **ENTER**. If you did not know the appropriate number to add, you could use the Help window available for this field. Compare your screen with Figure 4-21.

Figure 4-21 Edit Ailment Detail Screen

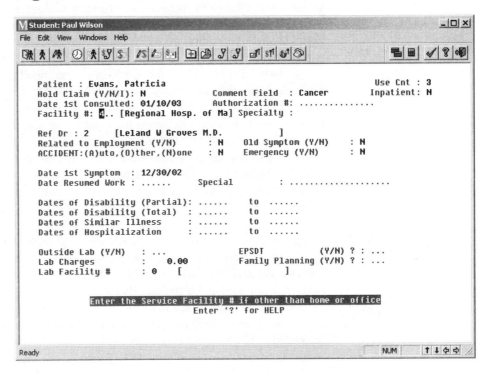

Because Ms. Evans entered the hospital on January 27, 2003 (01/27/03), and left on January 31, 2003 (01/31/03), enter these dates in the Hospitalization fields.

STEP 3

Once you have entered both hospitalization dates, press **F1** or click on the PROCESS button ('√') to process.

Press **ESCAPE** twice or click twice on the EXIT button on the top toolbar to return to the File Maintenance Menu (Menu 2).

UNIT 4 SUMMARY

It is frequently necessary to update information about patients. Patients may change their last name, address, employer, insurance companies, or add new dependents. You can modify account and dependent information by using the Edit Patient option on the File Maintenance menu. Once you retrieve a patient's account, the Guarantor

Information screen will be displayed. If the guarantor is the patient whose information you wish to change, you may choose 'Modify' and edit that information. Changing the guarantor's last name will not change the last name of other dependents on the account.

To edit or change dependent information, select '**D**' for dependents on the Guarantor screen to access a list of dependents on the account. Select the desired dependent and press **ENTER**. You may modify any of the information displayed on the Dependent screen.

To modify a patient's insurance information, from the Guarantor screen choose '**I**' for Insurance and a list of insurance policies on that account will be displayed. To change information about the policy select the desired insurance policy and choose '**M**' to modify. To change the patient's insurance coverage, choose '**S**' to set coverage, and select the desired dependent. You will not change plan address information or insured party address information from Edit Patient. Insurance Plans and Insured Parties are support files, which are edited from Support File Maintenance.

To change Extended Information for a guarantor, choose '**E**' from the Guarantor screen to access 'Extended Information' and then '**M**' to modify. To change Extended Information for a dependent, first choose '**D**' for dependent, then select the dependent, then choose '**E**' to access Extended Information for that dependent, and finally '**M**' to modify. To add Extended Information for either a dependent or a guarantor, follow the same steps to display Extended Information. If Extended Information has not previously been added, the screen will prompt you to choose '**A**' for Add.

To add new dependents to an existing account, select the account. From the Guarantor Information screen, choose '**D**' for Dependent, then choose '**A**' to Add.

Posting errors can be corrected from the File Maintenance menu as well. To edit a charge select option **2** 'Edit Activity Records' and retrieve the appropriate account. A list of activity records (charges) will be displayed. The Edit Level column of the list will display a status of unclosed, closed, unbilled, or billed. The edit level determines what fields may be edited and if the activity can be deleted.

Select the activity record to be modified and choose '**M**' to modify. Make any necessary corrections. Duplicate activity charges erroneously entered into the system can be deleted if they have not been daily closed or have not been billed. Select the activity record to be modified and choose '**D**' to delete.

Once an item is daily closed a copy of some of the charge information is written into the Procedure History file. When editing an activity record that has been daily closed, you will also have to go to option **8** 'Edit Procedure History' on the File Maintenance menu and make similar corrections in the corresponding item in the procedure history file.

Ailment information may also be edited by selecting option **9** 'Edit Ailment Records' on the File Maintenance menu. Retrieve the desired patient and select the desired ailment record. Choose '**M**' to modify. After the ailment information is edited, the edits will apply to insurance bills for all items that are associated with that particular ailment.

Nonpatient information may also be edited in the system. To change information about a referring doctor, from the File Maintenance menu select Support File Maintenance then Referring Doctor Maintenance. Locate the referring doctor by entering the referring doctor number or by using the referring doctor Help window. Once the appropriate doctor is displayed choose '**M**' to modify. Other types of support files can be edited in a similar fashion.

TESTING YOUR KNOWLEDGE

1. Describe any two methods of retrieving an account.

2. Describe how you would change a guarantor's last name. Describe how you would change a dependent's last name.

3. A patient reports that the address for their insurance company has changed. Where would you go to change the company's address?

(continues)

4. List two conditions that would prevent you from editing all of the fields on a charge.

5. Why is insurance coverage order important when adding insurance for dependents?

6. List the steps you would take to change the procedure code on a charge that has been posted and daily closed.

Unit 4

2 methods of retrieving an account? 1

Describe how u would change guarantor's
last name. How 2 change dependent's lastname. 2

List 2 conditions that would prevent you from editing 4 X
all of the fields on a charge.

why's ins. coverage order imp when adding ins. for 5. X
dependents.

List the steps you would take 2 change the procedure
code on a charge that has been posted + daily closed. 6

1) Enter account #. Enter a '/'.

→ Opt. 1 → Edit Pt. Records + retrieve their
account. key in Modify then enter.

3) Go to 1 for Ins. under Edit pt. record
also under opt. 7 file maintenance.

4) 6) File Maintenance.
Option Edit Activity Records
Retrieve Account
Choose Code, then Modify → Enter.

Unit 4 p.189.

2 methods of retrieving an account are

UNITS 1-4 CONCEPTS EVALUATION

I. Match the terms from Column 1 with a related phrase from Column 2.

Column 1

1. ___ Medicare
2. ___ 99213
3. ___ ICD-9
4. ___ Password
5. ___ HMO
6. ___ Guarantor
7. ___ Dependent
8. ___ Insurance plan
9. ___ Insured party
10. ___ Overbooking
11. ___ Encounter form
12. ___ Medicaid
13. ___ 541.2
14. ___ Default

Column 2

a. sample diagnosis code

b. health protection for the poor

c. party responsible for paying the medical account

d. sometimes called carrier or claim center

e. scheduling more than one patient in a time slot

f. individual covered by another's insurance

g. code for secure software access

h. printed device used for communicating treatment and financial information

i. health protection for the elderly and disabled population

j. procedure code

k. built-in, automatic response

l. pay-in-advance health care instead of traditional insurance

m. person covered by insurance

n. universal coding system recognized by insurers

II. Give a one- or two-sentence explanation of the following concepts:

15. Backup copy

16. Default

(continues)

17. Basic insurance coverage

18. Major medical coverage

19. CPT-4

20. ICD-9

III. Outline the flow of information in a medical office using an encounter form as both the beginning and the end of the flow of information.

Office Management/ Appointment Scheduling

LEARNING OUTCOMES

After completing this unit, you should be able to:

◆ Explain the procedure for scheduling and canceling individual and multiple appointments.

◆ Make follow-up appointments from encounter forms.

◆ Explain the (J)ump command.

◆ Discuss the purpose and importance of the daily list of appointments and print this list.

◆ Explain the importance of the Hospital Rounds report and enter the Hospital Rounds information.

◆ Print Hospital Rounds reports.

◆ Use help windows to locate procedure and diagnosis codes for hospital charges.

◆ Explain how the Hospital Rounds reports can be used in place of an encounter form for posting purposes.

Efficient operation of the medical office depends on correct scheduling of appointments. The entire staff depends on a smooth flow of patient traffic in order to maintain a workable schedule. Appointments must allow sufficient time for each patient's medical condition to be treated thoroughly, yet without wasteful time gaps.

MAKING AND CANCELING APPOINTMENTS

One of the most common functions you will perform in the medical office is appointment scheduling. Every day you will schedule appointments for established patients who are already part of the practice, and for new patients who wish to become part of the practice. The appointment schedule shows the names of the patients to be seen each day, the time of each patient's appointment, each patient's telephone number, and reasons for each patient's visit.

The Appointments Toolbar

The Appointments Toolbar (Figure 5-1) contains many shortcut buttons that may be used during appointment scheduling. It is important that you become familiar with the basic function of each button on the Appointments Toolbar before proceeding.

Using the Appointments Toolbar

The Appointments toolbar appears across the top of the Appointments window when Appointment Entry is selected. The shortcuts available on this toolbar are used to save both time and keystrokes when scheduling or modifying an appointment. The toolbar contains the most frequently used Appointment options, and appears as follows:

Figure 5-1 Appointments Toolbar

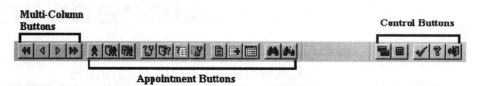

Multicolumn Buttons.

Reading from left to right, the multicolumn buttons on the Appointments Toolbar allow the user to do the following:

Button	Function
Scroll Page Left	Page left to view four additional resources or days
Scroll Column Left	Scroll one column to the left to view one additional resource or day
Scroll Column Right	Scroll one column to the right to view one additional resource or day
Scroll Page Right	Page right to view four additional resources or days

Appointment Buttons.

The appointment buttons allow the user to do the following:

Button	Function
Get Patient	Select another patient for appointment scheduling
Add Patient	Access the New Patient Entry module from within the appointment scheduler
Temporary Patient	Access the Temporary Patient Entry module from within the appointment scheduler
Doctor Help	Select an appointment schedule for a given doctor
Room Help	Select an appointment schedule for a given room
Mode Help	Select the display mode of the appointment schedule
Multiple Resource Set-Up	Select the doctors, rooms, or days to be displayed in multicolumn modes
Waiting List	Display the patient waiting list

Add to Waiting List	Add a patient to the waiting list
Calendar	Jump to a specific day from a full month calendar
Search	Searches for available or existing appointments
Advanced Search	Defines multiple resources required for an appointment (such as a team of physicians, nurses, and therapists whose services are needed within a specific time sequence of one another), searches for them in the schedule, and posts appointments automatically; requires the Advanced Multi-Resource Scheduling Option.
Control	The functions of the control buttons were discussed previously in Unit 1.

Entering Appointments

(J)ump allows you to move through the scheduling calendar.

Appointments for patients and other visitors are scheduled from the Appointments/Recall Menu and by using the Appointments Toolbar. You may make, cancel, and view appointments for any day, doctor, or room. You can also jump any number of days, weeks, months, or years backward or forward. A search function allows you to locate the next available group of free time slots or to search for a specific reason for an appointment.

Mrs. Sharon Carlson calls for an appointment for a General Check-Up in 2 weeks. She would like to come after lunch, around 1:00 P.M., if possible. Complete the following example to understand how appointments are entered into the system.

STEP 1

Using the keyboard or the mouse, select option **8**, OFFICE Management at the Main Menu (Menu 1). Select option **1**, APPOINTMENTS/Recall; the screen shown in Figure 5-2 will appear.

Figure 5-2 Appointments/Recall Menu Screen

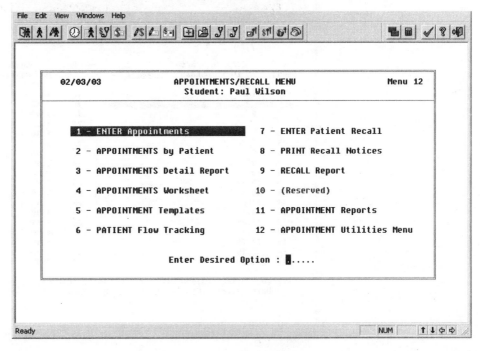

From the Appointments/Recall Menu (Menu 12), select option **1**, ENTER Appointments. The screen shown in Figure 5-3 will appear.

Figure 5-3 Appointment Routine Screen

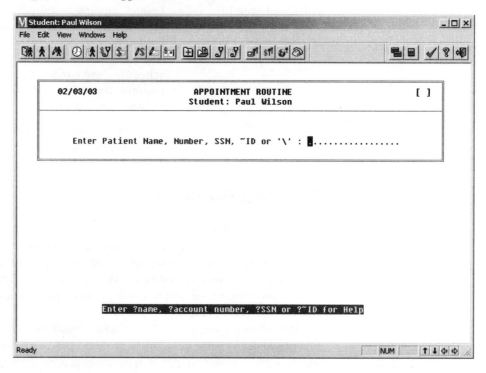

STEP 2

Enter the patient's last name or patient number at the prompt: '**Carlson**'. Then, use the highlight bar to select 'Sharon Carlson' and press **ENTER** or using the mouse, double-click on Sharon Carlson to highlight and select her account. The Appointment screen shown in Figure 5-4 will appear.

Figure 5-4 Appointment Screen

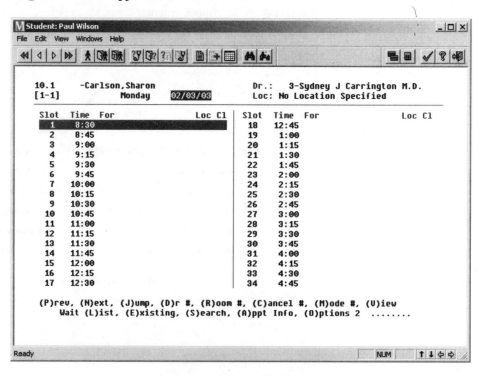

STEP 3

Look at the two command lines at the bottom of the screen. Key '**J**' for (J)ump and press **ENTER**. Note that the screen will automatically default to the number of the patient's primary care physician. Press **ENTER** to accept the default doctor # 3, and the message "Sydney J. Carrington M.D." will appear on the last line of the screen.

You can use (**J**)ump any time you want to schedule a specific appointment date. You can also use the mouse to click on the Calendar button on the top toolbar to choose a specific date.

STEP 4

At the "Weeks from Now" prompt, key the number of weeks until the patient will be seen: '**2**', and press **ENTER**.

Notice that after you press ENTER, the command line changes and the date two weeks ahead (02/17/03) appears in the Date field. Look for the day, date, and doctor at the top of the screen.

STEP 5

Select an available time slot. Each time slot has been assigned a number. Because the patient requested 1:00 P.M., and the slot is available, schedule her for that time. Type '**19**', and press **ENTER** OR using the mouse, double-click in slot 19 to select it.

The command line changes again to display information about the appointment. The first field on the new command line is Reason #. You need to supply a number here that indicates the reason for the appointment.

?Help displays a list of reasons for the visit.

You can use the '?help' feature or click on the Help button ('**?**') on the top toolbar to display the list of Appointment Reason Codes shown in Figure 5-5. In this example, '**1**' is the default reason code since it is the code for a General Check-Up.

Figure 5-5 Appointment Reason Code Help Window

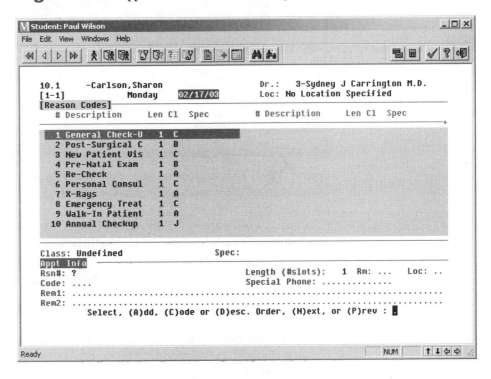

STEP 6

Press **ENTER** to accept the default reason code for a General Check-Up. Note that the appointment information again appears at the bottom of the screen. Press **ENTER** or use the mouse to move the cursor to the Length (# Slots) field. This field is used to indicate the length of the appointment. Mrs. Carlson's appointment is for one 15-minute time slot. Since '1' is the default, press **ENTER** at this field. Press **ENTER** to bypass the remaining fields until you see the message "Make: Dr#3 to see Carlson, Sharon at 1:00

for 15 min." At this point, if you made a mistake, you could press **ESCAPE** or click on the EXIT button on the top toolbar and begin the scheduling process again. However, if your screen is correct, press **F1** or click on the PROCESS button ('√') on the top toolbar to process. Notice that the word "Exists" appears next to Mrs. Carlson's name. This message indicates that an appointment now exists in **The Medical Manager** system for Mrs. Carlson. Your screen should be identical to Figure 5-6.

Press **ESCAPE** or click on the EXIT button on the top toolbar to return to the Appointment Routine Patient Retrieval screen and begin the next exercise.

Figure 5-6 Scheduled Appointment Screen for Sharon Carlson

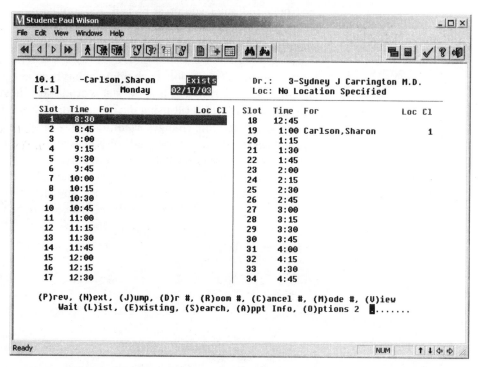

APPLYING YOUR KNOWLEDGE

Several typical appointment situations are given below. Schedule each appointment using the information given. Note that you can use the keyboard or the mouse to complete the instructions shown for each exercise. Additionally, for the Appointment Scheduling exercises, you may also use the functions available through the Appointments Toolbar, explained earlier in this unit.

EXERCISE 1: Portia D. Edwards

An Appointment with Multiple Slots

Mrs. Portia Edwards calls for an appointment for a Personal Consultation (also called a Personal Consult) in two weeks. She would like to come in the late morning. A Personal Consult routinely takes 30 minutes. Therefore, you will need to schedule this appointment to cover two 15-minute time slots.

STEP 1 At the Appointment Routine Patient Retrieval screen, key '**Edwards,Portia**' and press **ENTER**. The lightbar should be on Mrs. Edwards; press **ENTER** or double-click with the mouse to select her from the list. At the first line of the prompts at the bottom of the screen, choose (**J**)ump, and press **ENTER**. Press **ENTER** to accept the default doctor # 3, and the message "Sydney J. Carrington M.D." will appear on the last line. Enter that

Mrs. Edwards wants an appointment '**2**' weeks from now. When the schedule appears, notice that the 1:00 P.M. appointment you made for Sharon Carlson will be displayed on Dr. Carrington's schedule for 2/17/03. Now schedule Mrs. Edwards's appointment to start at 11:30 A.M. (Slot #**13**) and press **ENTER**.

STEP 2

At the Reason # field, key '?' for help or click on the Help button ('?') on the top toolbar. Look for Personal Consult and the reason number that accompanies it. Figure 5-5 shows that the Appointment Reason Code for Personal Consult is reason number 6. Highlight reason code **6**, Personal Consult, and press **ENTER** or using the mouse, double-click on reason code 6 to highlight it and select it.

STEP 3

Now the cursor rests in the "Length (# Slots)" field. Remember, this field is used to indicate the length of the appointment. For Portia Edwards, the *length* of the appointment is equivalent to two 15-minute time slots. Therefore, you enter the number '**2**' in this field, and press **ENTER** until you see the message "Make: Dr#3 to see Edwards,Portia at 11:30 for 30 min." If your screen matches this, press **F1** or click on the PROCESS button ('√') on the top toolbar to process.

Mrs. Edwards's appointment is now set to cover two time slots for a total time of 30 minutes, starting at 11:30 A.M. and ending at noon. Your screen should be similar to Figure 5-7.

Figure 5-7 Scheduled Half-Hour Appointment Screen for Portia Edwards

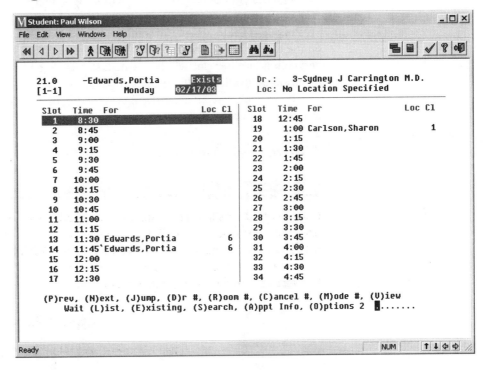

Note: Appointment length is based on the specific reason code selected. Unless an appointment will require extra time, there is no need to change the Length (# Slots) field, since the default = 1.

EXERCISE 2: Deborah A. Evans

An Appointment Conflict

If you are beginning this exercise immediately on completion of Exercise 1, your screen will contain the Appointment Scheduler and the top left corner will show that the last patient for whom you made an appointment was Portia Edwards. In order to make an appointment for a different patient, you need to first retrieve that patient by name. There are two ways to do this: (1) You can ESCAPE back to the Patient Retrieval screen and start from there, or, (2) at the bottom of the current screen, you can choose (O)ptions, then (**G**)et Another Patient, then press **ENTER**. The (**G**)et Another Patient option is especially useful when you want to schedule several patients very quickly.

Mrs. Deborah Evans calls to schedule a General Check-Up at 11:45 A.M. two weeks from now.

STEP 1

At the Appointment Routine Patient Retrieval screen, retrieve Mrs. Evans's account. Check the top of the Appointment Scheduler screen to be sure the date is 02/17/03. Schedule the appointment as you have learned in the previous exercise. You will notice that the time Mrs. Evans has requested is in conflict with Portia Edwards's appointment. However, **The Medical Manager** software allows you to "double book" appointments. That means you can schedule two patients for the same time slot.

STEP 2

Schedule Mrs. Evans's appointment for 11:45 by typing '**14**' at the prompt, then pressing the **ENTER** key. Using the mouse, you could also double-click on slot 14 to highlight and select it simultaneously. Enter the Reason Code '**1**', Length of Slot '**1**', and press **ENTER** through the remaining fields.

A warning message will appear:

Appointment Conflict for Doctor Slot #14: <Enter> or <Exit>

Press **ENTER** to accept the conflict. Press **F1** or click on the PROCESS button ('√') on the top toolbar to process, and the appointment will be assigned to the same time period, but another slot will be created, slot 14.1, which indicates multiple appointments are scheduled for that same time slot.

Check your screen against Figure 5-8 to be sure the appointment has been processed correctly.

Figure 5-8 Screen Showing Double-Booked Appointments

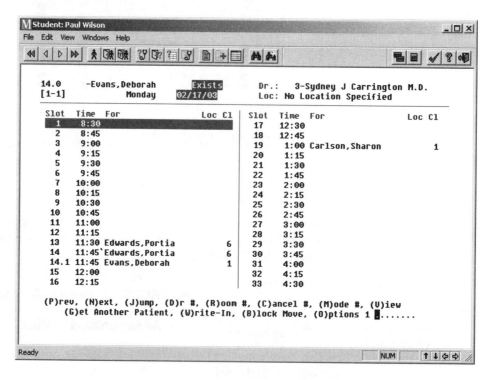

EXERCISE 3: Timothy R. Davis

An Appointment with a Different Doctor

Instead of leaving the Appointment Scheduler screen to retrieve the next patient, you can key (**O**)ptions, then key '**G**' for (G)et Another Patient. This will display the Patient Retrieval screen.

STEP 1
Use the highlight bar or the mouse to select Timothy Davis. The scheduler now returns to the same date and doctor you were previously working with.

STEP 2
Choose (**J**)ump to schedule with Doctor # **2**, Frances Simpson. The appointment is for a General Check-Up on February 17, 2003. Press **ENTER** to (J)ump 0 weeks from now (i.e., February 17) and **ENTER** again to bypass the Location field.

As you schedule this appointment, you will notice that the appointments scheduled previously are not displayed. This is because the schedule currently displayed is for Doctor 2, Frances Simpson, the physician who was assigned to this patient during New Patient Entry.

STEP 3
Key Mr. Davis's appointment at 10:00 A.M. (slot **7**), and press **F1** or click on the PROCESS button ('√') on the top toolbar to process. Compare your screen with Figure 5-9, and you will see Dr. Simpson's name in the upper right corner, as well as the scheduled appointment for Mr. Davis.

Figure 5-9 Different Doctor's Schedule Screen

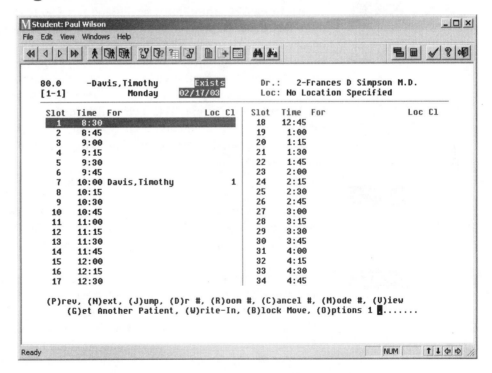

Making Follow-up Appointments

Follow-up appointments are often required by the physician.

Follow-up appointments are scheduled when the physician thinks the patient should be seen again. The reason for the follow-up might be a continuing illness, a recheck of an existing condition, or removal of a cast.

At the time of check out, it is typical for you to post procedure and charge information from the encounter form to the patient's account and then schedule a follow-up appointment for the patient to return. This means you must move often between the Procedure Entry screen and Appointment screen. You may do this through the menus or by using direct chaining. From any menu or retrieval screen, you can key in '/**APP**' and press **ENTER**, or click on the Appointments button (clock face icon) on the top toolbar and the system will take you to Enter Appointments. Keying '/**PRO**' and pressing **ENTER** will take you directly to Procedure Entry. For a list of direct chaining codes, type '/?' and press **ENTER** at any prompt line.

In the following exercises, you will first post a series of charges for patients, using the encounter forms that are given. Then read the doctor's note about a follow-up appointment on the lower right corner of the encounter form and make the appointment as indicated.

APPLYING YOUR KNOWLEDGE

EXERCISE 4: Claire E. League

Posting Procedures and Scheduling an Appointment

Ms. Claire League's encounter form (Figure 5-10) shows two procedure codes and charges. In the lower right corner of the form, it also indicates that she needs a follow-up appointment.

STEP 1   Return to the Procedure Entry screen and post the first charge from her encounter form. Designate '**Medicare**' as her primary insurance and '**Medicare Plus**' as her secondary insurance. Because Ms. League was not seen by her regular doctor, be very careful to not accept the default doctor. Before you process the data for the first procedure compare your screen with Figure 5-11. If all information is correct, press **F1** or click the PROCESS button ('√') on the top toolbar to process. Answer '**0**' for 'None' to the Ailment Detail prompt. When you finish posting the first procedure and are ready to begin posting the second procedure, you will see that the cursor has returned to the Procedure field and that the bottom of the screen lets you know that one procedure has already been processed.

STEP 2   Continue using the encounter form as a guide and post the information for the second procedure. Before processing the data, compare your screen with Figure 5-12. If all information is correct, press **F1** or click on the PROCESS button ('√') to process. Answer '**0**' for 'None' to the Ailment Detail prompt.

STEP 3   Now you will exit by pressing **ESCAPE** or by clicking on the EXIT button on the top toolbar so that you can make an appointment for Ms. League's follow-up visit in 2 weeks. Once you have exited Procedure Entry and are on the Patient Retrieval screen, type '/**APP**' and press **ENTER** or use the mouse to click on the Appointment button (clock face icon) on the top toolbar to directly chain to Entering Appointments.

Notice that the heading on the Patient Retrieval screen indicates "APPOINTMENT ROUTINE" and that the account number in square brackets in the upper right corner is Ms. League's. Because you were just posting to Ms. League's account, **The Medical Manager** system assumes that she is also the patient who requires an appointment; therefore, the screen defaults to her patient number. Press **ENTER** to accept the default.

Figure 5-10 Claire League's Encounter Form—Voucher 1060

Sydney Carrington & Associates P.A.
34 Sycamore Street Suite 300
Madison, CA 95653

Date: 02/03/2003

Voucher No.: 1060

Time: 10:30

Patient: Claire League
Guarantor: Claire E. League

Patient No: 30.0
Doctor: 3 - S. Carrington

□ CPT	DESCRIPTION	FEE
OFFICE/HOSPITAL CONSULTS		
□ 99201	Office New:Focused Hx-Exam	
□ 99202	Office New:Expanded Hx-Exam	
□ 99211	Office Estb:Min/None Hx-Exa	
□ 99212	Office Estb:Focused Hx-Exam	
X 99213	Office Estb:Expanded Hx-Exa	$40.00
□ 99214	Office Estb:Detailed Hx-Exa	
□ 99215	Office Estb:Comprhn Hx-Exam	
□ 99221	Hosp. Initial:Comprh Hx-	
□ 99223	Hosp.Ini:Comprh Hx-Exam/Hi	
□ 99231	Hosp. Subsequent: S-Fwd	
□ 99232	Hosp. Subsequent: Comprhn Hx	
□ 99233	Hosp. Subsequent: Ex/Hi	
□ 99238	Hospital Visit Discharge Ex	
□ 99371	Telephone Consult - Simple	
□ 99372	Telephone Consult - Intermed	
□ 99373	Telephone Consult - Complex	
□ 90843	Counseling - 25 minutes	
□ 90844	Counseling - 50 minutes	
□ 90865	Counseling - Special Interview	
IMMUNIZATIONS/INJECTIONS		
□ 90585	BCG Vaccine	
□ 90659	Influenza Virus Vaccine	
□ 90701	Immunization-DTP	
□ 90702	DT Vaccine	
□ 90703	Tetanus Toxoids	
□ 90732	Pneumococcal Vaccine	
□ 90746	Hepatitis B Vaccine	
□ 90749	Immunization; Unlisted	

□ CPT	DESCRIPTION	FEE
LABORATORY/RADIOLOGY		
□ 81000	Urinalysis	
□ 81002	Urinalysis; Pregnancy Test	
□ 82951	Glucose Tolerance Test	
□ 84478	Triglycerides	
□ 84550	Uric Acid: Blood Chemistry	
□ 84830	Ovulation Test	
□ 85014	Hematocrit	
X 85031	Hemogram, Complete Blood Wk	$15.00
□ 86403	Particle Agglutination Test	
□ 86485	Skin Test; Candida	
□ 86580	TB Intradermal Test	
□ 86585	TB Tine Test	
□ 87070	Culture	
□ 70190	X-Ray; Optic Foramina	
□ 70210	X-Ray Sinuses Complete	
□ 71010	Radiological Exam Ent Spine	
□ 71020	X-Ray Chest Pa & Lat	
□ 72050	X-Ray Spine, Cerv (4 views)	
□ 72090	X-Ray Spine; Scoliosis Ex	
□ 72110	Spine, lumbosacral; a/p & Lat	
□ 73030	Shoulder-Comp, min w/ 2vws	
□ 73070	Elbow, anteropost & later vws	
□ 73120	X-Ray; Hand, 2 views	
□ 73560	X-Ray, Knee, 1 or 2 views	
□ 74022	X-Ray; Abdomen, Complete	
□ 75552	Cardiac Magnetic Res Img	
□ 76020	X-Ray; Bone Age Studies	
□ 76088	Mammary Ductogram Complete	
□ 78465	Myocardial Perfusion Img	

□ CPT	DESCRIPTION	FEE
PROCEDURES/TESTS		
□ 00452	Anesthesia for Rad Surgery	
□ 11100	Skin Biopsy	
□ 15852	Dressing Change	
□ 29075	Cast Appl. - Lower Arm	
□ 29530	Strapping of Knee	
□ 29705	Removal/Revis of Cast w/Exa	
□ 53670	Catheterization Incl. Suppl	
□ 57452	Colposcopy	
□ 57505	ECC	
□ 69420	Myringotomy	
□ 92081	Visual Field Examination	
□ 92100	Serial Tonometry Exam	
□ 92120	Tonography	
□ 92552	Pure Tone Audiometry	
□ 92567	Tympanometry	
□ 93000	Electrocardiogram	
□ 93015	Exercise Stress Test (ETT)	
□ 93017	ETT Tracing Only	
□ 93040	Electrocardiogram - Rhythm	
□ 96100	Psychological Testing	
□ 99000	Specimen Handling	
□ 99058	Office Emergency Care	
□ 99070	Surgical Tray - Misc.	
□ 99080	Special Reports of Med Rec	
□ 99195	Phlebotomy	
□		
□		
□		
□		

□ ICD-9 CODE DIAGNOSIS	
□ 009.0	Ill-defined Intestinal Infect
□ 133.2	Establish Baseline
□ 174.9	Breast Cancer
□ 185.0	Prostate Cancer
□ 250	Diabetes Mellitus
□ 272.4	Hyperlipidemia
□ 282.5	Anemia - Sickle Trait
□ 282.60	Anemia - Sickle Cell
X 285.9	Anemia, Unspecified
□ 300.4	Neurotic Depression
□ 340	Multiple Sclerosis
□ 342.9	Hemiplegia - Unspecified
□ 346.9	Migraine Headache
□ 352.9	Cranial Neuralgia
□ 354.0	Carpal Tunnel Syndrome
□ 355.0	Sciatic Nerve Root Lesion
□ 366.9	Cataract
□ 386.0	Vertigo
□ 401.1	Essential Hypertension
□ 414.9	Ischemic Hearth Disease
□ 428.0	Congestive Heart Failure

□ ICD-9 CODE DIAGNOSIS	
□ 435.0	Basilar Artery Syndrome
□ 440.0	Atherosclerosis
□ 442.81	Carotid Artery
□ 460.0	Common Cold
□ 461.9	Acute Sinusitis
□ 474.0	Tonsillitis
□ 477.9	Hay Fever
□ 487.0	Flu
□ 496	Chronic Airway Obstruction
□ 522	Low Red Blood Count
□ 524.6	Temporo-Mandibular Jnt Synd
□ 538.8	Stomach Pain
□ 553.3	Hiatal Hernia
□ 564.1	Spastic Colon
□ 571.4	Chronic Hepatitis
□ 571.5	Cirrhosis of Liver
□ 573.3	Hepatitis
□ 575.2	Obstruction of Gallbladder
□ 648.2	Anemia - Compl. Pregnancy
□ 715.90	Osteoarthritis - Unspec
□ 721.3	Lumbar Osteo/Spondylarthrit

□ ICD-9 CODE DIAGNOSIS	
□ 724.2	Pain: Lower Back
□ 727.6	Rupture of Achilles Tendon
□ 780.1	Hallucinations
□ 780.3	Convulsions
□ 780.5	Sleep Disturbances
□ 783.0	Anorexia
□ 783.1	Abnormal Weight Gain
□ 783.2	Abnormal Weight Loss
□ 830.6	Dislocated Hip
□ 830.9	Dislocated Shoulder
□ 841.2	Sprained Wrist
□ 842.5	Sprained Ankle
□ 891.2	Fractured Tibia
□ 892.0	Fractured Fibula
□ 919.5	Insect Bite, Nonvenomous
□ 921.1	Contus Eyelid/Perioc Area
□ v16.3	Fam. Hist of Breast Cancer
□ v17.4	Fam. Hist of Cardiovasc Dis
□ v20.2	Well Child
□ v22.0	Pregnancy - First Normal
□ v22.1	Pregnancy - Normal

Previous Balance	Today's Charges	Total Due	Amount Paid	New Balance
_____	_____	_____	_____	_____

Follow Up

PRN _____ Weeks __2__ Months _____ Units _____

Next Appointment Date: Feb 17   Time: 10:30

I hereby authorize release of any information acquired in the course of examination or treatment and allow a photocopy of my signature to be used.

Figure 5-11 Procedure 1 Screen for Claire League

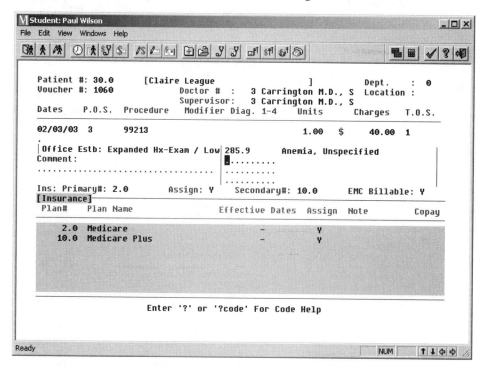

Figure 5-12 Procedure 2 Screen for Claire League

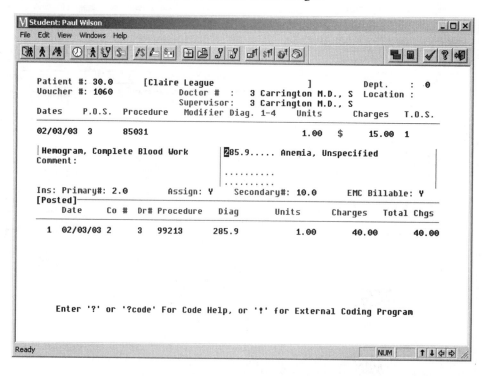

STEP 4

Use the (J)ump command to make an appointment for Ms. League at 10:30 A.M. on February 17, 2003 for a Re-Check with Dr. #3 - Carrington. *Because Ms. League was seen by Dr. Carrington who is not her regular doctor, be very careful that you do not accept the default doctor.* Be sure to list the correct reason, '5', for the visit. Press **F1** or click the PROCESS button ('√') to process, then compare your screen with Figure 5-13.

In order to proceed to Exercise 5, press **ESCAPE** or click on the EXIT button on the top toolbar. Then, key '/**PRO**' at the Patient Retrieval screen, and press **ENTER**. This will take you back to the Procedure Entry Patient Retrieval screen so you can retrieve Mr. Gene Evans's account.

Figure 5-13 Making a Follow-Up Appointment

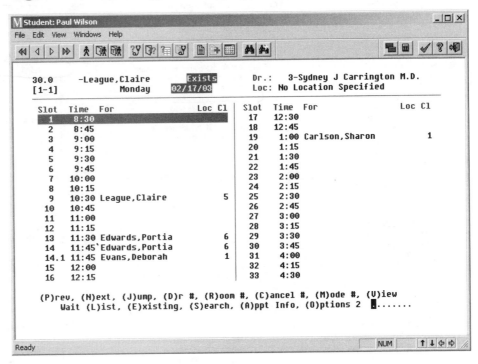

EXERCISE 5: Gene S. Evans

Posting Procedures and Scheduling an Appointment

By studying the encounter form shown in Figure 5-14, you will see that two procedures were performed during Gene Evans's visit on 02/03/03, and that a return visit should be scheduled for February 17 at 11:00 A.M.

STEP 1

From Procedure Entry, first post the two procedures shown on the encounter form.

Note: There is no Ailment Detail.

STEP 2

Then, using the information provided at the bottom right of the encounter form, make an appointment for Mr. Evans to see Dr. Carrington for a general check-up.

Figure 5-14 Gene Evans's Encounter Form—Voucher 1061

Sydney Carrington & Associates P.A.
34 Sycamore Street   Suite 300
Madison, CA 95653

Date: 02/03/2003

Time: 10:30

Patient: Gene Evans
Guarantor: Deborah A. Evans

Voucher No.: 1061

Patient No: 14.1
Doctor: 3 - S. Carrington

	CPT	DESCRIPTION	FEE
	OFFICE/HOSPITAL CONSULTS		
☐	99201	Office New:Focused Hx-Exam	
☐	99202	Office New:Expanded Hx-Exam	
☐	99211	Office Estb:Min/None Hx-Exa	
☐	99212	Office Estb:Focused Hx-Exam	
☒	99213	Office Estb:Expanded Hx-Exa	$40.00
☐	99214	Office Estb:Detailed Hx-Exa	
☐	99215	Office Estb:Comprhn Hx-Exam	
☐	99221	Hosp. Initial:Comprh Hx-	
☐	99223	Hosp.Ini:Comprh Hx-Exam/Hi	
☐	99231	Hosp. Subsequent: S-Fwd	
☐	99232	Hosp. Subsequent: Comprhn Hx	
☐	99233	Hosp. Subsequent: Ex/Hi	
☐	99238	Hospital Visit Discharge Ex	
☐	99371	Telephone Consult - Simple	
☐	99372	Telephone Consult - Intermed	
☐	99373	Telephone Consult - Complex	
☐	90843	Counseling - 25 minutes	
☐	90844	Counseling - 50 minutes	
☐	90865	Counseling - Special Interview	
	IMMUNIZATIONS/INJECTIONS		
☐	90585	BCG Vaccine	
☐	90659	Influenza Virus Vaccine	
☐	90701	Immunization-DTP	
☐	90702	DT Vaccine	
☐	90703	Tetanus Toxoids	
☐	90732	Pneumococcal Vaccine	
☐	90746	Hepatitis B Vaccine	
☒	90749	Immunization; Unlisted	$12.00

	CPT	DESCRIPTION	FEE
	LABORATORY/RADIOLOGY		
☐	81000	Urinalysis	
☐	81002	Urinalysis; Pregnancy Test	
☐	82951	Glucose Tolerance Test	
☐	84478	Triglycerides	
☐	84550	Uric Acid: Blood Chemistry	
☐	84830	Ovulation Test	
☐	85014	Hematocrit	
☐	85031	Hemogram, Complete Blood Wk	
☐	86403	Particle Agglutination Test	
☐	86485	Skin Test; Candida	
☐	86580	TB Intradermal Test	
☐	86585	TB Tine Test	
☐	87070	Culture	
☐	70190	X-Ray; Optic Foramina	
☐	70210	X-Ray Sinuses Complete	
☐	71010	Radiological Exam Ent Spine	
☐	71020	X-Ray Chest Pa & Lat	
☐	72050	X-Ray Spine, Cerv (4 views)	
☐	72090	X-Ray Spine; Scoliosis Ex	
☐	72110	Spine, lumbosacral; a/p & Lat	
☐	73030	Shoulder-Comp, min w/ 2vws	
☐	73070	Elbow, anteropost & later vws	
☐	73120	X-Ray; Hand, 2 views	
☐	73560	X-Ray, Knee, 1 or 2 views	
☐	74022	X-Ray; Abdomen, Complete	
☐	75552	Cardiac Magnetic Res Img	
☐	76020	X-Ray; Bone Age Studies	
☐	76088	Mammary Ductogram Complete	
☐	78465	Myocardial Perfusion Img	

	CPT	DESCRIPTION	FEE
	PROCEDURES/TESTS		
☐	00452	Anesthesia for Rad Surgery	
☐	11100	Skin Biopsy	
☐	15852	Dressing Change	
☐	29075	Cast Appl. - Lower Arm	
☐	29530	Strapping of Knee	
☐	29705	Removal/Revis of Cast w/Exa	
☐	53670	Catheterization Incl. Suppl	
☐	57452	Colposcopy	
☐	57505	ECC	
☐	69420	Myringotomy	
☐	92081	Visual Field Examination	
☐	92100	Serial Tonometry Exam	
☐	92120	Tonography	
☐	92552	Pure Tone Audiometry	
☐	92567	Tympanometry	
☐	93000	Electrocardiogram	
☐	93015	Exercise Stress Test (ETT)	
☐	93017	ETT Tracing Only	
☐	93040	Electrocardiogram - Rhythm	
☐	96100	Psychological Testing	
☐	99000	Specimen Handling	
☐	99058	Office Emergency Care	
☐	99070	Surgical Tray - Misc.	
☐	99080	Special Reports of Med Rec	
☐	99195	Phlebotomy	
☐			
☐			
☐			
☐			

	ICD-9 CODE DIAGNOSIS	
☐	009.0	Ill-defined Intestinal Infect
☐	133.2	Establish Baseline
☐	174.9	Breast Cancer
☐	185.0	Prostate Cancer
☐	250	Diabetes Mellitus
☐	272.4	Hyperlipidemia
☐	282.5	Anemia - Sickle Trait
☐	282.60	Anemia - Sickle Cell
☐	285.9	Anemia, Unspecified
☐	300.4	Neurotic Depression
☐	340	Multiple Sclerosis
☐	342.9	Hemiplegia - Unspecified
☐	346.9	Migraine Headache
☐	352.9	Cranial Neuralgia
☐	354.0	Carpal Tunnel Syndrome
☐	355.0	Sciatic Nerve Root Lesion
☐	366.9	Cataract
☐	386.0	Vertigo
☐	401.1	Essential Hypertension
☐	414.9	Ischemic Hearth Disease
☐	428.0	Congestive Heart Failure

	ICD-9 CODE DIAGNOSIS	
☐	435.0	Basilar Artery Syndrome
☐	440.0	Atherosclerosis
☐	442.81	Carotid Artery
☐	460.0	Common Cold
☒	461.9	Acute Sinusitis
☐	474.0	Tonsillitis
☐	477.9	Hay Fever
☐	487.0	Flu
☐	496	Chronic Airway Obstruction
☐	522	Low Red Blood Count
☐	524.6	Temporo-Mandibular Jnt Synd
☐	538.8	Stomach Pain
☐	553.3	Hiatal Hernia
☐	564.1	Spastic Colon
☐	571.4	Chronic Hepatitis
☐	571.5	Cirrhosis of Liver
☐	573.3	Hepatitis
☐	575.2	Obstruction of Gallbladder
☐	648.2	Anemia - Compl. Pregnancy
☐	715.90	Osteoarthritis - Unspec
☐	721.3	Lumbar Osteo/Spondylarthrit

	ICD-9 CODE DIAGNOSIS	
☐	724.2	Pain: Lower Back
☐	727.6	Rupture of Achilles Tendon
☐	780.1	Hallucinations
☐	780.3	Convulsions
☐	780.5	Sleep Disturbances
☐	783.0	Anorexia
☐	783.1	Abnormal Weight Gain
☐	783.2	Abnormal Weight Loss
☐	830.6	Dislocated Hip
☐	830.9	Dislocated Shoulder
☐	841.2	Sprained Wrist
☐	842.5	Sprained Ankle
☐	891.2	Fractured Tibia
☐	892.0	Fractured Fibula
☐	919.5	Insect Bite, Nonvenomous
☐	921.1	Contus Eyelid/Perioc Area
☐	v16.3	Fam. Hist of Breast Cancer
☐	v17.4	Fam. Hist of Cardiovasc Dis
☐	v20.2	Well Child
☐	v22.0	Pregnancy - First Normal
☐	v22.1	Pregnancy - Normal

Previous Balance	Today's Charges	Total Due	Amount Paid	New Balance

Follow Up

PRN _____ Weeks __2__ Months _____ Units _____

Next Appointment Date: Feb 17   Time: 11:00
General Checkup

I hereby authorize release of any information acquired in the course of examination or treatment and allow a photocopy of my signature to be used.

Figure 5-15 Appointment Screen Before Reschedule for Gene Evans

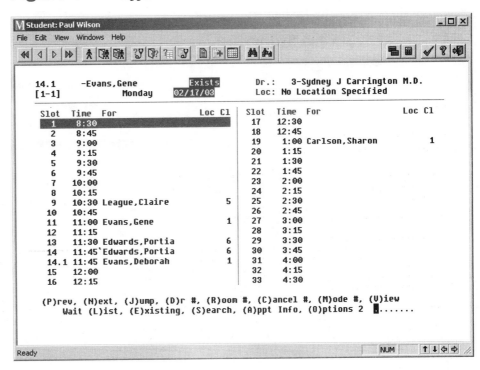

Carefully review each screen as you complete your work. Review Figure 5-15 after you have scheduled the appointment.

EXERCISE 6: Gene S. Evans

Rescheduling an Appointment

Mr. Gene Evans calls back later in the day and asks to move his 11:00 A.M. appointment with Dr. Carrington to 2:00 P.M. on February 17, 2003.

STEP 1   If you have already exited the Appointment Scheduler, reenter and retrieve Mr. Evans's account, then (J)ump to the correct doctor and day. Locate the appointment Mr. Evans scheduled with Dr. Carrington. Among the prompts at the bottom of the screen, you will notice the (E)xisting command. Key 'E' for (E)xisting and press **ENTER** to display all existing appointments for this patient. The appointment Mr. Evans has scheduled with Dr. Carrington will appear (Figure 5-16).

STEP 2   From the prompts at the bottom of the screen, key '**R**' for (R)eschedule and press **ENTER**. You will be prompted to enter a Reschedule Reason Code, the reason for the patient needing to reschedule the appointment. Key '?' and press **ENTER** to invoke a help window for this field. Remember that you can also use the mouse to click on the Help button ('?') on the top toolbar. Use the keyboard or the mouse to select '**CALLED**' as the Reschedule Reason Code, and press **ENTER**. Press **F1** or click the PROCESS button ('√') to process without entering anything into the Remark field. Press **F1** or click the PROCESS button ('√') again to proceed to reschedule the displayed appointment for Mr. Evans.

Figure 5-16 Existing Appointment Screen for Gene Evans

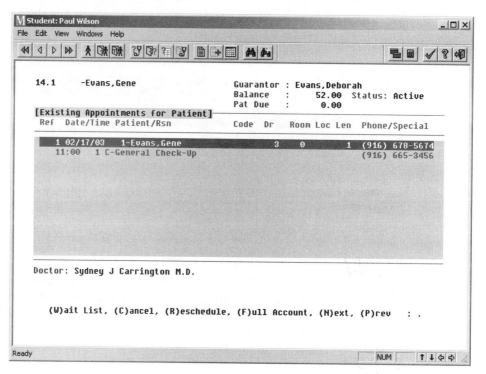

STEP 3 To reschedule Mr. Evans's appointment for 2:00 P.M., key slot '**23**' and press **ENTER**. Press **ENTER** again to accept the default Appointment Reason Code of 1, General Check-Up. Press **ENTER** until you see the prompt "Make: Dr # 3 to see Evans, Gene at 2:00 for 15 min." Then, press **F1** or click the PROCESS button ('√') to complete the appointment rescheduling process. Your screen should be similar to Figure 5-17.

Figure 5-17 Rescheduled Appointment Screen for Gene Evans

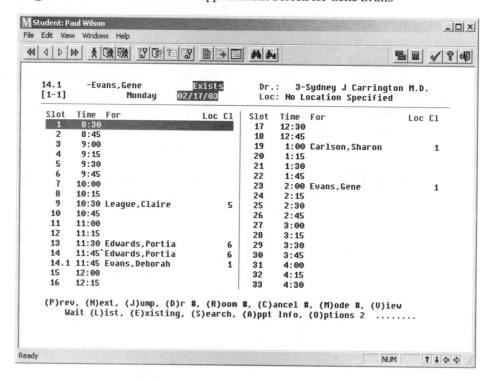

EXERCISE 7: Patricia G. Evans

Making a Recheck Appointment

Due to the serious nature of Ms. Patricia Evans's condition, breast cancer, Dr. Carrington has asked his medical assistant to call Ms. Evans and schedule an appointment for a Recheck within one week. Ms. Evans agrees to come in and has requested an appointment time of 10:00 A.M.

You should already be at the Appointment Routine Patient Retrieval screen. If not, from any menu screen or patient retrieval prompt, key '/**APP**' and press **ENTER**. Remember that you may also use the mouse to click on the Appointment button (clock face icon) on the top toolbar.

STEP 1 Key '**Evans,Patricia**' at the Appointment Routine Patient Retrieval screen and press **ENTER** to retrieve Ms. Evans's account. Press **ENTER** again to proceed with scheduling Ms. Evans's appointment.

STEP 2 From the prompt lines at the bottom of the screen, choose to (**J**)ump and press **ENTER**. Press **ENTER** again to accept Dr. # 3, Dr. Carrington, as Ms. Evans's default doctor. Key that you would like to schedule an appointment '**1**' week from now and press **ENTER**. Key '**7**' and press **ENTER** or using the mouse, double-click in slot 7 to schedule Ms. Evans's appointment at 10:00 A.M.; the time she requested for the appointment.

STEP 3 At the Appointment Reason Code field, key '?' and press **ENTER** or using the mouse, click on the Help button ('?') on the top toolbar to invoke a Help window of Appointment Reason Codes. Using the keyboard or mouse, choose code **5**, Recheck. Press **ENTER** until you see the message "Make: Dr # 3 to see Evans,Patricia at 10:00 for 15 min." Check the information on your screen carefully as there is no comparison screen provided for this exercise. Then, press **F1** or click the PROCESS button ('√') to complete the appointment scheduling process.

DAILY LIST OF APPOINTMENTS

The daily list of appointments determines each staff member's schedule.

Each morning, a daily list of appointments is prepared for the physician, the nurses, and the medical assistants. A copy is also maintained at the receptionist's desk. The daily list is the time schedule around which staff members plan their day.

The Medical Manager allows you to view daily appointments on the screen, or you may print a report. Three types of daily list reports are available to you.

1. *Appointments by Patient.* This report provides appointment information for requested patients. The report is printed by account number, date, and time sequence and is useful when you need to see when a patient's next appointment is scheduled.

2. *Appointments Detail Report.* This report provides appointment information for each patient; the information can be selected by doctor number, room number, date, or time. Also included is abbreviated financial information as well as two phone numbers for all patients with scheduled appointments. This report is useful each day because it shows which patients are coming in, the reasons for their appointments, and whether they need to have their financial accounts discussed.

3. *Appointments Worksheet.* This report provides the only appointment report that includes blank space for unused time slots.

Figure 5-18 Appointments Worksheet Selection Screen

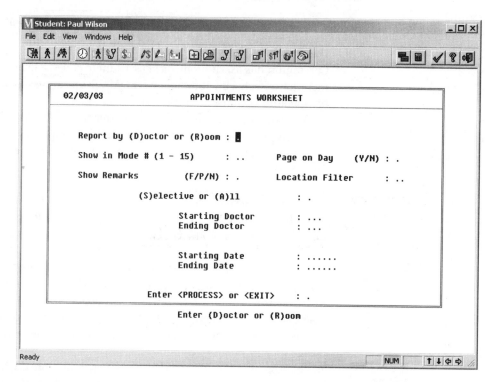

This exercise demonstrates one type of report, the Appointments Worksheet. However, you may also practice printing a report of appointments by patient, and appointments by detail if you wish.

STEP 1

Using the keyboard or mouse, select option **8**, OFFICE Management, at the Main Menu (Menu 1). Then select option **1**, APPOINTMENTS/Recall. Finally, select option **4**, APPOINTMENTS Worksheet, from the APPOINTMENTS/Recall menu (Menu 12).

Press **ENTER**, and a Report screen similar to Figure 5-18 appears.

STEP 2

You may print appointments for each doctor, for each examining room, by date, or by a range of dates. For this demonstration, key in the following information:

Order: **D** (for Doctor No. order)
Mode: **1**
Page on Day: **Y**
Show Remarks: **F**
Location Filter: (Press **ENTER** to default to all locations)
Selective or All: **S**
Starting Doctor: **1**
Ending Doctor: **3**
Starting Date: **021703**
Ending Date: **021703**

Note: Make sure that you do NOT accept the default date!

Key 'Y' if you want to print each day's appointments on a separate page. You may also print appointments in a continuous listing for consecutive days without page breaks by pressing 'N'.

Make sure your printer is on, has paper in it, and is online. Press **F1** or click the PROCESS button ('√') to process the screen, and reports for Dr. James Monroe, Dr.

Figure 5-19 Appointments Worksheet for Dr. Sydney Carrington

```
02/03/03                    APPOINTMENTS WORKSHEET REPORT BY DOCTOR                    Page    3
                                     Student: Paul Wilson
                                 (3) Sydney J Carrington M.D.
                                   Dates 02/17/03 - 02/17/03

 Slot   Time     Patient              Len Reason (Class # Desc.)      Rm Loc   (Remarks Follow Appointment)
 =======================================================================================================
 -------------------------------------------------------------------------------------------------------
 02/17/03  Monday        (1) Full Day Patient Information
 -------------------------------------------------------------------------------------------------------
   1     8:30
   2     8:45
   3     9:00
   4     9:15
   5     9:30
   6     9:45
   7    10:00
   8    10:15
   9    10:30      30.0  League,Claire      1  A  5   -Re-Check               0
  10    10:45
  11    11:00
  12    11:15
  13    11:30      21.0  Edwards,Portia     2  C  6   -Personal Consult       0
  14    11:45      21.0  Edwards,Portia     -  C  6   -Personal Consult       0
  14.1  11:45      14.0  Evans,Deborah      1  C  1   -General Check-Up        0
  15    12:00
  16    12:15
  17    12:30
  18    12:45
  19     1:00      10.1  Carlson,Sharon     1  C  1   -General Check-Up        0
  20     1:15
  21     1:30
  22     1:45
  23     2:00      14.1  Evans,Gene         1  C  1   -General Check-Up        0
  24     2:15
  25     2:30
  26     2:45
  27     3:00
  28     3:15
  29     3:30
  30     3:45
  31     4:00
  32     4:15
  33     4:30
  34     4:45
  35     5:00
```

Frances Simpson, and Dr. Sydney Carrington will be generated. You may abort the report at any time by pressing **ESCAPE** or by clicking on the EXIT button on the top toolbar. Only Dr. Carrington's Appointments Worksheet is shown in Figure 5-19.

ENTERING AND PRINTING HOSPITAL ROUNDS AND REPORTS

Hospital rounds refer to the visits the doctor makes to hospitalized patients.

Hospitalized patients are visited by the physician each day during hospital rounds. A record must be kept of which patients are in the hospital, their room numbers, their estimated length of stay, their referring doctor's name and phone number, their diagnosis, and any remarks or comments the physician wants to remember.

The hospital record ensures that the physician is informed about which patients are hospitalized or have been dismissed from the hospital. It also allows the doctor to check off names as patients are visited. By returning the list to the billing clerk after rounds are complete, the physician provides a procedure charges voucher, much like the encounter form, that can be used to post patient accounts for the hospital visit charges.

Two types of reports are available in **The Medical Manager** system to show the status of hospitalized patients: the Hospital Rounds Report and the Patient In-Hospital Report (not addressed in the Student Edition course).

Hospital Rounds Entry

The Medical Manager allows complete information about a patient's hospital stay to be stored in the patient's record. A Hospital Rounds Entry screen permits you to key and process these data. In the following exercises, you will build on your prior knowledge as you use the Hospital Rounds Entry function and print a Hospital Rounds Report.

APPLYING YOUR KNOWLEDGE

EXERCISE 8: Patricia G. Evans
Canceling an Appointment

Dr. Carrington has evaluated Ms. Patricia Evans's condition and has decided to admit her to the hospital for further evaluation and treatment, rather than wait for her scheduled Recheck appointment in a week. Therefore, you will need to cancel her previously scheduled appointment with Dr. Carrington.

From the Main Menu (Menu 1), use the keyboard or mouse to select option **8**, OFFICE Management. From the Office Management menu (Menu 9), choose option **1**, APPOINTMENTS/Recall. At the Appointments/Recall menu (Menu 12), choose option **1**, ENTER Appointments, and the Appointment Routine Patient Retrieval screen will appear.

STEP 1   Key Ms. Evans's complete patient number, '**110.0**' at the Patient Retrieval screen and press **ENTER** to retrieve her account. Use the (**J**)ump command to locate the appointment already scheduled for Ms. Evans. Using the keyboard or the mouse, highlight slot '**7**', in which Ms. Evans's appointment is scheduled.

STEP 2   Among the prompts at the bottom of the screen, you will notice the (C)ancel command. This can be used in two ways. To cancel only one slot (in this case, slot #7), you can enter 'C7' at the bottom of the screen, press ENTER, enter the Cancel Reason Code (there is a help window available for this field) then PROCESS. If you have more than one consecutive slot to cancel, you can press 'C', then ENTER and complete the "Starting Slot _____ through Ending Slot _____" prompt. For appointments occupying more than one slot, the entire appointment will be removed using this procedure.

For this exercise, key '**C7**' at the bottom of the screen, press **ENTER**, and the following prompt appears: "Cancel: Dr # 3 to see Evans, Patricia at 10:00 for 15 min." At the Cancel Reason Code field, key '?' and press **ENTER** or click on the Help button ('?') on the top toolbar to invoke a help window for this field. Using the keyboard or mouse, you will choose cancel code '**ECARE**' (Emergency Care Given) because Dr. Carrington has arranged to admit Ms. Evans to the hospital. Press **F1** or click the PROCESS button ('√') on the top toolbar to process the change. You have completed canceling Ms. Evans's appointment.

EXERCISE 9: Patricia G. Evans
Adding a Patient to Hospital Rounds Entry

Because Dr. Carrington is so concerned about Ms. Patricia Evans, he arranged to have her admitted to Regional Hospital of Madison, service facility 4, on January 27, 2003, for her cancer condition. She is expected to be in the hospital for five days.

STEP 1   From the Main Menu (Menu 1), select option **8**, OFFICE Management, then option **6**, HOSPITAL Tracking, then option **1**, HOSPITAL Rounds Entry by using either the keyboard or mouse. Retrieve Ms. Evans's account by keying her account number, '**110.0**', and pressing **ENTER**. A screen for entering hospital information will appear.

STEP 2   Because no previous Hospital Rounds information exists, 'Rounds Not Found' appears on the screen. Select the (**A**)dd option to add the following data. If some information had been entered previously, you would select (**M**)odify, then enter the new data. Enter the following information:

- a. Show on Report (Y/N): (**Y**)es

  This field is used to indicate that this Hospital Rounds entry is to appear on the doctor's rounds report. The field is set to (**N**)o when the patient is still in the hospital but the doctor will no longer be visiting the patient during their rounds. An example of this would be a specialist who did a single-visit consult in a multipractice specialty when another doctor was visiting the patient regularly.

- b. Doctor #: **3**

  The Doctor # field is the doctor who is responsible for making rounds and on whose rounds report this center would print.

- c. Referring Dr.: **2**

  Press enter to default to the patient's normal referring doctor or enter a '?' to display a Help window of referring doctors in the practice.

- d. Remark: **Admit**

  The practice can enter any free text remark. This remark will appear on the report. In this case you will type in the word admit.

- e. Diagnosis: **174.9** (Breast Cancer)

  Diagnosis is the admitting diagnosis (why the patient is being admitted to the hospital).

- f. Serv. Facility: **4**

  Facility is the hospital to which the patient is being admitted.

- g. Room No.: **E-308**

  Room No. allows the practice to enter the patient's room number and the Hospital Rounds Report will include the room number in the order that it prints information on the report. This information might not be available to the office until after the patient has actually been admitted to the hospital.

- h. Hospital Patient No.: **RH345667**

  Enter the hospital's medical record or I.D. number for the patient to facilitate easy communication between the practice and the hospital.

- i. Admit Date: **01272003**

  Enter the date on which the patient is to be admitted or was admitted to the hospital.

- j. Est. Days Stay: **5**

  If the doctor has estimated a number of days that the patient will be staying in the hospital that number can be entered here. In this case, it is estimated that Ms. Evans will be in the hospital 5 days.

- k. Admissions Source: **1**

  The source of the patient's admission in this case is the physician who is admitting the patient. Select number 1.

- l. Type (**1** Emergency, **2** Urgent, **3** Elective, **4** Newborn): **2**

  This field allows you to indicate whether the type of admission is an emergency, an urgent admission, or an elective procedure.

  Similar information will be completed at the time the patient is discharged. These fields do not have to be completed at this time. Compare your screen with Figure 5-20. Press **F1** or click on the PROCESS button ('√') on the top toolbar to process. Press **EXIT** to leave the Hospital Rounds screen and return to the Hospital Tracking Menu (Menu 33).

Figure 5-20 Hospital Rounds Entry Screen

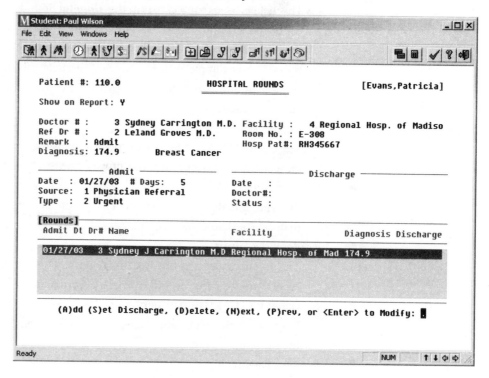

EXERCISE 10: Patricia G. Evans

Printing the Hospital Rounds Report

Doctors normally take the Hospital Rounds Report to the hospital with them, make any additional notes, then return the report to the front desk to be used as a posting voucher in lieu of an encounter form as they make their rounds. The report normally lists all hospitalized patients. However, your report is smaller because only one patient, Ms. Evans, has been entered.

STEP 1 From the Office Management Menu (Menu 9), select option **6**, HOSPITAL Tracking then option **7**, HOSPITAL Rounds Report by using either the keyboard or mouse. This option will allow you to request a Hospital Rounds Report by Service Facility.

STEP 2 Select (**P**)rinter, (**Y**)es Include Tomorrow's Admissions, (**D**) Sort by Doctor, (**A**)ll Selected Doctors, (**A**)ll Selected Facilities. Compare your report with Figure 5-21.

Figure 5-21 Hospital Rounds Report

```
02/03/03                        HOSPITAL ROUNDS REPORT BY SERVICE FACILITY                      Page    1
                                        Student: Paul Wilson
                                    (3)Sydney J Carrington M.D.
                                           All Facilities

   Patient                      Pat #   DOB        Admit Info                 Referring Dr.        Remark
================================================================================================================
---------------------------------------
Regional Hosp. of Madison  (4)
---------------------------------------
   Evans,Patricia                110.0   12/13/1951   Date  : 01/27/03  Days: 5   Leland W Groves M.D.    Admit
                                                      Source: Physician Referral  Phone: (916) 678-9012
       Room: E-308      Hosp ID: RH345667             Type  : Urgent             Notes:
       Diag: 174.9      Breast Cancer
                                           ---------------------------
```

FINDING PROCEDURE CODES
FOR HOSPITAL VISITS

When hospital visit charges are posted to a patient's account, procedure codes are not given on the Hospital Round Report. You will need to use the procedure code help window to locate codes. Several options for using the help window are given below. Read the information carefully, so you can process the correct codes in the upcoming *Applying Your Knowledge* exercise.

1. You may enter '?' and press **ENTER** at a prompt or click on the Help button ('?') on the top toolbar to select the type of procedure code help you need. Press **ENTER** at the prompt, and a list of the procedure codes will appear in numerical code order. You have the option to see the list in either code or description order, and you may page through the listing by using (N)ext or (P)revious, or by using the mouse to click on the right ('→') and left ('←') arrow buttons on the bottom toolbar.

2. You may enter '?' plus a code or part of a code and press **ENTER** at the prompt or click on the Help button ('?') on the top toolbar, and the closest match to the code will appear followed by other codes. This is most useful if you have an idea as to which code is needed.

A sample procedure code file list in description order is shown in Figure 5-22. The procedure code, description, standard charge, profile amount, and the pay level is displayed. Remember that the highlight bar or the mouse can be used to select the appropriate code. *For detailed information about the Procedure Code field, refer to Unit 2.*

Figure 5-22 Procedure Code Help Window

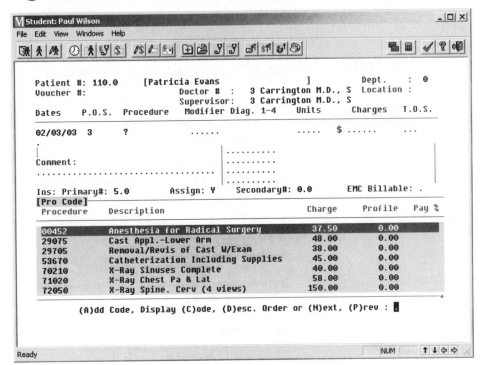

EXERCISE 11: Patricia G. Evans

Finding Codes for Posting Hospitalization

The doctor has discharged Ms. Patricia Evans from the hospital, and you will use the Hospital Rounds Report to post her account. The Hospital Rounds Report providing posting information is shown in Figure 5-23.

Figure 5-23 Hospital Rounds Report as Posting Voucher

```
02/03/03                          HOSPITAL ROUNDS REPORT BY SERVICE FACILITY                   Page   1
                                            Student: Paul Wilson
                                        (3)Sydney J Carrington M.D.
                                             All Facilities

   Patient                    Pat #   DOB        Admit Info              Referring Dr.        Remark
======================================================================================================
-----------------------------------
Regional Hosp. of Madison  (4)
-----------------------------------
   Evans,Patricia            110.0   12/13/1951  Date : 01/27/03  Days: 5  Leland W Groves M.D.    Admit
                                                 Source: Physician Referral  Phone: (916) 678-9012
     Room: E-308      Hosp ID: RH345667          Type : Urgent            Notes:
     Diag: 174.9      Breast Cancer
                                                 ------------------------

Discharge 1/31/03
S. J. Carrington
```

Before attempting any data entry, study the Hospital Rounds Report and answer the following questions:

1. What is the name of the hospital listed?

2. What is the date of admission for Ms. Evans?

3. What is the date of discharge for Ms. Evans?

4. Who is Ms. Evans's referring physician?

5. Which doctor cared for Ms. Evans during her hospital stay?

During a typical hospital stay, the following procedures may occur:

Admission History and Comprehensive Physical Exam—This is done on the day of the patient's admission to the hospital.

Hospital Visit Expanded—This procedure is done between the date of the patient's admission to the hospital and the date of the patient's discharge from the hospital.

Hospital Visit Discharge Exam—This is done on the day the patient will be discharged from the hospital.

Accordingly, Patricia Evans's hospitalization charges will include:

One Procedure: Admission History and Comprehensive Physical Exam (1/27).

Four Procedures: Hospital Visit Expanded (1/28, 1/29, 1/30, and 1/31).

One Procedure: Hospital Visit Discharge Exam (1/31).

Follow the instructions provided below and post the charges appropriate to Ms. Evans's hospitalization. First, return to the Procedure Entry screen. Then you will post the admission, daily visit, and discharge charges to Ms. Evans's account using the Hospital

Rounds Report. Do not become confused even though you are posting admission charges after Ms. Evans has been discharged.

STEP 1

The Hospital Rounds Report serves as an encounter form for all hospital charges. The primary insurance plan is plan '**5**', assignment is accepted, and there is no secondary insurance.

Enter '**HOSP**' for the voucher number, '**3**' for the doctor number, '01272003' as the date of service, and '**1**' for place of service. The resulting charge will have the current date for the Date of Post and will appear on today's Daily Close; however, it will show the correct date of service. Compare your screen with Figure 5-24 before proceeding.

Figure 5-24 First Procedure Code Entry Screen

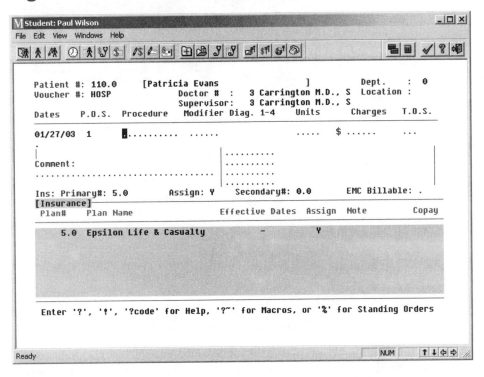

STEP 2

Because you are using the Hospital Rounds Report as the posting voucher, you do not have the codes conveniently listed; therefore, use the procedure code help window to locate the correct codes. At the Procedure Code field, key '?' and press **ENTER** OR using the mouse, you can also click on the Help button ('?') on the top toolbar. Look at the prompt and select '**D**' to list the codes in (D)escription order. Press **ENTER** to start at the beginning of the alphabet. Notice that the Hospital Rounds Report tells you that this patient is to be admitted. This means your first procedure code will refer to admitting the patient to the hospital.

Locate procedure code '**99223**' for 'Hospital Initial: Comprh Hx-Exam/Hi' for Admission History & Physical Comprehensive; use the highlight bar or mouse to select it; then, key the diagnosis, '**174.9**', which is also listed on the Hospital Rounds Report. Press **F1** or click on the PROCESS button ('√') on the top toolbar to process and the ailment help window will appear listing ailments that were previously created. The first ailment, Ailment 1, is highlighted so press **ENTER** to link this ailment to this procedure.

STEP 3

When the Ailment Detail is entered, the posted window will appear, and the Procedure Code field will clear. Again key '?' and press **ENTER** or click on the Help button ('?') on the top toolbar to invoke the procedure code help window and choose to search in

(**D**)escription order for the Hospital Visit Discharge Exam. This time, limit the search by beginning with the letters '**hosp**'. The list of procedures will appear beginning with "Hosp. Subsequent: Comprhn Hx-Exam/Hi." Locate the correct code, **99238**, highlight it and press **ENTER** or double-click on procedure code **99238** to highlight it and select it simultaneously. *Now use the up arrow key or the mouse to move the cursor back to the Date of Service field.* Look at the Hospital Rounds Report to determine the date the patient was discharged (01312003). Key the correct date. Compare your screen with Figure 5-25. Press **F1** or click the PROCESS button ('√') to process. The Ailment Detail is (**S**)ame.

Figure 5-25 Second Procedure Code Entry Screen

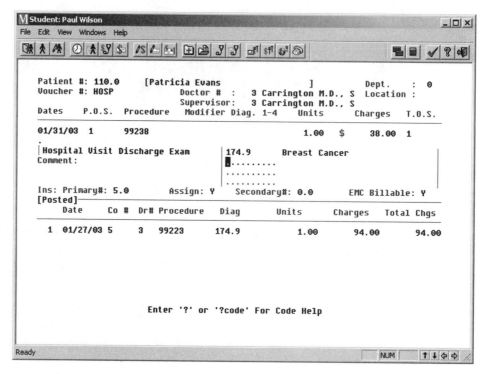

STEP 4

The final entry will be for Ms. Evans's daily visits. Use the From Date/To Date for entering data. First, use the help window to locate the correct code for Hosp. Subsequent: Comprhn Hx - Exam/Mod. Enter the procedure code. *Use the up arrow or the mouse to move the cursor to the Date of Service field.* Enter the date '**012703**', because Ms. Evans's first hospital visit from the doctor occurred the day after she was admitted. Press **ENTER** to move to the To Date field, one line below, and enter the date '**013103**'. This date range indicates a series of continuous visits.

Position the cursor at the Units field. Count the number of days from January 27 through January 30. Type '**4**' in the Units field to indicate four days' service and press **ENTER**. Notice that the charges are automatically multiplied by the number of units entered. Your final screen should be similar to Figure 5-26. Press **F1** or click the PROCESS button ('√') on the top toolbar to process. The ailment is (**S**)ame. This completes posting of hospital charges for Ms. Evans.

The Diagnosis Code Help Window works in the same manner as the Procedure Code Help Window.

Figure 5-26 From Date/To Date Procedure Entry Screen

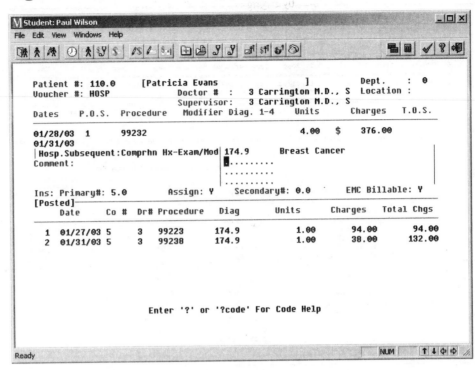

EXERCISE 12: Performing a Final Daily Close for February 3

STEP 1

Perform a Daily Close for February 3, 2003, following the instructions in Unit 4. Remember that the first step in performing a Daily Close is to run the Trial Daily Report; check your work carefully, and make any necessary corrections using File Maintenance (Menu 2). Check the numbers in your Trial Daily Report using the information contained in the Final Daily Close Report, shown in Figures 5-27 through 5-32.

Note: Notice that several adjustments appear on your Trial Daily Report. These are HMO write-offs, which are calculated automatically by The Medical Manager software. These adjustments do not represent student entries. In addition, some adjustments in the net A/R (Accounts Receivable) occur as a result of other automatic calculations by the software. If your figures differ from what is shown below, check with your instructor.

STEP 2

When you have checked your Trial Daily Report and are sure all entries are correct, run the Final Daily Close. Remember to request a check register for the practice and press '0' at the Appointment Purge prompt (no purge). Make sure your printer is ready and print your reports. Hand in your reports in to your instructor.

Figure 5-27 Daily Report for 02/03/03—James Monroe, M.D

```
02/03/03                              DAILY REPORT FOR 02/03/03                              Page    1
                                        James T Monroe MD (1)


                                                                [to Vchr   Total   Ref Date]
Account   Patient Name      Dt Post    Type Dates of Service  Dept Voucher Proc Code  Units  Pri/Sec Ail  Loc  Exc   Amount
========================================================================================================================
120.4     Williams,Janet    02/03/03   CHG  02/03/03-          0    1058   99212       1.00    11/    0   N            30.00
120       Williams,Terry    02/03/03   A05  HMO Adj & Write-O  0           [1058               30.00          02/03/03]  -30.00
120.3     Williams,Thomas   02/03/03   CHG  02/03/03-          0    1059   99212       1.00    11/    0   N            30.00
120       Williams,Terry    02/03/03   A05  HMO Adj & Write-O  0           [1059               30.00          02/03/03]  -30.00

Exception Codes:
overrides: c= charge, p= profile, w= writedown, o= overpay, i= pmt not from resp. ins, e= item edited, x= rebuilt dlyfile.tmp used


                                    Summary for : James T Monroe MD
                    --------------------------------------------------------------
                       Item          Today      Period-to-Date        Year-to-Date
                    Description     02/03/03   01/01/03 - 02/03/03   01/01/03 - 02/03/03
                    --------------------------------------------------------------
                    Total Charges        60.00          182.00            182.00
                    Total Receipts        0.00            0.00              0.00
                    Refunds               0.00            0.00              0.00
                    Cross-Alloc Unapplied 0.00            0.00              0.00
                    Total Adjustments    60.00          120.00            120.00
                    Accounts Receivable  62.00           62.00             62.00
                    Total # Procedures       2               7                 7
                    Service Charges       0.00            0.00              0.00
                    Tax Charges           0.00            0.00              0.00
                    Copay Expected        0.00             ---               ---
                    Copay Paid            0.00             ---               ---
                    Deposit Amount        0.00             ---               ---
                           Checks   0.00
                           Cash     0.00
                           Other    0.00
                    --------------------------------------------------------------
```

Figure 5-28 Daily Report for 02/03/03—Sydney Carrington, M.D.

```
02/03/03                              DAILY REPORT FOR 02/03/03                              Page    2
                                      Sydney J Carrington M.D. (3)


                                                                [to Vchr   Total   Ref Date]
Account   Patient Name      Dt Post    Type Dates of Service  Dept Voucher Proc Code  Units  Pri/Sec Ail  Loc  Exc   Amount
========================================================================================================================
30.0      League,Claire     02/03/03   CHG  02/03/03-          0    1060   99213       1.00     2/   10   N            40.00
30.0      League,Claire     02/03/03   CHG  02/03/03-          0    1060   85031       1.00     2/   10   N            15.00
14.1      Evans,Gene        02/03/03   CHG  02/03/03-          0    1061   99213       1.00     7/    0   N            40.00
14.1      Evans,Gene        02/03/03   CHG  02/03/03-          0    1061   90749       1.00     7/    0   N            12.00
110.0     Evans,Patricia    02/03/03   CHG  01/27/03-          0    HOSP   99223       1.00     5/    0   Y            94.00
110.0     Evans,Patricia    02/03/03   CHG  01/31/03-          0    HOSP   99238       1.00     5/    0   Y            38.00
110.0     Evans,Patricia    02/03/03   CHG  01/28/03-01/31/03  0    HOSP   99232       4.00     5/    0   Y           376.00

Exception Codes:
overrides: c= charge, p= profile, w= writedown, o= overpay, i= pmt not from resp. ins, e= item edited, x= rebuilt dlyfile.tmp used


                                 Summary for : Sydney J Carrington M.D.
                    --------------------------------------------------------------
                       Item          Today      Period-to-Date        Year-to-Date
                    Description     02/03/03   01/01/03 - 02/03/03   01/01/03 - 02/03/03
                    --------------------------------------------------------------
                    Total Charges       615.00         1,304.00          1,304.00
                    Total Receipts        0.00             0.00              0.00
                    Refunds               0.00             0.00              0.00
                    Cross-Alloc Unapplied 0.00             0.00              0.00
                    Total Adjustments     0.00             0.00              0.00
                    Accounts Receivable 1,304.00       1,304.00          1,304.00
                    Total # Procedures      10               22                22
                    Service Charges       0.00             0.00              0.00
                    Tax Charges           0.00             0.00              0.00
                    Copay Expected        0.00              ---               ---
                    Copay Paid            0.00              ---               ---
                    Deposit Amount        0.00              ---               ---
                           Checks   0.00
                           Cash     0.00
                           Other    0.00
                    --------------------------------------------------------------
```

Figure 5-29 Cash Analysis Report for 02/03/03

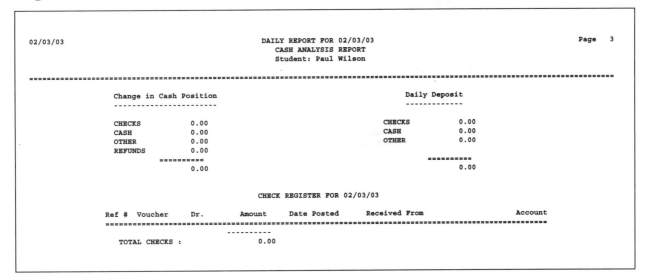

```
02/03/03                        DAILY REPORT FOR 02/03/03                       Page   3
                                   CASH ANALYSIS REPORT
                                   Student: Paul Wilson

=================================================================================

        Change in Cash Position                        Daily Deposit
        -----------------------                        -------------

        CHECKS          0.00                    CHECKS          0.00
        CASH            0.00                    CASH            0.00
        OTHER           0.00                    OTHER           0.00
        REFUNDS         0.00
                   ==========                              ==========
                        0.00                                    0.00


                              CHECK REGISTER FOR 02/03/03

    Ref #   Voucher    Dr.      Amount   Date Posted   Received From          Account
=================================================================================
                              ----------
        TOTAL CHECKS :          0.00
```

Figure 5-30 Daily Report Totals for 02/03/03

handwritten: .1359 −1304 / 0955

```
02/03/03                        DAILY REPORT FOR 02/03/03                       Page   4
                                   Student: Paul Wilson

=================================================================================


                              TOTALS FOR 02/03/03

-----------------------------------------------------------------------------------
Doctor                   Charges   Receipts  Adjustments   Net A/R   Total A/R  # Proc.  Serv Chg  Tax Chg
-----------------------------------------------------------------------------------
  1. James T Monroe MD     60.00      0.00      60.00        0.00      62.00       2      0.00     0.00
  3. Sydney J Carrington M.D.  615.00  0.00      0.00      615.00    1,304.00      10      0.00     0.00
-----------------------------------------------------------------------------------
TOTAL                     675.00      0.00      60.00      615.00    1,366.00      12      0.00     0.00


            PERIOD-TO-DATE TOTALS FOR 01/01/03 - 02/03/03

-----------------------------------------------------------------------------------
Doctor                   Charges   Receipts  Adjustments   Net A/R   Total A/R  # Proc.  Serv Chg  Tax Chg
-----------------------------------------------------------------------------------
  1. James T Monroe MD    182.00      0.00     120.00       62.00      62.00       7      0.00     0.00
  2. Frances D Simpson M.D. 128.00     0.00       0.00      128.00     128.00       3      0.00     0.00
  3. Sydney J Carrington M.D. 1,304.00 0.00       0.00    1,304.00   1,304.00      22      0.00     0.00
-----------------------------------------------------------------------------------
TOTAL                   1,614.00      0.00     120.00    1,494.00   1,494.00      32      0.00     0.00


            YEAR-TO-DATE TOTALS FOR 01/01/03 - 02/03/03

-----------------------------------------------------------------------------------
Doctor                   Charges   Receipts  Adjustments   Net A/R   Total A/R  # Proc.  Serv Chg  Tax Chg
-----------------------------------------------------------------------------------
  1. James T Monroe MD    182.00      0.00     120.00       62.00      62.00       7      0.00     0.00
  2. Frances D Simpson M.D. 128.00     0.00       0.00      128.00     128.00       3      0.00     0.00
  3. Sydney J Carrington M.D. 1,304.00 0.00       0.00    1,304.00   1,304.00      22      0.00     0.00
-----------------------------------------------------------------------------------
TOTAL                   1,614.00      0.00     120.00    1,494.00   1,494.00      32      0.00     0.00
```

handwritten annotations throughout: 670, 1359, 1356, 1549, 34, 1669, 670/55/615

Figure 5-31 GL Daily Distribution Report for 02/03/03

```
02/03/03                    GL DAILY DISTRIBUTION REPORT - FULL DETAIL                 Page   1
                                     Student: Paul Wilson
                                          02/03/03

  GL Account      Description      Dr   Pat #     Procedure   Date Post   Voucher      Debit           Credit
=========================================================================================================
    15001.00
                 Accounts Rec       1   120.4                 02/03/03     1058         30.00
                 Accounts Rec       1   120.0                 02/03/03                                   30.00
                 Accounts Rec       1   120.3                 02/03/03     1059         30.00
                 Accounts Rec       1   120.0                 02/03/03                                   30.00
                                                                                    -----------      -----------
    15003.00                                  POST TO ACCOUNT   15001.00               60.00            60.00
                 Accounts Rec       3    30.0                 02/03/03     1060         40.00
                 Accounts Rec       3    30.0                 02/03/03     1060         15.00
                 Accounts Rec       3    14.1                 02/03/03     1061         40.00
                 Accounts Rec       3    14.1                 02/03/03     1061         12.00
                 Accounts Rec       3   110.0                 02/03/03     HOSP         94.00
                 Accounts Rec       3   110.0                 02/03/03     HOSP         38.00
                 Accounts Rec       3   110.0                 02/03/03     HOSP        376.00
                                                                                    -----------      -----------
    60001.00                                  POST TO ACCOUNT   15003.00              615.00             0.00
                 Revenue            1   120.4     99212       02/03/03     1058                          30.00
                 Revenue            1   120.3     99212       02/03/03     1059                          30.00
                                                                                    -----------      -----------
    60003.00                                  POST TO ACCOUNT   60001.00                0.00            60.00
                 Revenue            3    30.0     99213       02/03/03     1060                          40.00
                 Revenue            3    30.0     85031       02/03/03     1060                          15.00
                 Revenue            3    14.1     99213       02/03/03     1061                          40.00
                 Revenue            3    14.1     90749       02/03/03     1061                          12.00
                 Revenue            3   110.0     99223       02/03/03     HOSP                          94.00
                 Revenue            3   110.0     99238       02/03/03     HOSP                          38.00
                 Revenue            3   110.0     99232       02/03/03     HOSP                         376.00
                                                                                    -----------      -----------
    60061.00                                  POST TO ACCOUNT   60003.00                0.00           615.00
            A05- HMO Adj & Write-Off  1   120.0   99212       02/03/03                  30.00
            A05- HMO Adj & Write-Off  1   120.0   99212       02/03/03                  30.00
                                                                                    -----------      -----------
                                             POST TO ACCOUNT   60061.00                60.00             0.00
                                                                                    ============      ============
                                                                                     735.00          -735.00
```

Figure 5-32 Daily Close Status Report for 02/03/03

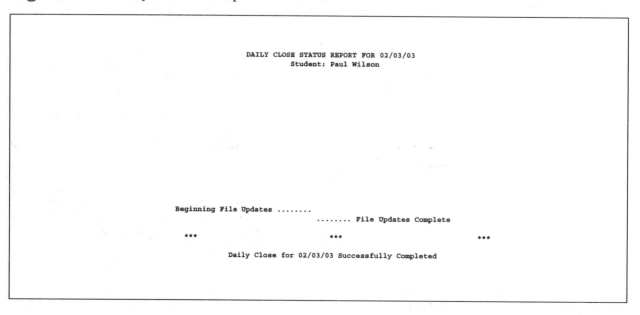

```
                          DAILY CLOSE STATUS REPORT FOR 02/03/03
                                   Student: Paul Wilson







                 Beginning File Updates ........
                                        ........ File Updates Complete

                      ***                  ***                  ***

                     Daily Close for 02/03/03 Successfully Completed
```

TESTING YOUR KNOWLEDGE

1. How are appointments scheduled within **The Medical Manager** system?

2. What is a daily list of appointments? How is this list used in the daily operation of the practice?

3. How is the (J)ump command used in scheduling appointments?

(continues)

4.   Why is the Hospital Rounds Report important? Describe how the doctor uses this report.

5.   How is the Hospital Rounds Report used in place of an encounter form for posting hospital charges?

6.   Describe how a user could use a help window to locate procedure and diagnosis codes.

U N I T 6

Practice Management

LEARNING OUTCOMES

After completing this unit, you should be able to:

◆ Describe why insurance billing is important.
◆ Explain why an Insurance Billing Worksheet should be prepared in advance of billing.
◆ Prepare an Insurance Billing Worksheet.
◆ Interpret the information on an Insurance Billing Worksheet.
◆ Print claim forms for insurance companies.
◆ Post payments from patients and insurance carriers.
◆ Make posting adjustments from the Procedure Entry screen.
◆ Make posting adjustments from the Payment Entry screen.
◆ Describe why the system date should not be advanced except after a daily close or when instructed to in the text.
◆ Locate and interpret information from an insurance plan's Explanation of Benefits.
◆ Describe the information to be processed at each portion of the Payment Entry screen.

You have already learned how to set up patient files, schedule appointments, post accounts, and develop assorted reports. In this unit, you will learn how to manage insurance and billing.

BILLING ROUTINES

Billing routines are for the generation of bills and statements sent to guarantors and their insurance companies. Six different tasks that you may complete within **The Medical Manager** system as you bill patient fees are (1) patient billing, (2) patient statements, (3) insurance billing worksheet, (4) trial insurance billing, (5) insurance billing process, and (6) electronic media claims (EMC). EMC refers to claims sent electronically by the computer over telephone lines using a modem.

Insurance companies require specific preprinted forms. These forms are called *Physical Forms* in **The Medical Manager** software's terminology. Insurance companies also require specific methods of form completion, called *Format Files* by **The Medical Manager** system. The numbers 1 to 99 indicate which versions of an insurance claim form are to be used in the printer. A second group of numbers, 1 to 99, is also used to indicate which of 99 different arrangements for printing information on the form should be used.

For example, most government and private insurance companies accept the standard American Medical Association Health Insurance Claim Form (CMS-1500 claim); yet each plan may want the form completed in a slightly different way. Medicare requires a physician's Medicare provider number; other insurance carriers require a Worker's Compensation number, Medicaid number, or state identification number. Therefore, the standard CMS-1500 claim could have as many as 99 different formats in **The Medical Manager** system.

Insurance format files are set up through the File Maintenance Menu (Menu 2). **The Medical Manager** software comes supplied with ready to use insurance format files.

Return to the Main Menu (Menu 1) and select option **6**, BILLING & EDI (EDI stands for Electronic Data Interchange). The screen shown in Figure 6-1 will appear. In the next exercises, you will use the Insurance Billing Worksheet and insurance billing items.

Figure 6-1   Billing & EDI Menu Screen

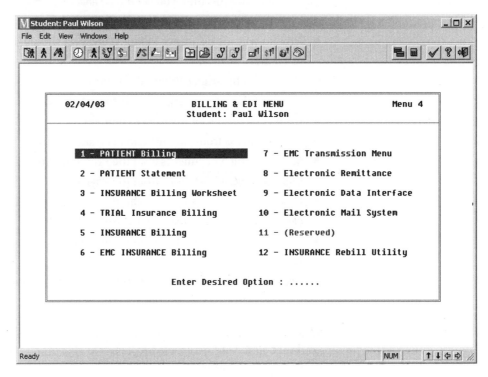

INSURANCE BILLING WORKSHEET

Verification of billing ensures prompt payment.

The Insurance Billing Worksheet allows you to verify that previous information was entered correctly. For example, you should determine that procedure charges were assigned to the proper primary and secondary insurance companies and that procedure codes and ailment information match. You should check all related information to make sure it is correct. By eliminating mistakes at this point, you can expect faster payment from the insurance plan.

You should always run the Insurance Billing Worksheet before printing a large number of insurance bills because it is your last opportunity to edit insurance-related information. The question marks ('?') that appear on this worksheet can be ignored. They refer to EMC billing that will not be covered in the following exercises, but will be covered in a subsequent course, **The Medical Manager** software's *Managed Care System—Student Edition.*

Note: It is a wise practice to back up your data before creating an Insurance Billing Worksheet. However, if you already completed a backup at the end of Unit 5, you do not need to do so now.

Complete the following exercises in insurance billing.

STEP 1   Select option **3**, INSURANCE Billing Worksheet, at the Billing & EDI Menu (Menu 4). The Insurance Billing Worksheet screen is shown in Figure 6-2.

Figure 6-2   Insurance Billing Worksheet Screen

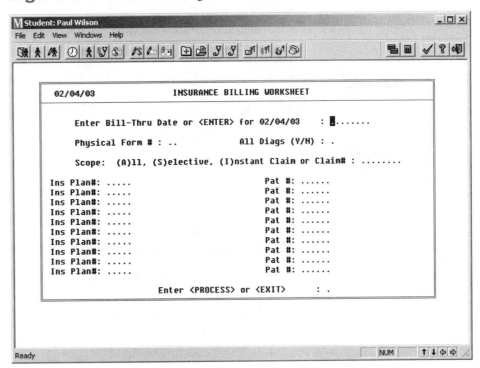

- ◆ a.   Enter a Bill-Thru Date: **020303** (Yesterday's date)

    This represents the last posting date for which charges will be reported on the billing worksheet.

    Because you will want to see the last complete day of charges, it is generally recommended that you enter the day *prior* to the current system date as the bill-through date.

- ◆ b.   Enter a Physical Form #: **1**

    This refers to the billing form used for the insurance plan. Only companies using the selected physical form identified by the number '1' will be considered for billing.

- ◆ c.   All Diags: (**N**)o

    Choosing (N)o will print only the primary diagnosis codes. Choosing (Y)es would print all diagnoses for each item.

- ◆ d.   Choose (**A**)ll claims to be billed.

The other possible option at this prompt is (S)elective. This option allows you to enter up to ten selections. The options for (S)elective claims are

1. *To report all claims for a specific insurance plan:* Select an insurance plan but do not select the corresponding patient account. All billable items for this insurance plan will be reported. You may press the F1 key or click on the PROCESS button ('√') on the top toolbar to process without going through any further selections.

2. *To report all claims for a specific patient account:* Press **ENTER** to default to '0' for the insurance plan, then key a patient account. All billable items for this account against all insurance plans will be reported.

3. *To report all claims for a specific insurance plan for a specific patient:* Key in an insurance plan and the corresponding patient account. Items for the selected account billable to the selected insurance plan will be reported.

STEP 2

Make sure your printer is ready. Press **F1** or click on the PROCESS button ('√') on the top toolbar to process, and the billing worksheet will be generated. If necessary, the printing of the worksheet can be aborted by pressing ESCAPE or by clicking on the EXIT button on the top toolbar.

STEP 3

Review the screen in Figure 6-3 that will be displayed only during the time the report is running.

Figure 6-3 Insurance Billing Worksheet Monitor Screen

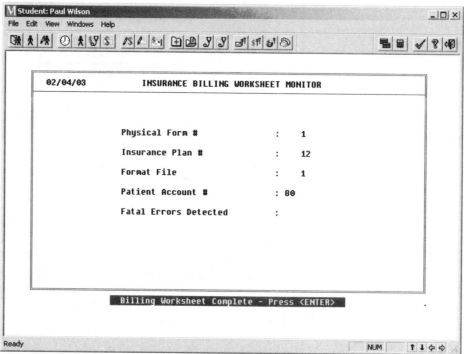

1. Physical Form # identifies which form will be used when you actually print bills.

2. Insurance Plan # refers to the insurance plan currently being processed.

3. Format File # identifies the method used to print information on the page.

4. Patient Account # refers to the account being processed.

UNIT 6 Practice Management

5. Fatal Errors Detected lists the number of fatal errors discovered and reported on the worksheet.

Compare your Insurance Prebilling Worksheet; it should look like Figure 6-4a and b.

Figure 6-4a Insurance Prebilling Worksheet Sample

```
02/04/03                          INSURANCE PREBILLING WORKSHEET                        Page   1
                                        Student: Paul Wilson
                                 Form # 1 - Thru 02/03/03 - All Claims

Ins Plan Dates of Service Diag Code  Proc Code  Mod  Voucher  POS/TOS    Units  Dr/Al/As  2nd Plan Bill Amt  Receipts     Net
==============================================================================================================================
    2 - Medicare               Fmt : A:ins0101a.fmt   Bill Amt = Adjusted
      10.0 - Carlson, Steven
        01/10/03 -       564.1      99214             1050      3/1      1.00   3/ N/ Y       5     50.00      0.00       50.00
                                                                                                ----------  ----------  ----------
                                                                            Totals       :         50.00      0.00       50.00

      30.0 - League, Claire
        01/10/03 -       285.9      99213             1054      3/1      1.00   1/ N/ Y      10     40.00      0.00       40.00
        01/10/03 -       571.5      85014             1054      3/1      1.00   1/ N/ Y      10     18.00      0.00       18.00
        02/03/03 -       285.9      99213             1060      3/1      1.00   3/ N/ Y      10     40.00      0.00       40.00
        02/03/03 -       285.9      85031             1060      3/1      1.00   3/ N/ Y      10     15.00      0.00       15.00
                                                                                                ----------  ----------  ----------
                                                                            Totals       :        113.00      0.00      113.00
                                                                                                                        ==========
                                      TOTAL TO BE BILLED FOR INSURANCE PLAN #      2 :                                  163.00
    5 - Epsilon Life & Casualty   Fmt : A:ins0101a.fmt   Bill Amt = Adjusted
      21.2 - Edwards, Andrea
        01/10/03 -       783.0      99214             1057      3/1      1.00   3/ Y/ Y       0     40.00      0.00       40.00
        01/10/03 -       783.0      81000             1057      3/1      1.00   3/ Y/ Y       0      8.00      0.00        8.00
        01/10/03 -       783.0      85014             1057      3/1      1.00   3/ Y/ Y       0     18.00      0.00       18.00
                                                                                                ----------  ----------  ----------
                                                                            Totals       :         66.00      0.00       66.00

      110.0 - Evans, Patricia
        01/10/03 -       174.9      99214             1056      3/1      1.00   3/ Y/ Y       0     50.00      0.00       50.00
        01/10/03 -       174.9      71020             1056      3/1      1.00   3/ Y/ Y       0     58.00      0.00       58.00
        01/10/03 -       174.9      76088             1056      3/1      1.00   3/ Y/ Y       0    125.00      0.00      125.00
        01/27/03 -       174.9      99223             HOSP      1/1      1.00   3/ Y/ Y       0     94.00      0.00       94.00
        01/31/03 -       174.9      99238             HOSP      1/1      1.00   3/ Y/ Y       0     38.00      0.00       38.00
        01/28/03 - 01/31/03 174.9  99232             HOSP      1/1      4.00   3/ Y/ Y       0    376.00      0.00      376.00
                                                                                                ----------  ----------  ----------
                                                                            Totals       :        741.00      0.00      741.00
                                                                                                                        ==========
                                      TOTAL TO BE BILLED FOR INSURANCE PLAN #      5 :                                  807.00
    6 - Cross and Shield Ins Plan  Fmt : A:ins0101a.fmt   Bill Amt = Adjusted
      34.0 - Dudley, Wayne
        01/10/03 -       346.9      99215             1053      3/1      1.00   3/ N/ Y       0     85.00      0.00       85.00
        01/10/03 -       346.9      81000             1053      3/1      1.00   3/ N/ Y       0      8.00      0.00        8.00
        01/10/03 -       346.9      72050             1053      3/1      1.00   3/ N/ Y       0    150.00      0.00      150.00
        01/10/03 -       346.9      93000             1053      3/1      1.00   3/ N/ Y       0     57.00      0.00       57.00
                                                                                                ----------  ----------  ----------
                                                                            Totals       :        300.00      0.00      300.00
                                                                                                                        ==========
                                      TOTAL TO BE BILLED FOR INSURANCE PLAN #      6 :                                  300.00
    7 - Pan American Health Ins.   Fmt : A:ins0101a.fmt   Bill Amt = Adjusted
      10.1 - Carlson, Sharon
        01/10/03 -       461.9      99213             1051      3/1      1.00   3/ N/ Y       0     40.00      0.00       40.00
                                                                                                ----------  ----------  ----------
                                                                            Totals       :         40.00      0.00       40.00

      14.1 - Evans, Gene
        02/03/03 -       461.9      99213             1061      3/1      1.00   3/ N/ Y       0     40.00      0.00       40.00
        02/03/03 -       461.9      90749             1061      3/1      1.00   3/ N/ Y       0     12.00      0.00       12.00
                                                                                                ----------  ----------  ----------
                                                                            Totals       :         52.00      0.00       52.00
```

Figure 6-4b Insurance Prebilling Worksheet Sample

```
02/04/03                          INSURANCE PREBILLING WORKSHEET                                    Page   2

Ins Plan Dates of Service Diag Code  Proc Code  Mod  Voucher  POS/TOS    Units  Dr/Al/As  2nd Plan Bill Amt    Receipts      Net
================================================================================================================================
   7 - Pan American Health Ins. (cont)
                                                                                                               ==========
                                                        TOTAL TO BE BILLED FOR INSURANCE PLAN #    7 :              92.00
  11 - Health Maint. Org.              Fmt : A:ins0101a.fmt    Bill Amt = Adjusted
  120.1 - Simmons, Laura
  + 01/10/03 -        v20.2            99211             WorkIn   3/1      1.00   1/ N/ N      0      0.00         0.00       0.00
                                                                                                  ----------   ----------  ----------
                                                                         Totals        :          0.00         0.00       0.00

  120.2 - Spivey, Alice
  + 01/10/03 -        v20.2            99211             1052     3/1      1.00   1/ N/ N      5      0.00         0.00       0.00
    01/10/03 -        v20.2            90701             1052     3/1      1.00   1/ N/ Y      5      4.00         0.00       4.00
                                                                                                  ----------   ----------  ----------
                                                                         Totals        :          4.00         0.00       4.00

  120.3 - Williams, Thomas
  + 02/03/03 -        487.0            99212             1059     3/1      1.00   1/ N/ N      0      0.00         0.00       0.00
                                                                                                  ----------   ----------  ----------
                                                                         Totals        :          0.00         0.00       0.00

  120.4 - Williams, Janet
  + 02/03/03 -        487.0            99212             1058     3/1      1.00   1/ N/ N      0      0.00         0.00       0.00
                                                                                                  ----------   ----------  ----------
                                                                         Totals        :          0.00         0.00       0.00
                                                                                                               ==========
                                                        TOTAL TO BE BILLED FOR INSURANCE PLAN #   11 :               4.00
  12 - Fringe Benefit Center          Fmt : A:ins0101a.fmt    Bill Amt = Adjusted
  80.0 - Davis, Timothy
    01/10/03 -        841.2            99213             1055     3/1      1.00   2/ Y/ Y      0     40.00         0.00      40.00
    01/10/03 -        841.2            29075             1055     3/1      1.00   2/ Y/ Y      0     48.00         0.00      48.00
                                                                                                  ----------   ----------  ----------
                                                                         Totals        :         88.00         0.00      88.00
                                                                                                               ==========
                                                        TOTAL TO BE BILLED FOR INSURANCE PLAN #   12 :              88.00
================================================================================================================================

                                                        TOTAL TO BE BILLED FOR ALL INSURANCE PLANS :             1454.00
```

Below is a brief explanation of the information reported on the worksheet. Compare this with your worksheet.

Ins Plan	Insurance plan number and name of insurance plan that will be sent the claim.
*	An asterisk preceding an item indicates that the item being billed has previously been billed to another insurance plan. The plan previously billed is now the secondary plan.
+	A plus sign preceding an item indicates that the item being billed is a nonassignment item and responsibility for payment will automatically be transferred to the patient.
?	A question mark preceding an item indicates that the item being billed necessitates special attention; for example, the item requires attached forms or is not EMC billable.
Dates of Service	Dates procedures were performed.
Diag Code	Diagnosis Code.
Proc Code	Procedure Code.
Mod	Modifier.
Voucher	Procedure charge voucher number.
POS/TOS	Place of Service/Type of Service.
Units	Number of times the procedure was performed.
Dr/Al/As	The number of the doctor who performed the procedure/Ailment Detail (Y/N)/Accept Assignment (Y/N).

2nd Plan	The insurance plan secondarily responsible.
Bill Amount	The procedure's charges minus adjustments. This will appear on the insurance form as the procedure charge.
Receipts	The total amount of payments applied to the charge to date. This will appear on the insurance form in the amount paid block.
Net	Bill amount minus receipts.

After the Insurance Billing Worksheet is generated, press **ENTER** to return to the Billing & EDI Menu (Menu 4). Check your worksheet. If any items are incorrect or missing, correct them through options available on the File Maintenance Menu (Menu 2).

Procedure code, diagnosis, or date information can be corrected through the Edit Procedure History option. Insurance information for a specific patient can be corrected through the Edit Patient Records option by choosing (I)ns. After making any necessary corrections, proceed to the next section in Insurance Billing.

INSURANCE BILLING PROCESS

Patients with insurance coverage must file a claim with their carrier that explains the services received and the fees charged. Sometimes the encounter form plus a handwritten or computerized claim form will suffice. Although patients are sometimes responsible for filing their own claims, many medical offices have found that the collection rate is better if the office produces and mails a computerized claim form to the insurance carrier. Medicare and most HMOs require the doctor to file the claim instead of the patient.

The health insurance claim form must be accurate and complete.

The claims examiner at the insurance plan evaluates the insurance form and determines whether the patient's benefits cover the services and fees listed. If the claim form is improperly filled out, incomplete, or unsigned by either the patient or physician, it will be returned unpaid or placed in a suspense file. The form can be resubmitted; however, payment for resubmissions takes longer and reduces a practice's cash flow.

APPLYING YOUR KNOWLEDGE

EXERCISE 1: Printing Insurance Forms

You are to submit claim forms for all patients listed on the prebilling worksheet from the previous demonstration. Review the prebilling worksheet to make corrections as needed before billing.

Note: Your school may have laser or dot matrix printers available for printing on blank CMS-1500 claims. For the purposes of checking your work in this exercise, you may print the information on a regular piece of blank paper. Note, however, that a dot matrix printer will not draw the boxes as on the form shown in Figure 6-5.

STEP 1

Load your blank paper or insurance forms, if provided by your instructor, in the printer. Return to the Billing & EDI Menu (Menu 4) and select option **5**, INSURANCE Billing. Enter the previous day's date ('**020303**') and Physical Form # **1**. Select (**A**)ll for claims. This is the same information you used to develop the prebilling worksheet, and it must match now that you are ready to print final insurance bills. Press **F1** or click on the PROCESS button ('√') on the top toolbar to process your data.

You may abort the billing routine at any time by pressing ESCAPE or by clicking on the EXIT button on the top toolbar. If a format file number is incorrect, you will get a fatal error message. To correct the format number, return to the Main Menu (Menu 1); then select menus in the following order: File Maintenance (Menu 2), Support Files Maintenance (Menu 13), and Insurance Plan Maintenance (option 3 in Support Files Maintenance Menu). The default format number is '1'.

STEP 2   **The Medical Manager** system allows you to check the alignment of information on the insurance forms. If you wish to check alignment, key 'Y' at the prompt "Do You Need A Form Alignment Pass (Y/N)." If you enter 'N', claim forms will print without an alignment check. Enter '**1**' in the Format Number prompt when you request an alignment check.

Accept the insurance billing by entering '**Y**' at the prompt "Do You Wish To Accept Insurance Billing?" Enter '**N**' if a problem has occurred, and you do not wish to accept this billing. A sample of a completed insurance claim form is shown in Figure 6-5. Hand in all your forms to your instructor.

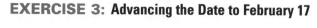

EXERCISE 2: Running a Final Daily Close for February 4

At the Main Menu (Menu 1), choose option **5**, REPORT Generation, then option **4**, DAILY Report.

STEP 1   Enter '**N**' to indicate you do not want a Trial Daily Report. Enter '**P**' to ask for a check register for the practice. Enter '**0**' to indicate that you do not wish to purge appointments. Press **F1** or click on the PROCESS button ('√') on the top toolbar to process, and the report will be generated.

STEP 2   When the report is complete, accept the Daily Close by entering 'Y' at the prompt.

EXERCISE 3: Advancing the Date to February 17

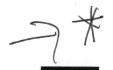

After you complete the Daily Close, the opening screen will appear so that you can change the date.

STEP 1   Enter '**02172003**.' Remember to enter the date very carefully. After you enter the date, you will receive the following warning message:

184: * WARNING * Skip>7 Days: Continue (Y/N)

In an office setting, you would never bypass such a warning. However, because these are practice sessions, you may key in '**Y**' and press **ENTER** to bypass the date warning message.

STEP 2   You will be prompted to reenter your password. Key '**ICAN**' and press **ENTER** to verify the date advance and return to the Main Menu (Menu 1).

When you complete the above-mentioned steps to change the date, you should see the new date, 02/17/03, appear in the upper left corner of the Main Menu (Menu 1). If this *exact* date does not appear, notify your instructor immediately so that your files may be restored from backup and the steps to change the date can be reentered. *If you proceed with an incorrect date, your data files will NOT be reliable.* Do not change the date again until you are specifically instructed to do so in the following lessons.

Figure 6-5 Completed Claim Form

PLEASE
DO NOT
STAPLE
IN THIS
AREA

Epsilon Life & Casualty
P.O. Box 189
Macon, GA 31298

CARRIER

☐☐ PICA   **HEALTH INSURANCE CLAIM FORM**   PICA ☐☐

1. MEDICARE MEDICAID CHAMPUS CHAMPVA GROUP HEALTH PLAN (SSN or ID) FECA BLK LUNG (SSN) OTHER	1a. INSURED'S I.D. NUMBER (FOR PROGRAM IN ITEM 1)
☐ (Medicare #) ☐ (Medicaid #) ☐ (Sponsor's SSN) ☐ (VA File #) ☐ (SSN or ID) ☐ (SSN) ☒ (ID)	756575675

2. PATIENT'S NAME (Last Name, First Name, Middle Initial)	3. PATIENT'S BIRTH DATE MM DD YY SEX	4. INSURED'S NAME (Last Name, First Name, Middle Initial)
Evans Patricia	12 13 51 M☐ F☒	Evans Patricia G

5. PATIENT'S ADDRESS (No., Street)	6. PATIENT RELATIONSHIP TO INSURED	7. INSURED'S ADDRESS (No., Street)
8907 Harbor Drive	Self ☒ Spouse ☐ Child ☐ Other ☐	8907 Harbor Drive

CITY	STATE	8. PATIENT STATUS	CITY	STATE
Madison	CA	Single ☐ Married ☐ Other ☐	Madison	CA

ZIP CODE	TELEPHONE (Include Area Code)		ZIP CODE	TELEPHONE (INCLUDE AREA CODE)
95653	( )	Employed ☐ Full-Time Student ☐ Part-Time Student ☐	95653	( )

9. OTHER INSURED'S NAME (Last Name, First Name, Middle Initial)	10. IS PATIENT'S CONDITION RELATED TO:	11. INSURED'S POLICY GROUP OR FECA NUMBER
a. OTHER INSURED'S POLICY OR GROUP NUMBER	a. EMPLOYMENT? (CURRENT OR PREVIOUS) ☐ YES ☒ NO	a. INSURED'S DATE OF BIRTH MM DD YY SEX M☐ F☐
b. OTHER INSURED'S DATE OF BIRTH MM DD YY SEX M☐ F☐	b. AUTO ACCIDENT? PLACE (State) ☐ YES ☐ NO	b. EMPLOYER'S NAME OR SCHOOL NAME
c. EMPLOYER'S NAME OR SCHOOL NAME	c. OTHER ACCIDENT? ☐ YES ☐ NO	c. INSURANCE PLAN NAME OR PROGRAM NAME
d. INSURANCE PLAN NAME OR PROGRAM NAME	10d. RESERVED FOR LOCAL USE	d. IS THERE ANOTHER HEALTH BENEFIT PLAN? ☐ YES ☐ NO If yes, return to and complete item 9 a-d.

READ BACK OF FORM BEFORE COMPLETING & SIGNING THIS FORM.

12. PATIENT'S OR AUTHORIZED PERSON'S SIGNATURE I authorize the release of any medical or other information necessary to process this claim. I also request payment of government benefits either to myself or to the party who accepts assignment below.

SIGNED Signature on File   DATE 02/04/03

13. INSURED'S OR AUTHORIZED PERSON'S SIGNATURE I authorize payment of medical benefits to the undersigned physician or supplier for services described below.

SIGNED Signature on File

14. DATE OF CURRENT: MM DD YY ◀ ILLNESS (First symptom) OR INJURY (Accident) OR PREGNANCY(LMP)	15. IF PATIENT HAS HAD SAME OR SIMILAR ILLNESS. GIVE FIRST DATE MM DD YY	16. DATES PATIENT UNABLE TO WORK IN CURRENT OCCUPATION
12 30 02		FROM MM DD YY TO MM DD YY

17. NAME OF REFERRING PHYSICIAN OR OTHER SOURCE	17a. I.D. NUMBER OF REFERRING PHYSICIAN	18. HOSPITALIZATION DATES RELATED TO CURRENT SERVICES
Leland W. Groves, M.D.		FROM 01 27 03 TO 01 31 03

19. RESERVED FOR LOCAL USE	20. OUTSIDE LAB? ☐ YES ☐ NO $ CHARGES

21. DIAGNOSIS OR NATURE OF ILLNESS OR INJURY. (RELATE ITEMS 1,2,3 OR 4 TO ITEM 24E BY LINE)	22. MEDICAID RESUBMISSION CODE ORIGINAL REF. NO.
1. 174.9 3. ___.___	23. PRIOR AUTHORIZATION NUMBER
2. ___.___ 4. ___.___	

24. A DATE(S) OF SERVICE From MM DD YY To MM DD YY	B Place of Service	C Type of Service	D PROCEDURES, SERVICES, OR SUPPLIES (Explain Unusual Circumstances) CPT/HCPCS MODIFIER	E DIAGNOSIS CODE	F $ CHARGES	G DAYS OR UNITS	H EPSDT Family Plan	I EMG	J COB	K RESERVED FOR LOCAL USE
1	01 10 03		3	99214	174.9	50 00	1				
2	01 10 03		3	76088	174.9	125 00	1				
3	01 10 03		3	71020	174.9	58 00	1				
4	01 27 03		3	99223	174.9	180 00	1				
5	01 31 03		3	99238	174.9	38 00	1				
6	01 27 03 01 31 03		3	99232	174.9	208 00	4				

25. FEDERAL TAX I.D. NUMBER SSN EIN	26. PATIENT'S ACCOUNT NO.	27. ACCEPT ASSIGNMENT? (For govt. claims, see back) ☒ YES ☐ NO	28. TOTAL CHARGE $ 659 00	29. AMOUNT PAID $ 00	30. BALANCE DUE $ 659 00

31. SIGNATURE OF PHYSICIAN OR SUPPLIER INCLUDING DEGREES OR CREDENTIALS (I certify that the statements on the reverse apply to this bill and are made a part thereof.) Signature on File SIGNED DATE	32. NAME AND ADDRESS OF FACILITY WHERE SERVICES WERE RENDERED (If other than home or office)	33. PHYSICIAN'S, SUPPLIER'S BILLING NAME, ADDRESS, ZIP CODE & PHONE # 9169876543 Sydney Carrington & Assoc. 34 Sycamore St. Suite 300 Madison, CA 95653 PIN# GRP#

(APPROVED BY AMA COUNCIL ON MEDICAL SERVICE 8/88)   **PLEASE PRINT OR TYPE**   APPROVED OMB-0938-0008 FORM CMS-1500 (12-90). FORM RRB-1500, APPROVED OMB-1215-0055 FORM OWCP-1500, APPROVED OMB-0720-0001 (CHAMPUS)

PATIENT AND INSURED INFORMATION

PHYSICIAN OR SUPPLIER INFORMATION

EXERCISE 4: Timothy R. Davis

Posting Charges for Worker's Compensation

Post two charges for Mr. Timothy Davis using the procedure code numbers indicated on his encounter form, shown in Figure 6-6. From the Main Menu (Menu 1), key '/**PRO**' and press **ENTER** to direct chain to Procedure Entry. At the Procedure Entry Patient Retrieval screen, key '**Davis,Timothy**' and press **ENTER** twice to retrieve his account.

STEP 1 Select plan '**12**' as Mr. Davis's primary coverage and the plan to be billed for this visit. Post the first charge shown on Mr. Davis's encounter form. If you have any difficulty, refer back to Unit 3 for specific instructions on how to post charges to a patient account. When the first charge is processed, key in '**1**' at the ailment prompt to signify that this charge refers to the previous ailment, his sprained wrist.

STEP 2 Post the second charge listed on Mr. Davis's encounter form. When the second charge is processed, select (**S**)ame ailment.

Figure 6-6 Timothy Davis's Encounter Form—Voucher 1062

Sydney Carrington & Associates P.A.
34 Sycamore Street   Suite 300
Madison, CA 95653

Date: 02/17/2003

Voucher No.: 1062

Time: 10:00

Patient: Timothy Davis
Guarantor: Timothy R. Davis

Patient No: 80.0
Doctor: 2 - F. Simpson

□ CPT	DESCRIPTION	FEE
OFFICE/HOSPITAL CONSULTS		
□ 99201	Office New:Focused Hx-Exam	_____
□ 99202	Office New:Expanded Hx-Exam	_____
□ 99211	Office Estb:Min/None Hx-Exa	_____
□ 99212	Office Estb:Focused Hx-Exam	_____
⊠ 99213	Office Estb:Expanded Hx-Exa	$40.00
□ 99214	Office Estb:Detailed Hx-Exa	_____
□ 99215	Office Estb:Comprhn Hx-Exam	_____
□ 99221	Hosp. Initial:Comprh Hx-	_____
□ 99223	Hosp.Ini:Comprh Hx-Exam/Hi	_____
□ 99231	Hosp. Subsequent: S-Fwd	_____
□ 99232	Hosp. Subsequent: Comprhn Hx	_____
□ 99233	Hosp. Subsequent: Ex/Hi	_____
□ 99238	Hospital Visit Discharge Ex	_____
□ 99371	Telephone Consult - Simple	_____
□ 99372	Telephone Consult - Intermed	_____
□ 99373	Telephone Consult - Complex	_____
□ 90843	Counseling - 25 minutes	_____
□ 90844	Counseling - 50 minutes	_____
□ 90865	Counseling - Special Interview	_____
IMMUNIZATIONS/INJECTIONS		
□ 90585	BCG Vaccine	_____
□ 90659	Influenza Virus Vaccine	_____
□ 90701	Immunization-DTP	_____
□ 90702	DT Vaccine	_____
□ 90703	Tetanus Toxoids	_____
□ 90732	Pneumococcal Vaccine	_____
□ 90746	Hepatitis B Vaccine	_____
□ 90749	Immunization; Unlisted	_____

□ CPT	DESCRIPTION	FEE
LABORATORY/RADIOLOGY		
□ 81000	Urinalysis	_____
□ 81002	Urinalysis; Pregnancy Test	_____
□ 82951	Glucose Tolerance Test	_____
□ 84478	Triglycerides	_____
□ 84550	Uric Acid: Blood Chemistry	_____
□ 84830	Ovulation Test	_____
□ 85014	Hematocrit	_____
□ 85031	Hemogram, Complete Blood Wk	_____
□ 86403	Particle Agglutination Test	_____
□ 86485	Skin Test; Candida	_____
□ 86580	TB Intradermal Test	_____
□ 86585	TB Tine Test	_____
□ 87070	Culture	_____
□ 70190	X-Ray; Optic Foramina	_____
□ 70210	X-Ray Sinuses Complete	_____
□ 71010	Radiological Exam Ent Spine	_____
□ 71020	X-Ray Chest Pa & Lat	_____
□ 72050	X-Ray Spine, Cerv (4 views)	_____
□ 72090	X-Ray Spine; Scoliosis Ex	_____
□ 72110	Spine, lumbosacral; a/p & Lat	_____
□ 73030	Shoulder-Comp, min w/ 2vws	_____
□ 73070	Elbow, anteropost & later vws	_____
□ 73120	X-Ray; Hand, 2 views	_____
□ 73560	X-Ray, Knee, 1 or 2 views	_____
□ 74022	X-Ray; Abdomen, Complete	_____
□ 75552	Cardiac Magnetic Res Img	_____
□ 76020	X-Ray; Bone Age Studies	_____
□ 76088	Mammary Ductogram Complete	_____
□ 78465	Myocardial Perfusion Img	_____

□ CPT	DESCRIPTION	FEE
PROCEDURES/TESTS		
□ 00452	Anesthesia for Rad Surgery	_____
□ 11100	Skin Biopsy	_____
□ 15852	Dressing Change	_____
□ 29075	Cast Appl. - Lower Arm	_____
□ 29530	Strapping of Knee	_____
⊠ 29705	Removal/Revis of Cast w/Exa	$38.00
□ 53670	Catheterization Incl. Suppl	_____
□ 57452	Colposcopy	_____
□ 57505	ECC	_____
□ 69420	Myringotomy	_____
□ 92081	Visual Field Examination	_____
□ 92100	Serial Tonometry Exam	_____
□ 92120	Tonography	_____
□ 92552	Pure Tone Audiometry	_____
□ 92567	Tympanometry	_____
□ 93000	Electrocardiogram	_____
□ 93015	Exercise Stress Test (ETT)	_____
□ 93017	ETT Tracing Only	_____
□ 93040	Electrocardiogram - Rhythm	_____
□ 96100	Psychological Testing	_____
□ 99000	Specimen Handling	_____
□ 99058	Office Emergency Care	_____
□ 99070	Surgical Tray - Misc.	_____
□ 99080	Special Reports of Med Rec	_____
□ 99195	Phlebotomy	_____
□	_____	_____
□	_____	_____
□	_____	_____
□	_____	_____

ICD-9 CODE DIAGNOSIS	
□ 009.0	Ill-defined Intestinal Infect
□ 133.2	Establish Baseline
□ 174.9	Breast Cancer
□ 185.0	Prostate Cancer
□ 250	Diabetes Mellitus
□ 272.4	Hyperlipidemia
□ 282.5	Anemia - Sickle Trait
□ 282.60	Anemia - Sickle Cell
□ 285.9	Anemia, Unspecified
□ 300.4	Neurotic Depression
□ 340	Multiple Sclerosis
□ 342.9	Hemiplegia - Unspecified
□ 346.9	Migraine Headache
□ 352.9	Cranial Neuralgia
□ 354.0	Carpal Tunnel Syndrome
□ 355.0	Sciatic Nerve Root Lesion
□ 366.9	Cataract
□ 386.0	Vertigo
□ 401.1	Essential Hypertension
□ 414.9	Ischemic Hearth Disease
□ 428.0	Congestive Heart Failure

ICD-9 CODE DIAGNOSIS	
□ 435.0	Basilar Artery Syndrome
□ 440.0	Atherosclerosis
□ 442.81	Carotid Artery
□ 460.0	Common Cold
□ 461.9	Acute Sinusitis
□ 474.0	Tonsillitis
□ 477.9	Hay Fever
□ 487.0	Flu
□ 496	Chronic Airway Obstruction
□ 522	Low Red Blood Count
□ 524.6	Temporo-Mandibular Jnt Synd
□ 538.8	Stomach Pain
□ 553.3	Hiatal Hernia
□ 564.1	Spastic Colon
□ 571.4	Chronic Hepatitis
□ 571.5	Cirrhosis of Liver
□ 573.3	Hepatitis
□ 575.2	Obstruction of Gallbladder
□ 648.2	Anemia - Compl. Pregnancy
□ 715.90	Osteoarthritis - Unspec
□ 721.3	Lumbar Osteo/Spondylarthrit

ICD-9 CODE DIAGNOSIS	
□ 724.2	Pain: Lower Back
□ 727.6	Rupture of Achilles Tendon
□ 780.1	Hallucinations
□ 780.3	Convulsions
□ 780.5	Sleep Disturbances
□ 783.0	Anorexia
□ 783.1	Abnormal Weight Gain
□ 783.2	Abnormal Weight Loss
□ 830.6	Dislocated Hip
□ 830.9	Dislocated Shoulder
⊠ 841.2	Sprained Wrist
□ 842.5	Sprained Ankle
□ 891.2	Fractured Tibia
□ 892.0	Fractured Fibula
□ 919.5	Insect Bite, Nonvenomous
□ 921.1	Contus Eyelid/Perioc Area
□ v16.3	Fam. Hist of Breast Cancer
□ v17.4	Fam. Hist of Cardiovasc Dis
□ v20.2	Well Child
□ v22.0	Pregnancy - First Normal
□ v22.1	Pregnancy - Normal

Previous Balance	Today's Charges	Total Due	Amount Paid	New Balance
_____	_____	_____	_____	_____

Follow Up

PRN _____ Weeks _____ Months _____ Units _____

Next Appointment Date: _____   Time: _____

I hereby authorize release of any information acquired in the course of examination or treatment and allow a photocopy of my signature to be used.

_____

(handwritten at top: 2:30 ✱ 10/21)

EXERCISE 5: Portia D. Edwards

Posting a Second Patient with Worker's Compensation

Portia Edwards is examined for an injury to her lower back. Use the encounter form shown in Figure 6-7 to post the procedure. *Remember to press ENTER to bypass any fields for which no information is given.*

From the Procedure Entry Patient Retrieval screen, retrieve Mrs. Edwards's account.

STEP 1 Post the information shown on Mrs. Edwards's encounter form. Select only her Worker's Compensation plan from the Procedure Entry Insurance help window, to *be sure her Worker's Compensation is solely billed.* Answer '0' at the Secondary Insurance field. Then press **F1** or click on the PROCESS button ('√') to process and choose to (**A**)dd an ailment.

STEP 2 Add Mrs. Edwards's Ailment Detail as given below.

Hold Insurance Bill (Y/N/I): (Press **ENTER** to accept the default of (N)ormal Billing)
Date First Consulted: **021703**
Facility #: (Press **ENTER** to leave blank)
Comment Field: **WC Back**
Prior Authorization #: (Press **ENTER** to leave blank)
Inpatient (Y/N): (**N**)o
Ref. Dr #: (Press **ENTER** to accept '0' to indicate there is no Referring Doctor)
Related to Employment (Y/N): (**Y**)es
Accident: (**O**)ther
Old Symptoms: (**N**)o
Emergency (Y/N): (**N**)o
Date First Symptom: **021403**

Note: Make sure you do not accept the current system date!

PROCESS and press **ESCAPE** until you are returned to the Procedure Entry Patient Retrieval screen.

Figure 6-7 Portia Edwards's Encounter Form—Voucher 1063

Sydney Carrington & Associates P.A.
34 Sycamore Street   Suite 300
Madison, CA 95653

Date: 02/17/2003

Time: 11:30

Patient: Portia Edwards
Guarantor: Portia D. Edwards

Voucher No.: 1063

Patient No: 21.0
Doctor: 3 - S. Carrington

□ CPT	DESCRIPTION	FEE
OFFICE/HOSPITAL CONSULTS		
□ 99201	Office New:Focused Hx-Exam	
□ 99202	Office New:Expanded Hx-Exam	
□ 99211	Office Estb:Min/None Hx-Exa	
□ 99212	Office Estb:Focused Hx-Exam	
□ 99213	Office Estb:Expanded Hx-Exa	
⊠ 99214	Office Estb:Detailed Hx-Exa	$50.00
□ 99215	Office Estb:Comprhn Hx-Exam	
□ 99221	Hosp. Initial:Comprh Hx-	
□ 99223	Hosp.Ini:Comprh Hx-Exam/Hi	
□ 99231	Hosp. Subsequent: S-Fwd	
□ 99232	Hosp. Subsequent: Comprhn Hx	
□ 99233	Hosp. Subsequent: Ex/Hi	
□ 99238	Hospital Visit Discharge Ex	
□ 99371	Telephone Consult - Simple	
□ 99372	Telephone Consult - Intermed	
□ 99373	Telephone Consult - Complex	
□ 90843	Counseling - 25 minutes	
□ 90844	Counseling - 50 minutes	
□ 90865	Counseling - Special Interview	
IMMUNIZATIONS/INJECTIONS		
□ 90585	BCG Vaccine	
□ 90659	Influenza Virus Vaccine	
□ 90701	Immunization-DTP	
□ 90702	DT Vaccine	
□ 90703	Tetanus Toxoids	
□ 90732	Pneumococcal Vaccine	
□ 90746	Hepatitis B Vaccine	
□ 90749	Immunization; Unlisted	

□ CPT	DESCRIPTION	FEE
LABORATORY/RADIOLOGY		
□ 81000	Urinalysis	
□ 81002	Urinalysis; Pregnancy Test	
□ 82951	Glucose Tolerance Test	
□ 84478	Triglycerides	
□ 84550	Uric Acid: Blood Chemistry	
□ 84830	Ovulation Test	
□ 85014	Hematocrit	
□ 85031	Hemogram, Complete Blood Wk	
□ 86403	Particle Agglutination Test	
□ 86485	Skin Test; Candida	
□ 86580	TB Intradermal Test	
□ 86585	TB Tine Test	
□ 87070	Culture	
□ 70190	X-Ray; Optic Foramina	
□ 70210	X-Ray Sinuses Complete	
□ 71010	Radiological Exam Ent Spine	
□ 71020	X-Ray Chest Pa & Lat	
□ 72050	X-Ray Spine, Cerv (4 views)	
□ 72090	X-Ray Spine; Scoliosis Ex	
□ 72110	Spine, lumbosacral; a/p & Lat	
□ 73030	Shoulder-Comp, min w/ 2vws	
□ 73070	Elbow, anteropost & later vws	
□ 73120	X-Ray; Hand, 2 views	
□ 73560	X-Ray, Knee, 1 or 2 views	
□ 74022	X-Ray; Abdomen, Complete	
□ 75552	Cardiac Magnetic Res Img	
□ 76020	X-Ray; Bone Age Studies	
□ 76088	Mammary Ductogram Complete	
□ 78465	Myocardial Perfusion Img	

□ CPT	DESCRIPTION	FEE
PROCEDURES/TESTS		
□ 00452	Anesthesia for Rad Surgery	
□ 11100	Skin Biopsy	
□ 15852	Dressing Change	
□ 29075	Cast Appl. - Lower Arm	
□ 29530	Strapping of Knee	
□ 29705	Removal/Revis of Cast w/Exa	
□ 53670	Catheterization Incl. Suppl	
□ 57452	Colposcopy	
□ 57505	ECC	
□ 69420	Myringotomy	
□ 92081	Visual Field Examination	
□ 92100	Serial Tonometry Exam	
□ 92120	Tonography	
□ 92552	Pure Tone Audiometry	
□ 92567	Tympanometry	
□ 93000	Electrocardiogram	
□ 93015	Exercise Stress Test (ETT)	
□ 93017	ETT Tracing Only	
□ 93040	Electrocardiogram - Rhythm	
□ 96100	Psychological Testing	
□ 99000	Specimen Handling	
□ 99058	Office Emergency Care	
□ 99070	Surgical Tray - Misc.	
□ 99080	Special Reports of Med Rec	
□ 99195	Phlebotomy	
□		
□		
□		
□		

ICD-9 CODE DIAGNOSIS	
□ 009.0	Ill-defined Intestinal Infect
□ 133.2	Establish Baseline
□ 174.9	Breast Cancer
□ 185.0	Prostate Cancer
□ 250	Diabetes Mellitus
□ 272.4	Hyperlipidemia
□ 282.5	Anemia - Sickle Trait
□ 282.60	Anemia - Sickle Cell
□ 285.9	Anemia, Unspecified
□ 300.4	Neurotic Depression
□ 340	Multiple Sclerosis
□ 342.9	Hemiplegia - Unspecified
□ 346.9	Migraine Headache
□ 352.9	Cranial Neuralgia
□ 354.0	Carpal Tunnel Syndrome
□ 355.0	Sciatic Nerve Root Lesion
□ 366.9	Cataract
□ 386.0	Vertigo
□ 401.1	Essential Hypertension
□ 414.9	Ischemic Hearth Disease
□ 428.0	Congestive Heart Failure

ICD-9 CODE DIAGNOSIS	
□ 435.0	Basilar Artery Syndrome
□ 440.0	Atherosclerosis
□ 442.81	Carotid Artery
□ 460.0	Common Cold
□ 461.9	Acute Sinusitis
□ 474.0	Tonsillitis
□ 477.9	Hay Fever
□ 487.0	Flu
□ 496	Chronic Airway Obstruction
□ 522	Low Red Blood Count
□ 524.6	Temporo-Mandibular Jnt Synd
□ 538.8	Stomach Pain
□ 553.3	Hiatal Hernia
□ 564.1	Spastic Colon
□ 571.4	Chronic Hepatitis
□ 571.5	Cirrhosis of Liver
□ 573.3	Hepatitis
□ 575.2	Obstruction of Gallbladder
□ 648.2	Anemia - Compl. Pregnancy
□ 715.90	Osteoarthritis - Unspec
□ 721.3	Lumbar Osteo/Spondylarthrit

ICD-9 CODE DIAGNOSIS	
⊠ 724.2	Pain: Lower Back
□ 727.6	Rupture of Achilles Tendon
□ 780.1	Hallucinations
□ 780.3	Convulsions
□ 780.5	Sleep Disturbances
□ 783.0	Anorexia
□ 783.1	Abnormal Weight Gain
□ 783.2	Abnormal Weight Loss
□ 830.6	Dislocated Hip
□ 830.9	Dislocated Shoulder
□ 841.2	Sprained Wrist
□ 842.5	Sprained Ankle
□ 891.2	Fractured Tibia
□ 892.0	Fractured Fibula
□ 919.5	Insect Bite, Nonvenomous
□ 921.1	Contus Eyelid/Perioc Area
□ v16.3	Fam. Hist of Breast Cancer
□ v17.4	Fam. Hist of Cardiovasc Dis
□ v20.2	Well Child
□ v22.0	Pregnancy - First Normal
□ v22.1	Pregnancy - Normal

Previous Balance	Today's Charges	Total Due	Amount Paid	New Balance

Follow Up

PRN _____ Weeks _____ Months _____ Units _____

Next Appointment Date: _____   Time: _____

I hereby authorize release of any information acquired in the course of examination or treatment and allow a photocopy of my signature to be used.

POSTING PAYMENTS AND ADJUSTMENTS

Payments may be made in a variety of ways.

Because both patients and insurance companies pay the doctor's fees, you will receive payment in a variety of forms. Payments can be entered into **The Medical Manager** in two ways. One method allows posting from the Procedure Entry screen, and the other allows posting from the Payment Entry screen.

Posting Payments from the Procedure Entry Screen

The easiest method of posting payments for patients who pay at the time of their visit is through the Procedure Entry screen. Deborah Evans will pay in full for her visit today. Therefore, the insurance plan will not be billed for today's charges.

STEP 1 Retrieve Deborah Evans's account so you can post charges and payments. Be sure to enter '**0**' at the Primary Ins # field since Mrs. Evans plans to pay in full for today's visit. Therefore, the insurance plan will *not* be billed for today's charges.

STEP 2 Post both charges shown on the encounter form in Figure 6-8. When you EXIT after posting the last procedure, the screen will prompt you to choose the method of payment allocation or to EXIT if the patient will not be making a payment at this time.

Figure 6-8 Deborah Evans's Encounter Form—Voucher 1064

Sydney Carrington & Associates P.A.
34 Sycamore Street   Suite 300
Madison, CA 95653

Date: 02/17/2003

Time: 11:45

Patient: Deborah Evans
Guarantor: Deborah A. Evans

Voucher No.: 1064

Patient No: 14.0
Doctor: 3 - S. Carrington

☐ CPT	DESCRIPTION	FEE
OFFICE/HOSPITAL CONSULTS		
☐ 99201	Office New:Focused Hx-Exam	
☐ 99202	Office New:Expanded Hx-Exam	
☐ 99211	Office Estb:Min/None Hx-Exa	
☐ 99212	Office Estb:Focused Hx-Exam	
☒ 99213	Office Estb:Expanded Hx-Exa	$40.00
☐ 99214	Office Estb:Detailed Hx-Exa	
☐ 99215	Office Estb:Comprhn Hx-Exam	
☐ 99221	Hosp. Initial:Comprh Hx-	
☐ 99223	Hosp.Ini:Comprh Hx-Exam/Hi	
☐ 99231	Hosp. Subsequent: S-Fwd	
☐ 99232	Hosp. Subsequent: Comprhn Hx	
☐ 99233	Hosp. Subsequent: Ex/Hi	
☐ 99238	Hospital Visit Discharge Ex	
☐ 99371	Telephone Consult - Simple	
☐ 99372	Telephone Consult - Intermed	
☐ 99373	Telephone Consult - Complex	
☐ 90843	Counseling - 25 minutes	
☐ 90844	Counseling - 50 minutes	
☐ 90865	Counseling - Special Interview	
IMMUNIZATIONS/INJECTIONS		
☐ 90585	BCG Vaccine	
☐ 90659	Influenza Virus Vaccine	
☐ 90701	Immunization-DTP	
☐ 90702	DT Vaccine	
☐ 90703	Tetanus Toxoids	
☐ 90732	Pneumococcal Vaccine	
☐ 90746	Hepatitis B Vaccine	
☐ 90749	Immunization; Unlisted	

☐ CPT	DESCRIPTION	FEE
LABORATORY/RADIOLOGY		
☐ 81000	Urinalysis	
☐ 81002	Urinalysis; Pregnancy Test	
☐ 82951	Glucose Tolerance Test	
☐ 84478	Triglycerides	
☐ 84550	Uric Acid: Blood Chemistry	
☐ 84830	Ovulation Test	
☐ 85014	Hematocrit	
☐ 85031	Hemogram, Complete Blood Wk	
☐ 86403	Particle Agglutination Test	
☐ 86485	Skin Test; Candida	
☐ 86580	TB Intradermal Test	
☐ 86585	TB Tine Test	
☒ 87070	Culture	$31.00
☐ 70190	X-Ray; Optic Foramina	
☐ 70210	X-Ray Sinuses Complete	
☐ 71010	Radiological Exam Ent Spine	
☐ 71020	X-Ray Chest Pa & Lat	
☐ 72050	X-Ray Spine, Cerv (4 views)	
☐ 72090	X-Ray Spine; Scoliosis Ex	
☐ 72110	Spine, lumbosacral; a/p & Lat	
☐ 73030	Shoulder-Comp, min w/ 2vws	
☐ 73070	Elbow, anteropost & later vws	
☐ 73120	X-Ray; Hand, 2 views	
☐ 73560	X-Ray, Knee, 1 or 2 views	
☐ 74022	X-Ray; Abdomen, Complete	
☐ 75552	Cardiac Magnetic Res Img	
☐ 76020	X-Ray; Bone Age Studies	
☐ 76088	Mammary Ductogram Complete	
☐ 78465	Myocardial Perfusion Img	

☐ CPT	DESCRIPTION	FEE
PROCEDURES/TESTS		
☐ 00452	Anesthesia for Rad Surgery	
☐ 11100	Skin Biopsy	
☐ 15852	Dressing Change	
☐ 29075	Cast Appl. - Lower Arm	
☐ 29530	Strapping of Knee	
☐ 29705	Removal/Revis of Cast w/Exa	
☐ 53670	Catheterization Incl. Suppl	
☐ 57452	Colposcopy	
☐ 57505	ECC	
☐ 69420	Myringotomy	
☐ 92081	Visual Field Examination	
☐ 92100	Serial Tonometry Exam	
☐ 92120	Tonography	
☐ 92552	Pure Tone Audiometry	
☐ 92567	Tympanometry	
☐ 93000	Electrocardiogram	
☐ 93015	Exercise Stress Test (ETT)	
☐ 93017	ETT Tracing Only	
☐ 93040	Electrocardiogram - Rhythm	
☐ 96100	Psychological Testing	
☐ 99000	Specimen Handling	
☐ 99058	Office Emergency Care	
☐ 99070	Surgical Tray - Misc.	
☐ 99080	Special Reports of Med Rec	
☐ 99195	Phlebotomy	
☐		
☐		
☐		

ICD-9 CODE DIAGNOSIS		
☐ 009.0	Ill-defined Intestinal Infect	
☐ 133.2	Establish Baseline	
☐ 174.9	Breast Cancer	
☐ 185.0	Prostate Cancer	
☐ 250	Diabetes Mellitus	
☐ 272.4	Hyperlipidemia	
☐ 282.5	Anemia - Sickle Trait	
☐ 282.60	Anemia - Sickle Cell	
☐ 285.9	Anemia, Unspecified	
☐ 300.4	Neurotic Depression	
☐ 340	Multiple Sclerosis	
☐ 342.9	Hemiplegia - Unspecified	
☐ 346.9	Migraine Headache	
☐ 352.9	Cranial Neuralgia	
☐ 354.0	Carpal Tunnel Syndrome	
☐ 355.0	Sciatic Nerve Root Lesion	
☐ 366.9	Cataract	
☐ 386.0	Vertigo	
☐ 401.1	Essential Hypertension	
☐ 414.9	Ischemic Hearth Disease	
☐ 428.0	Congestive Heart Failure	

ICD-9 CODE DIAGNOSIS		
☐ 435.0	Basilar Artery Syndrome	
☐ 440.0	Atherosclerosis	
☐ 442.81	Carotid Artery	
☐ 460.0	Common Cold	
☐ 461.9	Acute Sinusitis	
☒ 474.0	Tonsillitis	
☐ 477.9	Hay Fever	
☐ 487.0	Flu	
☐ 496	Chronic Airway Obstruction	
☐ 522	Low Red Blood Count	
☐ 524.6	Temporo-Mandibular Jnt Synd	
☐ 538.8	Stomach Pain	
☐ 553.3	Hiatal Hernia	
☐ 564.1	Spastic Colon	
☐ 571.4	Chronic Hepatitis	
☐ 571.5	Cirrhosis of Liver	
☐ 573.3	Hepatitis	
☐ 575.2	Obstruction of Gallbladder	
☐ 648.2	Anemia - Compl. Pregnancy	
☐ 715.90	Osteoarthritis - Unspec	
☐ 721.3	Lumbar Osteo/Spondylarthrit	

ICD-9 CODE DIAGNOSIS		
☐ 724.2	Pain: Lower Back	
☐ 727.6	Rupture of Achilles Tendon	
☐ 780.1	Hallucinations	
☐ 780.3	Convulsions	
☐ 780.5	Sleep Disturbances	
☐ 783.0	Anorexia	
☐ 783.1	Abnormal Weight Gain	
☐ 783.2	Abnormal Weight Loss	
☐ 830.6	Dislocated Hip	
☐ 830.9	Dislocated Shoulder	
☐ 841.2	Sprained Wrist	
☐ 842.5	Sprained Ankle	
☐ 891.2	Fractured Tibia	
☐ 892.0	Fractured Fibula	
☐ 919.5	Insect Bite, Nonvenomous	
☐ 921.1	Contus Eyelid/Perioc Area	
☐ v16.3	Fam. Hist of Breast Cancer	
☐ v17.4	Fam. Hist of Cardiovasc Dis	
☐ v20.2	Well Child	
☐ v22.0	Pregnancy - First Normal	
☐ v22.1	Pregnancy - Normal	

Previous Balance	Today's Charges	Total Due	Amount Paid	New Balance

Follow Up

PRN _____ Weeks _____ Months _____ Units _____

Next Appointment Date: _____   Time: _____

I hereby authorize release of any information acquired in the course of examination or treatment and allow a photocopy of my signature to be used.

_____

You will enter '**F**' because you know that Mrs. Evans plans to make (F)ull payment today. Mrs. Evans's check for $71.00 is shown in Figure 6-9.

Figure 6-9 Deborah Evans's Check

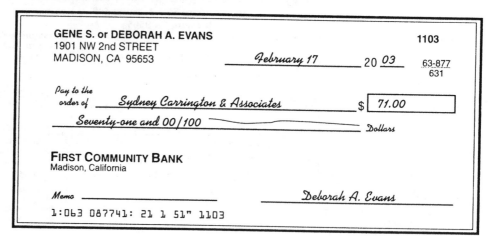

The screens in Figures 6-10 to 6-12 reflect the process of posting the first procedure, posting the second procedure, and selecting the (F)ull payment option for allocation of payment.

Figure 6-10 Post Two Procedures, Select Full Payment, Screen 1 of 3

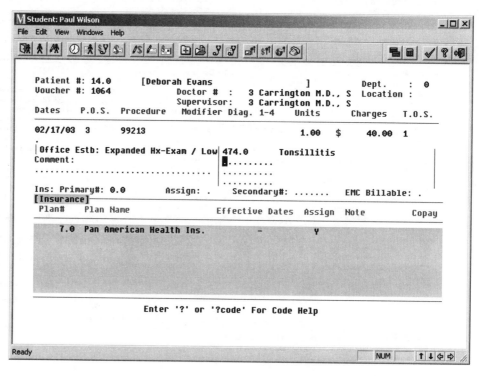

Figure 6-11 Post Two Procedures, Select Full Payment, Screen 2 of 3

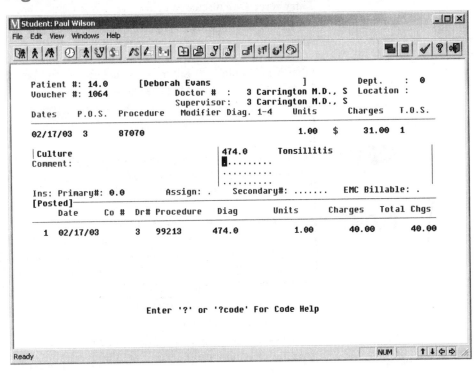

Figure 6-12 Post Two Procedures, Select Full Payment, Screen 3 of 3

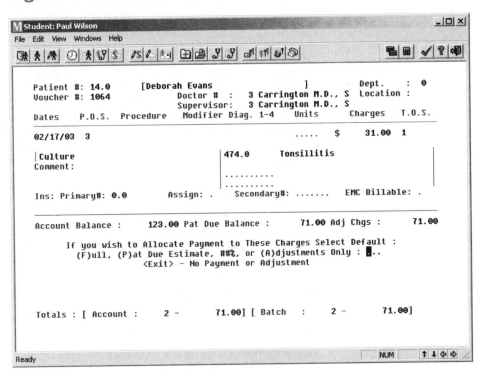

Other choices you could have made to allocate payment within the Procedure Entry screen are discussed below:

Exit
Press ESCAPE or click on the EXIT button on the top toolbar for no payment and return to the patient selection screen.

(P)at % of Profile
Enter 'P' to default to the percentage the patient pays of a Medicare approved amount.

##%
Enter the payment percentage (0–99) that represents the default amount that the patient will be paying.

STEP 3
Enter '**C**' for (C)heck, and enter the check number '**1103**' as the Voucher #. Press **ENTER** to leave the comment field blank, then press **ENTER** to accept the default amount of '0.00' for the remaining deductible.

STEP 4
Enter '**71.00**' (the whole payment amount) in the Pmt. Amount field. Enter '**40.00**' (amount of item 1) as the Pmt. Amount on line 1 (also highlighted). Press **F1** or click on the PROCESS button ('√') on the top toolbar to process. Notice that each time you credit an amount to an item and PROCESS, the next payment item in the list will automatically be highlighted. Enter '**31.00**' (amount of item 2) as the Pmt. Amount on line 2 (now highlighted). **PROCESS** to complete payment allocation, then compare your screen to Figure 6-13.

Figure 6-13 Patient Payment Allocation After Processing

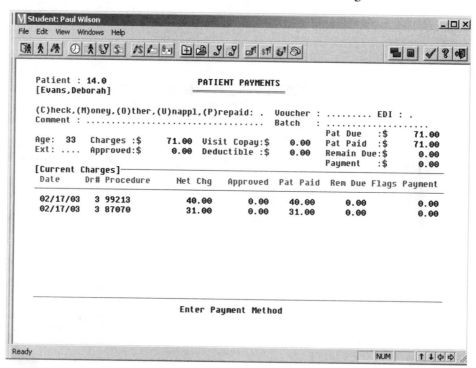

Press **ESCAPE** or click on the EXIT button on the top toolbar until you reach the Main Menu (Menu 1).

Charges may be posted and then paid later. Post the charges for the following patient.

EXERCISE 6: Sharon A. Carlson

Posting a Procedure and Payment Separately

Mrs. Sharon Carlson will pay for her visit, but you will post her payment later by another method.

STEP 1 Return to Procedure Entry and post the charge from the encounter form (Voucher 1065) shown in Figure 6-14. Refer to help windows for any additional information you need. Remember to enter '**0**' in the Primary Ins # field to indicate the insurance carrier will not be billed for this item.

STEP 2 When you have posted the procedure, press **ESCAPE** or click on the EXIT button on the top toolbar until you return to the Main Menu (Menu 1).

Posting Payments from the Payment Entry Screen

The Payment Entry screen is used whenever a payment, adjustment, or refund is to be posted to the patient's account. It can also be used to transfer the financial responsibility of a procedure or a claim to another insurance plan or to the patient. The Payment Entry routine is not used to edit payments or to edit adjustments.

The Payment Entry routine permits payments for procedures to be split between the patient and an insurance carrier. It also allows automatic posting of payments, monitoring payments from patient or insurance plan, posting adjustments, and handling of unapplied credits. You are permitted a variety of methods for handling partial payments including:

1. transferring responsibility to the same or a secondary insurance plan.

2. transferring responsibility to the patient.

3. accepting partial payment as a settlement of an account.

An example of the Payment Entry procedure is given below.

STEP 1 Select option **3**, PAYMENT Posting, at the Main Menu (Menu 1). Then, select option **1**, PAYMENT Entry at the Payment Posting Menu.

STEP 2 Retrieve Terry Williams's account, press **ENTER**, and the screen shown in Figure 6-15 (page 247) will appear.

Figure 6-14 Sharon Carlson's Encounter Form—Voucher 1065

Sydney Carrington & Associates P.A.
34 Sycamore Street   Suite 300
Madison, CA 95653

Date: 02/17/2003

Voucher No.:   1065

Time: 11:00

Patient: Sharon Carlson
Guarantor: Steven W. Carlson

Patient No: 10.1
Doctor: 3 - S. Carrington

	CPT	DESCRIPTION	FEE
OFFICE/HOSPITAL CONSULTS			
☐	99201	Office New:Focused Hx-Exam	
☐	99202	Office New:Expanded Hx-Exam	
☐	99211	Office Estb:Min/None Hx-Exa	
☐	99212	Office Estb:Focused Hx-Exa	
☒	99213	Office Estb:Expanded Hx-Exa	$40.00
☐	99214	Office Estb:Detailed Hx-Exa	
☐	99215	Office Estb:Comprhn Hx-Exam	
☐	99221	Hosp. Initial:Comprh Hx-	
☐	99223	Hosp.Ini:Comprh Hx-Exam/Hi	
☐	99231	Hosp. Subsequent: S-Fwd	
☐	99232	Hosp. Subsequent: Comprhn Hx	
☐	99233	Hosp. Subsequent: Ex/Hi	
☐	99238	Hospital Visit Discharge Ex	
☐	99371	Telephone Consult - Simple	
☐	99372	Telephone Consult - Intermed	
☐	99373	Telephone Consult - Complex	
☐	90843	Counseling - 25 minutes	
☐	90844	Counseling - 50 minutes	
☐	90865	Counseling - Special Interview	
IMMUNIZATIONS/INJECTIONS			
☐	90585	BCG Vaccine	
☐	90659	Influenza Virus Vaccine	
☐	90701	Immunization-DTP	
☐	90702	DT Vaccine	
☐	90703	Tetanus Toxoids	
☐	90732	Pneumococcal Vaccine	
☐	90746	Hepatitis B Vaccine	
☐	90749	Immunization; Unlisted	

	CPT	DESCRIPTION	FEE
LABORATORY/RADIOLOGY			
☐	81000	Urinalysis	
☐	81002	Urinalysis; Pregnancy Test	
☐	82951	Glucose Tolerance Test	
☐	84478	Triglycerides	
☐	84550	Uric Acid: Blood Chemistry	
☐	84830	Ovulation Test	
☐	85014	Hematocrit	
☐	85031	Hemogram, Complete Blood Wk	
☐	86403	Particle Agglutination Test	
☐	86485	Skin Test; Candida	
☐	86580	TB Intradermal Test	
☐	86585	TB Tine Test	
☐	87070	Culture	
☐	70190	X-Ray; Optic Foramina	
☐	70210	X-Ray Sinuses Complete	
☐	71010	Radiological Exam Ent Spine	
☐	71020	X-Ray Chest Pa & Lat	
☐	72050	X-Ray Spine, Cerv (4 views)	
☐	72090	X-Ray Spine; Scoliosis Ex	
☐	72110	Spine, lumbosacral; a/p & Lat	
☐	73030	Shoulder-Comp, min w/ 2vws	
☐	73070	Elbow, anteropost & later vws	
☐	73120	X-Ray; Hand, 2 views	
☐	73560	X-Ray, Knee, 1 or 2 views	
☐	74022	X-Ray; Abdomen, Complete	
☐	75552	Cardiac Magnetic Res Img	
☐	76020	X-Ray; Bone Age Studies	
☐	76088	Mammary Ductogram Complete	
☐	78465	Myocardial Perfusion Img	

	CPT	DESCRIPTION	FEE
PROCEDURES/TESTS			
☐	00452	Anesthesia for Rad Surgery	
☐	11100	Skin Biopsy	
☐	15852	Dressing Change	
☐	29075	Cast Appl. - Lower Arm	
☐	29530	Strapping of Knee	
☐	29705	Removal/Revis of Cast w/Exa	
☐	53670	Catheterization Incl. Suppl	
☐	57452	Colposcopy	
☐	57505	ECC	
☐	69420	Myringotomy	
☐	92081	Visual Field Examination	
☐	92100	Serial Tonometry Exam	
☐	92120	Tonography	
☐	92552	Pure Tone Audiometry	
☐	92567	Tympanometry	
☐	93000	Electrocardiogram	
☐	93015	Exercise Stress Test (ETT)	
☐	93017	ETT Tracing Only	
☐	93040	Electrocardiogram - Rhythm	
☐	96100	Psychological Testing	
☐	99000	Specimen Handling	
☐	99058	Office Emergency Care	
☐	99070	Surgical Tray - Misc.	
☐	99080	Special Reports of Med Rec	
☐	99195	Phlebotomy	
☐			
☐			
☐			

	ICD-9 CODE DIAGNOSIS	
☐	009.0	Ill-defined Intestinal Infect
☐	133.2	Establish Baseline
☐	174.9	Breast Cancer
☐	185.0	Prostate Cancer
☐	250	Diabetes Mellitus
☐	272.4	Hyperlipidemia
☐	282.5	Anemia - Sickle Trait
☐	282.60	Anemia - Sickle Cell
☐	285.9	Anemia, Unspecified
☐	300.4	Neurotic Depression
☐	340	Multiple Sclerosis
☐	342.9	Hemiplegia - Unspecified
☐	346.9	Migraine Headache
☐	352.9	Cranial Neuralgia
☐	354.0	Carpal Tunnel Syndrome
☐	355.0	Sciatic Nerve Root Lesion
☐	366.9	Cataract
☐	386.0	Vertigo
☐	401.1	Essential Hypertension
☐	414.9	Ischemic Hearth Disease
☐	428.0	Congestive Heart Failure

	ICD-9 CODE DIAGNOSIS	
☐	435.0	Basilar Artery Syndrome
☐	440.0	Atherosclerosis
☐	442.81	Carotid Artery
☐	460.0	Common Cold
☒	461.9	Acute Sinusitis
☐	474.0	Tonsillitis
☐	477.9	Hay Fever
☐	487.0	Flu
☐	496	Chronic Airway Obstruction
☐	522	Low Red Blood Count
☐	524.6	Temporo-Mandibular Jnt Synd
☐	538.8	Stomach Pain
☐	553.3	Hiatal Hernia
☐	564.1	Spastic Colon
☐	571.4	Chronic Hepatitis
☐	571.5	Cirrhosis of Liver
☐	573.3	Hepatitis
☐	575.2	Obstruction of Gallbladder
☐	648.2	Anemia - Compl. Pregnancy
☐	715.90	Osteoarthritis - Unspec
☐	721.3	Lumbar Osteo/Spondylarthrit

	ICD-9 CODE DIAGNOSIS	
☐	724.2	Pain: Lower Back
☐	727.6	Rupture of Achilles Tendon
☐	780.1	Hallucinations
☐	780.3	Convulsions
☐	780.5	Sleep Disturbances
☐	783.0	Anorexia
☐	783.1	Abnormal Weight Gain
☐	783.2	Abnormal Weight Loss
☐	830.6	Dislocated Hip
☐	830.9	Dislocated Shoulder
☐	841.2	Sprained Wrist
☐	842.5	Sprained Ankle
☐	891.2	Fractured Tibia
☐	892.0	Fractured Fibula
☐	919.5	Insect Bite, Nonvenomous
☐	921.1	Contus Eyelid/Perioc Area
☐	v16.3	Fam. Hist of Breast Cancer
☐	v17.4	Fam. Hist of Cardiovasc Dis
☐	v20.2	Well Child
☐	v22.0	Pregnancy - First Normal
☐	v22.1	Pregnancy - Normal

Previous Balance	Today's Charges	Total Due	Amount Paid	New Balance

Follow Up

PRN _____ Weeks _____ Months _____ Units _____

Next Appointment Date: _____   Time: _____

I hereby authorize release of any information acquired in the course of examination or treatment and allow a photocopy of my signature to be used.

Figure 6-15 Payment Entry Screen

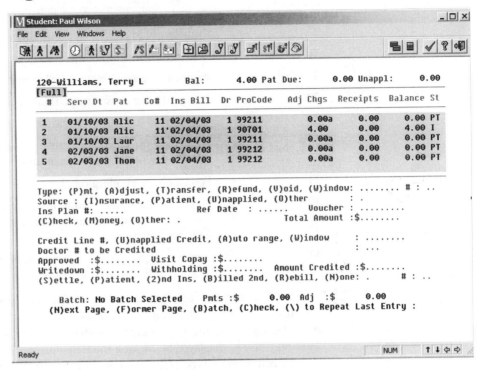

Note: In Guarantor/Dependent systems, all payments are received to the account as a whole, although the procedures credited refer to particular patients.

The Payment Entry screen is divided into three parts:

Part	Description
Top	A list of procedures ("open items") that have been posted to this account.
Middle	Information regarding the source of the payment (for example: Type, Source, Plan #, Voucher No., and Amount).
Bottom	Information regarding the allocation of the payment (for example: Line #, Dr #, Amount Credited, 2nd Ins, and balance information).

Open Items

The upper portion of the screen provides a display of items pertaining to the account. The screen displays the account's first six procedures, listing them in chronological order by date posted.

Each of the lines displayed on the upper part of the screen is prefaced with a reference number. This number is shown during Payment Entry to designate that the line is used for credit or adjustment. The line also contains the date of service, the patient's first name, insurance plan number, date billed, the number of the doctor who performed the procedure, the procedure code, the net adjusted charge for the line, receipts that have been posted to the line, and the balance due.

The apostrophe (') following the insurance plan number on line one indicates that a secondary plan shares responsibility for the payment but has not yet been billed.

The last column on each line is the status code, which shows who is currently responsible for payment. Status code definitions are, as follows:

Status Code	Definitions
P	Patient responsibility, never billed to insurance
PT	Transferred to patient responsibility
IU	Pending insurance billing
I	Insurance responsibility, billed to primary
IR	Insurance responsibility, pending rebill
IT	Transferred to insurance (either billed or unbilled)
F	Forced claim, billed to insurance and required to be subsequently maintained as a claim until transferred to patient
FR	Forced claim, pending rebill
FT	Forced claim, transferred to another insurance as a claim and required to be subsequently maintained as a claim until transferred to patient
FD	A forced claim completely adjusted or paid off and available for deletion at the next period close

Two other windows are displayed upon request in the upper portion of the payment screen. These Help windows appear when a question mark ('?') is entered in the appropriate field after the message "Enter ? for Help" appears at the bottom of the screen. They may also be displayed by clicking the Help button ('?') on the top toolbar.

The Adjustment Type Help Window displays the definitions of adjustment types that may be used for write-off, writedown, settlement, and general adjustments.

The Insurance Help Window displays the plan information for all insurance plans associated with the account and is helpful in matching a check to an insurance plan number or in transferring to third or fourth insurance billing.

Overall Transaction

The center portion of the Payment Entry screen accepts information regarding the overall transaction, including source, total amounts paid, voucher number, and method of payment. It also allows you to choose (N)ext or (F)ormer if you wish to page through the lines displayed within the window above, if there are more items than can be displayed in one window.

Individual Items

The bottom portion of the Payment Entry screen is used for the selection, allocation, settlement, and transfer of the items displayed at the top of the screen. You may also use the "Credit Line #" prompt for "paging" when more than seven items are displayed at the top. This is done by entering (N)ext or (F)ormer.

The batch total line that appears below the Payment Entry screen tells you the net payments (total payments less refunds) and total adjustments posted during this session. The batch totals include payments posted to all accounts during this session and will continue to accumulate until you exit the Payment Entry screen. The batch total is used to provide online verification when payments for multiple patients are received on a single check. This will be used in a later exercise.

STEP 3 Use the following information to complete the Payment Entry screen for Ms. Williams.

A private insurance carrier, insurance plan '11', sends the check for $4.00 shown in Figure 6-16 as payment for the immunization given to Alice Spivey during her Well-Child Check-Up on 01/10/03. As is often the case with managed care insurance plans,

Figure 6-16 Insurance Check for Terry Williams's Account

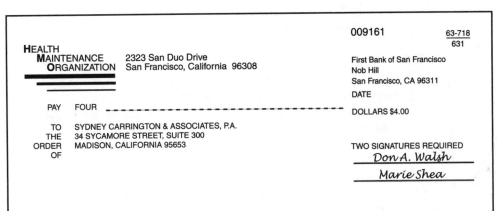

DATE	INVOICE NUMBER	AMOUNT	DISCOUNT	NET
02/03/03	(THOMAS WILLIAMS)	0.00		$ 0.00
02/03/03	(JANET WILLIAMS)	0.00		0.00
01/10/03	(ALICE SPIVEY)	4.00		4.00
01/10/03	(LAURA SIMMONS)	0.00		0.00

CONTROL NO. 6875	VENDOR NO. 1259	CHECK DATE	$ 4.00		$ 4.00

DETACH AND RETAIN THIS STATEMENT
THE ATTACHED CHECK IS IN PAYMENT OF ITEMS DESCRIBED
IF NOT CORRECT PLEASE NOTIFY US PROMPTLY

009161

Health Maintenance Organization pays for all normal physician visits made by Ms. Williams and her dependents. However, specific procedures performed in a physician's office, in this case, the application of an immunization for Alice Spivey, often require that the physician bill the plan for an additional amount. This check represents payment for the additional amount of $4.00 that was billed to plan 11 by Dr. Carrington's office.

Once you have selected option 3, PAYMENT Posting from the Main Menu (Menu 1), option 1, PAYMENT Entry from the Payment Posting Menu (Menu 3), and retrieved Terry Williams's account, post the insurance check shown in Figure 6-16.

Note: A full explanation of each field is provided after this posting exercise.

- ◆ a. Type: (**P**)ayment
- ◆ b. Source: (**I**)nsurance
- ◆ c. Insurance Plan #: **11**
- ◆ d. Ref. Date: (Press **ENTER** to default to system date of 02/17/03)

◆ e. Voucher No.: **009161**

◆ f. (**C**)heck

◆ g. Total Amount: **4.00**

When payment for multiple items is included, it is important to post the payments in the order provided on the insurance check, *not* in the order they appear on the Payment screen. To accomplish this, you would post one payment at a time from the Insurance Check (Figure 6-16) to its corresponding charge on the payment screen. It is important that you pay special attention to the date and patient ('Pat') field to match transactions. However, in this case, because the only payment amount received was for Alice's immunization, it is *not* necessary that you post the $0.00 payments for the other patients shown.

Use the arrow keys or the mouse to highlight line item **2** (90701 for Alice) and press **ENTER**. Press **ENTER** again to accept $4.00 as the Approved Amount. Press **F10** to clear the writedown field if it contains any data and press **ENTER**. Press **ENTER** again to accept $4.00 as the Amount Credited. Finally, press **ENTER** to accept (**N**)one because there will not be an item balance amount.

Note: If the message "238 WARNING: Entire Balance of Item Will Be Written Off," appears, press ENTER to bypass it.

Even though the insurance responsible amount of the charge shown on the screen is only an additional $4.00, the insurance plan may sometimes pay only a precalculated amount that can be set up as part of the system to appear automatically. In the future, if you receive an amount other than the precalculated amount, you can override it by typing in the new amount.

PROCESS to finish posting the $4.00 payment to Ms. Williams's account. Your screen should be similar to Figure 6-17.

[handwritten note in left margin: "Stuck!"]

Figure 6·17 Allocated Insurance Payment, After Processing

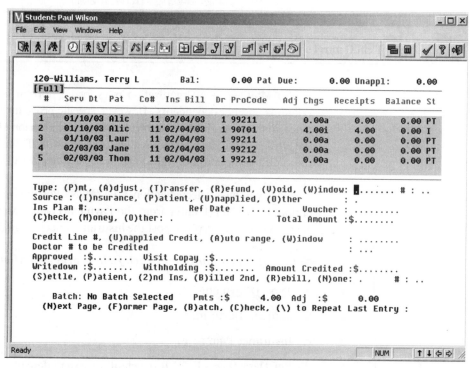

UNIT 6 Practice Management

For more information on how to post payments, read the following section before completing the next exercise.

Reference Guide for Payment Entry

The options available for the Type Prompt are listed below:

1. *(P)ayment:* Type 'P' and press ENTER if you wish to post a payment received, to allocate unapplied credits, or to transfer the responsibility of an item.

2. *(A)djust:* Type 'A' and press ENTER if you wish to adjust the charge on a procedure or to transfer the responsibility of payment for the procedure. Items paid off during the current period still remain available for adjustment.

Note: Adjustments for a charge normally reduce the net charge and the balance of the item. Therefore, negative adjustments will increase the net charge and the balance of the item. Zero adjustments are also permitted to transfer responsibility of an item.

3. *(R)efund:* Type 'R' if you wish to post a refund or remove funds from the doctor's period-to-date receipts. Refunds are always taken from Unapplied Credit.

4. *(V)oid:* Type 'V' if you wish to void a charge that has been processed through a Daily Close.

5. *(W)indow:* Windows are different ways of viewing the open items listed. The four windows available are Full (this is the default), Guarantor, Insurance Detail, and Claim.

6. *(N)ext or (F)ormer:* This is not displayed on the screen but using this will allow you to page up or down through the displayed items.

7. *Default option:* Press ENTER to default to (P)ayment as the type of transaction.

8. *(I)nsurance Source:* Type 'I' if the payment was received from an insurance plan.

9. *(P)atient source:* Type 'P' if the payment was received from the patient.

10. *(U)napplied credit source:* Type 'U' if the payment is to be moved from Unapplied Credit. The patient's Unapplied Credit, if there is any, is displayed at the top right of the screen. Unapplied Credits are payments credited to an account that are not specifically allocated to particular procedure charges. Payment from Unapplied Credits as the source is an internal transaction within the account and does not affect the doctor or practice cash position.

11. *(O)ther payment source:* Type 'O' if the payment is received from some other source.

12. *Default option:* Press ENTER to default to the (P)atient as source of payment.

The options available for posting partial payments are listed below:

1. *(S)ettle on payment received:* Type 'S' to settle for the amount of the payment received. An automatic adjustment will be posted, reducing the balance to zero. If (S)ettle is chosen, you may enter '?' or click on the Help button ('?') on the top toolbar to see an Adjustment Type Help Window.

2. *Balance transferred to patient:* Type 'P' to transfer all financial responsibility of this procedure strictly to the patient. It no longer will appear on any insurance plan reports, and all future statements will show it as the patient's responsibility.

3. *Balance transferred to secondary insurance plan:* Type '2' to transfer all financial responsibility for the procedure to a secondary insurance plan. Once selected, this option will request the insurance plan number that is to be billed. Enter the insurance plan number that will be billed and that will assume financial responsibility for the balance of the item. If '?' is entered at this field, a help window will list all insurance plans for the account. Using the mouse, you can also invoke a help window by clicking on the Help button ('?') on the top toolbar. If 'O' is entered at this field, the secondary plan selection will be aborted.

Once processed, this transfer will actually swap the primary and secondary insurance companies. The secondary plan becomes primarily responsible for the outstanding balance of the procedure, and the previous primary plan becomes the secondary plan. During insurance billing, the procedures that were partially paid by the previous plan can be marked on the form, the amount paid reported, and a note included explaining that those procedures were billed to a secondary plan. **The Medical Manager** system permits an unlimited number of billings to the same or different insurance companies and maintains data for the latest primary and secondary billings.

4. *Balance piggybacked to secondary insurance:* Type 'B' to indicate that the secondary insurance plan was already billed by the primary plan as a courtesy. This will transfer all financial responsibility for the procedure to the secondary insurance plan without billing this plan. Once selected, this option will request the insurance plan number that is to be held responsible.

5. *(R)ebilling an item:* Choosing 'R' indicates that another copy of the insurance form should be printed. Answer (N)o to the 'For Review?' question.

6. *(N)o change in status:* Type 'N' if responsibility for payment is not to be changed.

Patient Checkout Payments

Patient Checkout Payments is accessed from the Payment Posting Menu (Menu 31) and allows payments to be made for all of the charges posted on the current day for the current patient. It includes an estimate of the patient due portion of the day's charges, and allows precollected copay and other unapplied credit to be easily applied to today's charges.

Note: The Patient Payment module is normally accessed automatically from within Procedure Entry at the end of a posting session, and includes only charges posted during that session. If the user exits Procedure Entry without collecting the patient payment, then subsequently needs to post a patient payment for today's charges, the Patient Checkout Payments option may be used. This option is also used in offices that use a separate person to post payments.

When this option is selected, a help window displays all charges posted on the current system date for the current patient. The screen is then completed in the same way as during procedure entry. However, if the Patient Payments screen is accessed from Procedure Entry, the display lists only the charges for the current posting session, whereas if it is accessed via Payment Posting, the display lists all of today's charges.

Post the following payment through the Patient Checkout Payment screen.

EXERCISE 7: Sharon A. Carlson

Posting a Payment Using Patient Checkout Payments

At the end of her visit, Sharon Carlson gives you a $40.00 personal check, number 110, which is to be credited to her account (Figure 6-18). From the Main Menu (Menu 1), choose option **3**, PAYMENT Posting, then option **2**, PATIENT Checkout Payments. Retrieve Sharon Carlson's account by entering her name, '**Carlson**', at the Patient Retrieval prompt, moving the highlighted bar to '**Sharon A. Carlson**' and then pressing **ENTER**.

Figure 6-18   Sharon Carlson's Check—Voucher 110

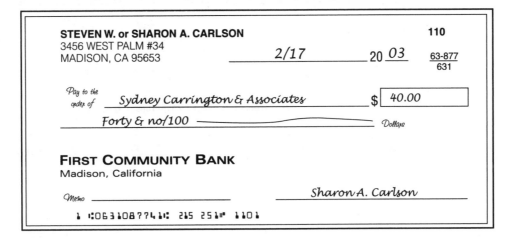

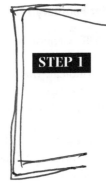

STEP 1   Select (**C**)heck as the type of payment. Record the voucher number ('**110**') in the voucher field. Press **ENTER** to bypass the Comment and Deductible fields. Key '**40.00**' in the Payment field, and press **ENTER**. Because the check is coming from a patient, it is appropriate to apply the payment to an item that is considered the patient's responsibility. Therefore, choose to make payment on the highlighted line and press **ENTER** to apply the full $40.00 credit toward today's charges for Mrs. Carlson.

STEP 2

Compare your screen to Figure 6-19 and press **F1** or click on the PROCESS button ('√') on the top toolbar to process. Notice that the Patient Paid balance will increase to $40.00, and the Remainder Due balance for today's visit will decrease to zero.

Figure 6-19 Completed Patient Checkout Payment Screen

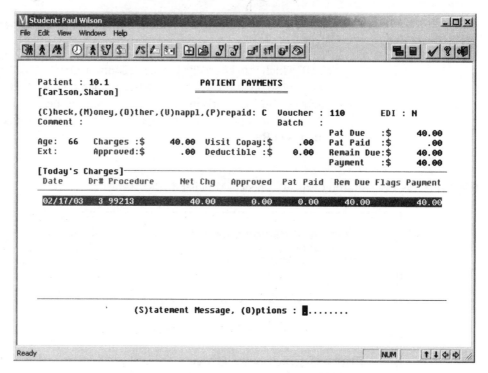

EXERCISE 8: Running a Trial Daily Close for February 17

Return to the Main Menu (Menu 1) and select option **5**, REPORT Generation.

STEP 1

At the Reports Menu, select option **4**, DAILY Report. Key **'Y'** to indicate that you desire a Trial Daily Report. Key **'P'** to request a check register for the practice. Press **ENTER** to leave the remaining Encounter Tracking Report field blank. Key **'A'** for (A)ll.

STEP 2

Make sure your printer is on, has paper in it, and is online. Press **F1** or click on the PROCESS button ('√') on the top toolbar to process and then print the Trial Daily Report. You may abort the report at any time by pressing ESCAPE or by clicking on the EXIT button on the top toolbar. Press **ENTER** at the prompt "Daily Close Not Performed" to return to the Reports Menu.

Check your work carefully and make any necessary corrections through File Maintenance. You may review File Maintenance in previous units, if necessary. Compare the information in your reports to Figures 6-20 through 6-24. When you are positive everything is accurate, run the Final Daily Close in Exercise 9.

Figure 6-20 Daily Report for 02/17/03—James Monroe, M.D.

```
02/17/03                         DAILY REPORT FOR 02/17/03                              Page   1
                                    James T Monroe MD (1)

                                                         [to Vchr  Total  Ref Date]
Account    Patient Name    Dt Post  Type Dates of Service Dept Voucher Proc Code  Units  Pri/Sec Ail Loc Exc  Amount
========================================================================================================================
120        Williams,Terry  02/17/03  PMT  Check Ins #11         009161 [1052      4.00           02/17/03]      -4.00

Exception Codes:
overrides: c= charge, p= profile, w= writedown, o= overpay, i= pmt not from resp. ins, e= item edited, x= rebuilt dlyfile.tmp used


                              Summary for : James T Monroe MD
               ----------------------------------------------------------------
                    Item          Today      Period-to-Date        Year-to-Date
                  Description     02/17/03  01/01/03 - 02/17/03  01/01/03 - 02/17/03
               ----------------------------------------------------------------
               Total Charges         0.00         182.00              182.00
               Total Receipts        4.00           4.00                4.00
               Refunds               0.00           0.00                0.00
               Cross-Alloc Unapplied 0.00           0.00                0.00
               Total Adjustments     0.00         120.00              120.00
               Accounts Receivable  58.00          58.00               58.00
               Total # Procedures       0              7                   7
               Service Charges       0.00           0.00                0.00
               Tax Charges           0.00           0.00                0.00
               Copay Expected        0.00            ---                 ---
               Copay Paid            0.00            ---                 ---
               Deposit Amount        4.00            ---                 ---
                     Checks    4.00
                     Cash      0.00
                     Other     0.00
               ----------------------------------------------------------------
```

Figure 6-21 Daily Report for 02/17/03—Frances Simpson, M.D.

```
02/17/03                         DAILY REPORT FOR 02/17/03                              Page   2
                                   Frances D Simpson M.D. (2)

                                                         [to Vchr  Total  Ref Date]
Account    Patient Name    Dt Post  Type Dates of Service Dept Voucher Proc Code  Units  Pri/Sec Ail Loc Exc  Amount
========================================================================================================================
80.0       Davis,Timothy   02/17/03  CHG  02/17/03-         0  1062   99213      1.00    12/     0   Y         40.00
80.0       Davis,Timothy   02/17/03  CHG  02/17/03-         0  1062   29705      1.00    12/     0   Y         38.00

Exception Codes:
overrides: c= charge, p= profile, w= writedown, o= overpay, i= pmt not from resp. ins, e= item edited, x= rebuilt dlyfile.tmp used


                            Summary for : Frances D Simpson M.D.
               ----------------------------------------------------------------
                    Item          Today      Period-to-Date        Year-to-Date
                  Description     02/17/03  01/01/03 - 02/17/03  01/01/03 - 02/17/03
               ----------------------------------------------------------------
               Total Charges        78.00         206.00              206.00
               Total Receipts        0.00           0.00                0.00
               Refunds               0.00           0.00                0.00
               Cross-Alloc Unapplied 0.00           0.00                0.00
               Total Adjustments     0.00           0.00                0.00
               Accounts Receivable 206.00         206.00              206.00
               Total # Procedures       2              5                   5
               Service Charges       0.00           0.00                0.00
               Tax Charges           0.00           0.00                0.00
               Copay Expected        0.00            ---                 ---
               Copay Paid            0.00            ---                 ---
               Deposit Amount        0.00            ---                 ---
                     Checks    0.00
                     Cash      0.00
                     Other     0.00
               ----------------------------------------------------------------
```

Figure 6-22 Daily Report for 02/17/03—Sydney Carrington, M.D.

```
02/17/03                          DAILY REPORT FOR 02/17/03                              Page    3
                                  Sydney J Carrington M.D. (3)

                                                              [to Vchr  Total  Ref Date]
Account   Patient Name    Dt Post  Type Dates of Service  Dept Voucher Proc Code  Units  Pri/Sec Ail Loc Exc  Amount
=================================================================================================================
21.0      Edwards,Portia  02/17/03  CHG  02/17/03-          0   1063   99214     1.00     9/    0   Y          50.00
14.0      Evans,Deborah   02/17/03  CHG  02/17/03-          0   1064   99213     1.00     0/    0   N          40.00
14.0      Evans,Deborah   02/17/03  CHG  02/17/03-          0   1064   87070     1.00     0/    0   N          31.00
14        Evans,Deborah   02/17/03  PMT  Check Patient          1103   [1064    71.00          02/17/03]      -40.00
14        Evans,Deborah   02/17/03  PMT  Check Patient          1103   [1064    71.00          02/17/03]      -31.00
10.1      Carlson,Sharon  02/17/03  CHG  02/17/03-          0   1065   99213     1.00     0/    0   N          40.00
10        Carlson,Steven  02/17/03  PMT  Check Patient          110    [1065    40.00          02/17/03]      -40.00

Exception Codes:
overrides: c= charge, p= profile, w= writedown, o= overpay, i= pmt not from resp. ins, e= item edited, x= rebuilt dlyfile.tmp used


                                  Summary for : Sydney J Carrington M.D.
                 ----------------------------------------------------------------------
                      Item           Today        Period-to-Date          Year-to-Date
                   Description      02/17/03    01/01/03 - 02/17/03     01/01/03 - 02/17/03
                 ----------------------------------------------------------------------
                 Total Charges        161.00          1,465.00              1,465.00
                 Total Receipts       111.00            111.00                111.00
                 Refunds                0.00              0.00                  0.00
                 Cross-Alloc Unapplied  0.00              0.00                  0.00
                 Total Adjustments      0.00              0.00                  0.00
                 Accounts Receivable 1,354.00          1,354.00              1,354.00
                 Total # Procedures       4                26                    26
                 Service Charges        0.00              0.00                  0.00
                 Tax Charges            0.00              0.00                  0.00
                 Copay Expected         0.00              ---                   ---
                 Copay Paid             0.00              ---                   ---
                 Deposit Amount       111.00              ---                   ---
                      Checks         111.00
                      Cash             0.00
                      Other            0.00
                 ----------------------------------------------------------------------
```

Figure 6-23 Cash Analysis Report for 02/17/03

```
02/17/03                          DAILY REPORT FOR 02/17/03                              Page    4
                                  CASH ANALYSIS REPORT
                                  Student: Paul Wilson
================================================================================================

          Change in Cash Position                               Daily Deposit
          -----------------------                               -------------

          CHECKS        115.00                    CHECKS        115.00
          CASH            0.00                    CASH            0.00
          OTHER           0.00                    OTHER           0.00
          REFUNDS         0.00
                      ==========                              ==========
                        115.00                                  115.00


                                  CHECK REGISTER FOR 02/17/03

          Ref #  Voucher   Dr.     Amount    Date Posted    Received From              Account
          ==========================================================================================
            1    1103       3       71.00     02/17/03      Evans, Deborah               14
            2    009161     1        4.00     02/17/03      Health Maint. Org.          120
            3    110        3       40.00     02/17/03      Carlson, Steven              10
                                 ----------
               TOTAL CHECKS :       115.00
```

Figure 6-24 Daily Report Totals for 02/17/03

```
02/17/03                          DAILY REPORT FOR 02/17/03                          Page   5
                                      Student: Paul Wilson

========================================================================================================


                                     TOTALS FOR 02/17/03

--------------------------------------------------------------------------------------------------------
Doctor                      Charges    Receipts   Adjustments    Net A/R    Total A/R   # Proc.  Serv Chg  Tax Chg
--------------------------------------------------------------------------------------------------------
  1. James T Monroe MD         0.00        4.00        0.00        -4.00       58.00        0      0.00     0.00
  2. Frances D Simpson M.D.    78.00        0.00        0.00        78.00      206.00        2      0.00     0.00
  3. Sydney J Carrington M.D. 161.00      111.00        0.00        50.00    1,354.00        4      0.00     0.00
--------------------------------------------------------------------------------------------------------
TOTAL                        239.00      115.00        0.00       124.00    1,618.00        6      0.00     0.00


                       PERIOD-TO-DATE TOTALS FOR 01/01/03 - 02/17/03

--------------------------------------------------------------------------------------------------------
Doctor                      Charges    Receipts   Adjustments    Net A/R    Total A/R   # Proc.  Serv Chg  Tax Chg
--------------------------------------------------------------------------------------------------------
  1. James T Monroe MD       182.00        4.00      120.00        58.00       58.00        7      0.00     0.00
  2. Frances D Simpson M.D.  206.00        0.00        0.00       206.00      206.00        5      0.00     0.00
  3. Sydney J Carrington M.D.1,465.00     111.00        0.00     1,354.00    1,354.00       26      0.00     0.00
--------------------------------------------------------------------------------------------------------
TOTAL                      1,853.00      115.00      120.00     1,618.00    1,618.00       38      0.00     0.00


                        YEAR-TO-DATE TOTALS FOR 01/01/03 - 02/17/03

--------------------------------------------------------------------------------------------------------
Doctor                      Charges    Receipts   Adjustments    Net A/R    Total A/R   # Proc.  Serv Chg  Tax Chg
--------------------------------------------------------------------------------------------------------
  1. James T Monroe MD       182.00        4.00      120.00        58.00       58.00        7      0.00     0.00
  2. Frances D Simpson M.D.  206.00        0.00        0.00       206.00      206.00        5      0.00     0.00
  3. Sydney J Carrington M.D.1,465.00     111.00        0.00     1,354.00    1,354.00       26      0.00     0.00
--------------------------------------------------------------------------------------------------------
TOTAL                      1,853.00      115.00      120.00     1,618.00    1,618.00       38      0.00     0.00


            ********** Daily Close Has NOT Been Performed for 02/17/03 **********
```

EXERCISE 9: Running a Final Daily Close for February 17

Note: Remember to make a backup of your data before performing the Final Daily Close.

STEP 1   Choose option **5**, REPORT Generation, at the Main Menu (Menu 1) and option **4**, DAILY Report, at the Reports Menu. Answer (**N**)o to indicate you do not want another Trial Daily Report, and answer '**P**' to ask for a check register for the practice. Enter '**0**' to not purge appointments.

STEP 2   Press **F1** or click the PROCESS button ('√') on the top toolbar to process, and the report will be generated. You may abort the report at any time by pressing ESCAPE or by clicking on the EXIT button on the top toolbar. Notice that, for the first time, the Cash Receipts Analysis and Check Register contain information.

When the report is complete, compare your reports with Figures 6-25 to 6-26.

Accept the Final Daily Close by entering '**Y**' at the prompt "Do You Wish To Accept Daily Close? (Y/N)." Hand in your reports to your instructor.

Press **ENTER** at the prompt "Daily Close is Complete. Returning to Log-On," so that you will be able to advance the date in Exercise 10.

Figure 6-25 GL Daily Distribution Report for 02/17/03

```
02/17/03                          GL DAILY DISTRIBUTION REPORT - FULL DETAIL                    Page   1
                                            Student: Paul Wilson
                                                 02/17/03

   GL Account     Description      Dr    Pat #      Procedure    Date Post   Voucher      Debit            Credit
==================================================================================================================
      10001.00
                  Cash             1    120.0                    02/17/03    009161         4.00
                                                                                        ------------     ------------
                                                  POST TO ACCOUNT   10001.00                4.00            0.00
      10003.00
                  Cash             3     14.0                    02/17/03    1103          40.00
                  Cash             3     14.0                    02/17/03    1103          31.00
                  Cash             3     10.0                    02/17/03    110           40.00
                                                                                        ------------     ------------
                                                  POST TO ACCOUNT   10003.00              111.00            0.00
      15001.00
                  Accounts Rec     1    120.0                    02/17/03    009161                          4.00
                                                                                        ------------     ------------
                                                  POST TO ACCOUNT   15001.00                0.00            4.00
      15002.00
                  Accounts Rec     2     80.0                    02/17/03    1062          40.00
                  Accounts Rec     2     80.0                    02/17/03    1062          38.00
                                                                                        ------------     ------------
                                                  POST TO ACCOUNT   15002.00               78.00            0.00
      15003.00
                  Accounts Rec     3     21.0                    02/17/03    1063          50.00
                  Accounts Rec     3     14.0                    02/17/03    1064          40.00
                  Accounts Rec     3     14.0                    02/17/03    1064          31.00
                  Accounts Rec     3     14.0                    02/17/03    1103                           40.00
                  Accounts Rec     3     14.0                    02/17/03    1103                           31.00
                  Accounts Rec     3     10.1                    02/17/03    1065          40.00
                  Accounts Rec     3     10.0                    02/17/03    110                            40.00
                                                                                        ------------     ------------
                                                  POST TO ACCOUNT   15003.00              161.00          111.00
      60002.00
                  Revenue          2     80.0      99213         02/17/03    1062                           40.00
                  Revenue          2     80.0      29705         02/17/03    1062                           38.00
                                                                                        ------------     ------------
                                                  POST TO ACCOUNT   60002.00                0.00           78.00
      60003.00
                  Revenue          3     21.0      99214         02/17/03    1063                           50.00
                  Revenue          3     14.0      99213         02/17/03    1064                           40.00
                  Revenue          3     14.0      87070         02/17/03    1064                           31.00
                  Revenue          3     10.1      99213         02/17/03    1065                           40.00
                                                                                        ------------     ------------
                                                  POST TO ACCOUNT   60003.00                0.00          161.00
                                                                                        ============     ============
                                                                                         354.00         -354.00
```

Figure 6-26 Daily Close Status Report for 02/17/03

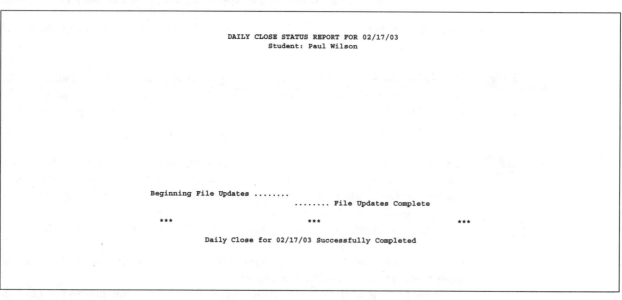

```
                              DAILY CLOSE STATUS REPORT FOR 02/17/03
                                        Student: Paul Wilson




                     Beginning File Updates ........
                                         ........ File Updates Complete

                ***                          ***                          ***

                     Daily Close for 02/17/03 Successfully Completed
```

EXERCISE 10: Advancing the Date to March 14

After you complete the Daily Close, the opening screen will appear so that you may change the date.

STEP 1   Key '**03142003**'. *Remember to enter the date very carefully.* After you enter the date, '03142003', you will receive the following warning message:

184: * WARNING * Skip > 7 Days: Continue (Y/N)

In an office setting you would *never* bypass such a warning. However, because these are practice sessions, you may press '**Y**' and then press **ENTER** to advance the date. You will be prompted to reenter your password to verify the date advance.

STEP 2   Key '**ICAN**' and press **ENTER** to verify the date advance.

When you complete the above steps to change the date, you should see the new date in the upper left corner of the Main Menu (Menu 1). If that date does not appear as '03/14/03', notify your instructor immediately so that your files may be restored from backup and the steps to change the date can be reentered. *If you proceed with an incorrect date, your data files will not be reliable.*

Help for the Future!

In an open-item accounting system such as **The Medical Manager** software it is important to allocate payments and adjustments to the individual patients shown on each charge line. **The Medical Manager** provides two methods of achieving this allocation. You may post to the item individually, or the system can be called upon to do automatic allocation through auto pay (addressed in Exercise 16). This section is intended to provide an understanding of the method used in the auto pay and auto adjust modes and the results that may be expected.

If you are provided with the amount the insurance plan paid toward each item within a claim, and if the total does not equal the entire amount billed, then allocation should be done on an item-by-item basis, as you saw in the previous exercise. On the other hand, if the amount paid for the claim is what is billed, or if the insurance plan does not provide itemized detail on a claim, auto pay allows automatic allocation based upon the remaining balance of the items.

Adjustment allocation or auto adjust is only used when you wish to write off the entire account. An adjustment will be posted for every item in the account. Upon completion, the total amount of the adjustment will appear in the Total Amount field.

EXERCISE 11: Running the Insurance Prebilling Worksheet

Because you have posted new items into the system, you should run the insurance billing again. From the Main Menu (Menu 1), select option **6**, BILLING & EDI, then option **3**, INSURANCE Billing Worksheet.

STEP 1   Press **ENTER** to accept the system date of 03/14/03 as the Bill-Thru Date. Press **ENTER** to accept the system default of '1' for the Physical Form number. Press **ENTER** to accept the system default of 'N' to not show all diagnoses. Press **ENTER** to accept the system default to run the worksheet for (A)ll Companies.

STEP 2 Press **F1** or click on the PROCESS button ('√') on the top toolbar to process. Your worksheet should be similar to Figure 6-27. Hand in your Insurance Prebilling Worksheet to your instructor.

Figure 6-27 Insurance Prebilling Worksheet

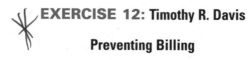

```
03/14/03                          INSURANCE PREBILLING WORKSHEET                                      Page    1
                                         Student: Paul Wilson
                               Form # 1 - Thru 03/14/03 - All Claims

Ins Plan Dates of Service Diag Code  Proc Code  Mod  Voucher  POS/TOS    Units  Dr/Al/As  2nd Plan Bill Amt  Receipts      Net
=================================================================================================================================
      9 - Worker's Compensation        Fmt : A:ins0101a.fmt   Bill Amt = Adjusted
      21.0 - Edwards, Portia
        02/17/03 -          724.2      99214                1063      3/1      1.00   3/ Y/ Y      0       50.00      0.00      50.00
                                                                                                      ----------  ---------- ----------
                                                                             Totals       :              50.00      0.00      50.00
                                                                                                                            ==========
                                                     TOTAL TO BE BILLED FOR INSURANCE PLAN #     9  :                        50.00
     12 - Fringe Benefit Center        Fmt : A:ins0101a.fmt   Bill Amt = Adjusted
      80.0 - Davis, Timothy
        02/17/03 -          841.2      99213                1062      3/1      1.00   2/ Y/ Y      0       40.00      0.00      40.00
        02/17/03 -          841.2      29705                1062      3/1      1.00   2/ Y/ Y      0       38.00      0.00      38.00
                                                                                                      ----------  ---------- ----------
                                                                             Totals       :              78.00      0.00      78.00
                                                                                                                            ==========
                                                     TOTAL TO BE BILLED FOR INSURANCE PLAN #    12  :                        78.00
=================================================================================================================================
                                                     TOTAL TO BE BILLED FOR ALL INSURANCE PLANS  :                         128.00
```

 EXERCISE 12: Timothy R. Davis

Preventing Billing

After running the insurance prebilling worksheet, you note that Mr. Timothy Davis should not be billed for *both* an office visit examination and a cast removal because the cost of the examination is included in the fee for a cast removal. Therefore, you must deal with the incorrectly posted procedure in two ways:

1. Prevent the insurance company from being billed for the incorrect procedure.

2. Remove the incorrect charge from the patient's account. (Because the item has already been daily closed, it cannot be deleted. However, it can be voided.)

STEP 1 From the Main Menu (Menu 1), choose option **7**, FILE Maintenance, then option **2**, EDIT Activity Records. Retrieve Mr. Davis's account, highlight the February 17, 2003 office visit (99213), and press **ENTER** to select it.

STEP 2 Enter (**M**)odify at the prompt at the bottom of the screen. Position the cursor over the Primary Ins # field and type '**00**' over the plan number. Press **F1** or click on the PROCESS button ('√') on the top toolbar to process. The item will remain on Mr. Davis's account but will not be billed to the insurance company. Press **ESCAPE** or click on the EXIT button on the top toolbar until you return to the Main Menu (Menu 1).

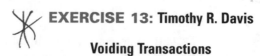 **EXERCISE 13: Timothy R. Davis**

Voiding Transactions

STEP 1 From the Main Menu (Menu 1), choose option **3**, PAYMENT Posting, then option **1**, PAYMENT Entry. Retrieve Mr. Davis's account. Choose (**V**)oid for the type of payment. Press **ENTER** at the Ref. Date field to accept the system date of 03/14/03.

STEP 2

Type '**ERROR**' in the Voucher field and press **ENTER**. Move the highlight bar over item 4 (procedure 99213 for 02/17/03) and press **ENTER** to select it. Answer '**Y**' to the prompt: "Voiding an Item is Irreversible, Continue? (Y/N)." Press **F1** or click on the PROCESS button ('√') on the top toolbar to process the screen. Press **ESCAPE** or click on the EXIT button on the top toolbar to leave the Payment Entry screen.

Return to Mr. Davis's account through Payment Entry. You will see that the voided line item is no longer present. Voiding an item will correct the patient's balance and ensure correct productivity reports. Your screen should be similar to Figure 6-28.

Figure 6-28 Corrected Account for Timothy Davis

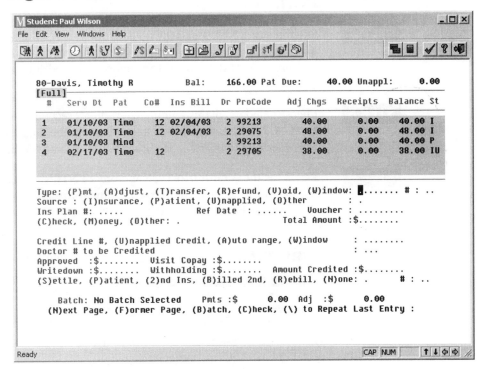

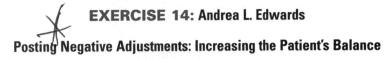

EXERCISE 14: Andrea L. Edwards

Posting Negative Adjustments: Increasing the Patient's Balance

Sometimes a patient's balance increases when an adjustment is made. In Unit 4, you altered the procedure code for Andrea Edwards from 99213 to 99214. This was performed through the Edit Activity and Edit History screens. Because changing a code does not alter the amount at which it was posted, you must also adjust the charge for Andrea's account.

The item has already been daily closed, so editing the amount of the charge is not possible. Instead, you must post a $10.00 adjustment to increase the amount. Although adjustments usually lower the amount to which they are applied, Andrea's adjustment will increase the amount due. This is called a *negative adjustment*, and the amount entered in the Total Amount field is preceded by a minus sign.

*A negative adjustment **increases** the patient amount due.*

STEP 1

From the Main Menu (Menu 1), choose option **3**, PAYMENT Posting, then option **1**, PAYMENT Entry. Key '**Edwards, Andrea**' at the Patient Retrieval screen and press **ENTER**. Highlight Andrea's name and press **ENTER** to select her.

STEP 2

Choose (**A**)djustment as the type of payment.

STEP 3 Choose (**I**)nsurance as the source of the payment because an "I," which represents insurance responsibility, follows the original charge of $40.00 for line 1 (99214 on 01/10/03).

STEP 4 Enter '**5**' as Andrea's Insurance Plan #. If you did not know the number, you could key '?' at the prompt and press ENTER or click on the Help button ('?') on the top toolbar to invoke a help window to display all insurance plans the patient has.

STEP 5 Press **ENTER** at the Ref. Date field to accept the system date of 03/14/03.

STEP 6 At the Voucher # field, key '**Dr. C**' to identify the reason for the adjustment and press **ENTER**.

STEP 7 Enter negative $10.00 ('**-10.00**') as the amount of the adjustment and press **ENTER**. Make sure the highlight bar is over item 1 (procedure 99214 for Andrea on 01/10/03) and press **ENTER** to apply this adjustment and increase the line item balance by $10.00.

STEP 8 Choose (**2**)nd to bill this amount to Andrea's secondary insurance and press **ENTER**. Enter '**5.1**' as the plan that is to be billed for the additional $10.00. At the prompt "Transfer Responsibility to Ins. Plan # 5.1," press **ENTER**.

STEP 9 Key '**1**' as the Adjustment Type and press **ENTER**. *Be careful not to accept the default type.* Check to see that your screen is similar to Figure 6-29, then press **F1** or click on the PROCESS button ('√') on the top toolbar to process.

Figure 6-29 Negative Adjustment for Andrea Edwards

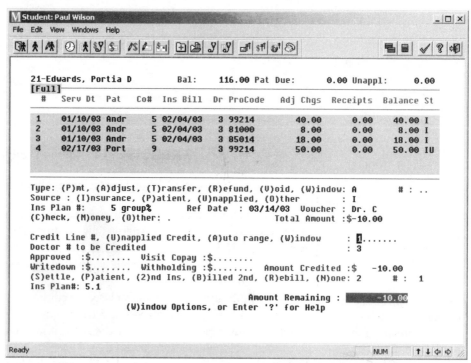

Once the payment information has been processed, the screen will change to reflect the adjustment. The adjusted charges column will increase by $10.00 for item 1, and the item balance will increase by $10.00. Insurance Plan 5.1 will be billed for the additional $10.00.

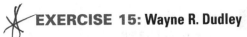

EXERCISE 15: Wayne R. Dudley

Using the Transfer Option to Change Responsibility without Affecting the Balance

The (T)ransfer option can also be used to transfer responsibility for an account. You receive a letter from Mr. Wayne Dudley's insurance plan stating the policy is no longer in effect (Figure 6-30). You must transfer responsibility on his account from insurance responsibility to patient responsibility. Because the items have already been billed to insurance, the primary plan number field cannot be edited via Edit Activity.

Figure 6-30 Letter from Wayne Dudley's Insurance Plan

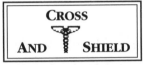

Individual Services Division
435 Embarcadero
San Francisco, California 95678

January 30, 2003

Wayne R. Dudley
Rt. 1 Box 23
Woodside, CA 98076

*Sydney Carrington & Associates P.A.
34 Sycamore St. Suite 300
Madison. CA 95653

Patient: W. R. Dudley
Cert. No.:   S678 75 4343
Group No.:   Hudson Construction
DCN No.:   88239 02 0286
Date of Service   1/10/03   Total Charges: $300.00

Dear Mr. Dudley:

We have received a claim for the service dates and amount listed above. We regret to inform you that no benefits are available for this claim as it was rendered after the termination date of your contract.

Please check your records for our notification to you regarding this termination.

If you have questions, please contact us at the telephone number listed below. We are also contacting your provider of our denial of benefits for these services.

Sincerely,
Your Dedicated Processing Unit
Individual Services Division
Cross and Shield

1204 0003 0719

For Customer Service   (800) 555-3883

STEP 1 From the Main Menu (Menu 1), select option **3**, PAYMENT Posting, then option **1**, PAYMENT Entry. At the Patient Retrieval screen, key '**Dudley, Wayne**' and press **ENTER**. (You could also type his account number, 34 and press **ENTER** twice to pull up his account.) Notice the difference between the account balance and the patient due portion at the top of the screen.

STEP 2 Enter '**T**' for Transfer and press **ENTER**. The Source and Referral Date Fields will automatically be completed by **The Medical Manager**.

STEP 3 Put an appropriate comment or reference in the Voucher field (for example, '**ins term**') and press **ENTER**.

STEP 4 Because you know all of Mr. Dudley's claims have been rejected, you must transfer responsibility for all of Mr. Dudley's charges to patient responsibility. Make sure the highlight bar is on line item '**1**' and press **ENTER**. Make sure the responsibility is marked to be transferred to (P)atient Responsibility. Note that (P)atient is the default entry for this field so you can just press **ENTER** to accept it. The message "Transfer Responsibility to Patient" will appear on the bottom line of your screen.

STEP 5 Compare your screen with Figure 6-31. Press **F1** or click on the PROCESS button ('√') on the top toolbar to process. The screen will change to reflect status 'PT', for patient responsibility.

Figure 6-31 Item Transfer Screen for Wayne Dudley

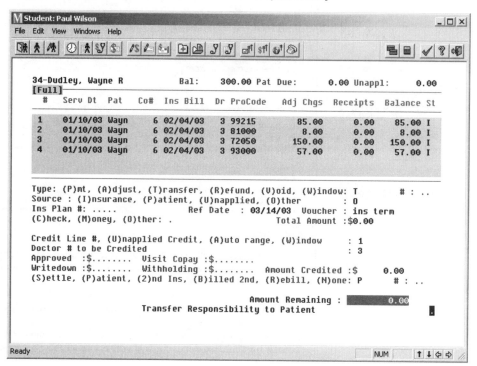

STEP 6 Because Mr. Dudley has multiple charges, it is necessary that you repeat this process with line items 2 to 4. *Double check that each item is being transferred to (P)atient Responsibility. Remember to PROCESS after each line item transfer.*

After you have repeated the process for all remaining items, notice that all line item statuses state "PT" to indicate that responsibility for each of these items has been successfully transferred to the patient.

EXERCISE 16: Wayne R. Dudley

Posting Patient Payment Using Automatic Crediting

When you call Mr. Dudley to explain that his insurance policy has expired, he comes in and pays his account in full (Figure 6-32). From the Main Menu (Menu 1), choose option **3**, PAYMENT Posting, then option **1**, PAYMENT Entry. Key '**34.0**' and press **ENTER** to retrieve Mr. Dudley's account.

Figure 6-32 Wayne Dudley's Check—Voucher 420

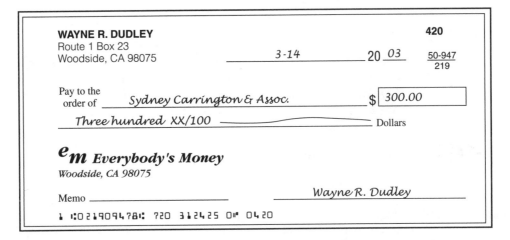

WAYNE R. DUDLEY Route 1 Box 23 Woodside, CA 98075	**420**

3-14 _____ 20 _03_   50-947 / 219

Pay to the order of _Sydney Carrington & Assoc._ $ | 300.00 |

Three hundred XX/100 ————————— Dollars

*e*_m_ **Everybody's Money**
Woodside, CA 98075

Memo _____   _Wayne R. Dudley_ _____

⑈ ⑆021909478⑆ 720 312425 0⑈ 0420

STEP 1 Choose (P)ayment, then (P)atient as the source of the payment. Press **ENTER** at the Ref. Date field to accept the current system date of 03/14/03. Key '**420**' as the Voucher # and (C)heck for Mr. Dudley's personal check. Key '**300.00**' as the Total Amount of the check and press **ENTER**.

STEP 2 Choose (A)uto to select Auto Pay and press **ENTER**. The message 'Auto Pay' will appear in the bottom portion of your screen. Press **ENTER** to accept the default response of (N)one since Mr. Dudley is paying the full balance of his account. Press **ENTER** to accept the default response (A1-4) as the lines to be credited with this payment.

STEP 3 Press **F1** or click on the PROCESS button ('√') on the top toolbar to process your information. Notice that the receipts column changes to reflect full payments made on each item. Accordingly, the balance for each item is decreased to $0.00. Your screen should be similar to Figure 6-33.

Figure 6-33 Auto Pay Patient Line Items

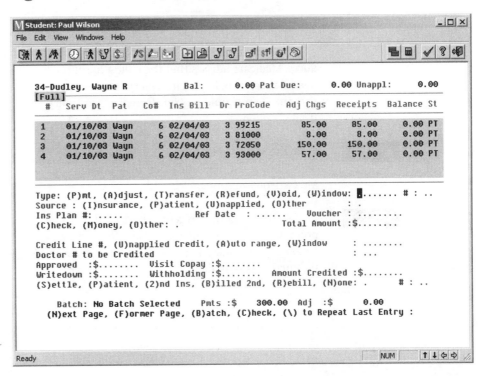

EXERCISE 17: Steven W. Carlson

Posting a Medicare Payment—Dual Insurance Coverage

You receive a $35.20 Medicare check, number 120720435, which is to be credited to Mr. Steven Carlson's account (Figure 6-34). Because the insurance plan is Medicare, the difference between the original charge and the approved charge must be adjusted; however, Medicare will actually pay only a percentage of the approved amount. The Automated Medicare Payment Handler will perform these calculations for you.

Figure 6-34 Steven Carlson's Medicare Check—Voucher 120720435

EXPLANATION OF MEDICARE PART I BENEFITS

THIS IS A STATEMENT OF ACTION TAKEN ON YOUR MEDICARE CLAIM

SERVICES WERE PROVIDED FOR NAME/NUMBER	CONTROL NO.	PROCEDURE CODE	MO. OF SERV.	POS	TOS	SERVICE DATES FROM MO. DAY YR.	SERVICE DATES TO MO. DAY YR.	CHARGES AMOUNT BILLED	CHARGES AMOUNT APPROVED	DEDUCTIBLE	NET PAY
Carlson, Steven 345653434A	B013840388061649320	99214	01 0	1	1	02 03 03	02 03 03	50 00	44 00	00	
PAT. NO. 10		TOTAL FOR THE ABOVE CLAIM						50 00	44 00	00	35 20

PROVIDER NUMBER	DATE	CHECK NUMBER	CHECK AMOUNT
		120720435	35 20

	CLAIMS PROCESSED	AMOUT PAYABLE	AMOUNT WITHHELD	NET PAYABLE	CREDITS	TOTAL MEDICARE EARNINGS
THIS EOMB•			00		00	
YEAR TO DATE•			00		00	

KEEP THIS NOTICE FOR YOUR RECORDS

The remaining balance on Medicare items must be transferred to secondary insurance. Medicare advises that the billing has already been forwarded to insurance plan 5, and a second bill is not necessary. However, to ensure accurate records for the practice, the item should be transferred to secondary insurance responsibility using the (B)illed option.

STEP 1 From the Main Menu (Menu 1), select option **3**, PAYMENT Posting, then option **1**, PAYMENT Entry. At the Patient Retrieval screen, key '**10.0**' and press **ENTER** to retrieve Mr. Carlson's account.

STEP 2 In the Type field of the center part of the screen, select (**P**)ayment. At the source prompt, choose (**I**)nsurance, then Plan # '**2**' (for Medicare). This invokes the Automated Medicare Payment Handler. Press **ENTER** at the Ref. Date field to accept the current system date of 03/14/03.

STEP 3 Since Medicare and many other insurance plans may use check numbers that are longer than the payment voucher field (9 digits), it may be necessary to use only the nine right digits. In this case, the check number is exactly nine digits and may be entered, in its entirety, in the Voucher field. Enter '**120720435**' into the Voucher field and press **ENTER**. Choose (**C**)heck, **ENTER**, then key '**35.20**' as the Total Amount field and press **ENTER**. Make sure item (**99214**) is highlighted, then press **ENTER** to select it as the line to be credited. The cursor will position itself at the Approved Amount field. Press **F10** to clear the field and key '**44.00**'. Press **ENTER** and '**6.00**' will appear as the writedown. Press **ENTER** again and the Automated Medicare Payment Handler will calculate the amount credited to be 80 percent of the approved amount or $35.20. Press **ENTER**, then enter '**B**' for (**B**)illed to transfer responsibility to secondary insurance without generating a second bill and press **ENTER**. Be careful that you do not accept the default for this field.

STEP 4 Press **ENTER** again to accept insurance plan 5 as the secondary plan to be billed. Compare your screen with Figure 6-35, and then press **F1** or click on the PROCESS button ('√') to process the information. The system will write an automatic adjusting entry that reduces the amount charged to the Medicare approved amount of $44.00. The receipts column will increase to $35.20 for item 1, and the balance will decrease to $8.80. Responsibility for 20 percent of the Medicare approved amount will be transferred to the secondary carrier. The insurance plan number will change to read '5', and the item status will indicate a transfer has occurred. The insurance bill column will continue to display a date, but no insurance bill will be printed.

Figure 6-35 Medicare Payment with Piggyback to Secondary Insurance

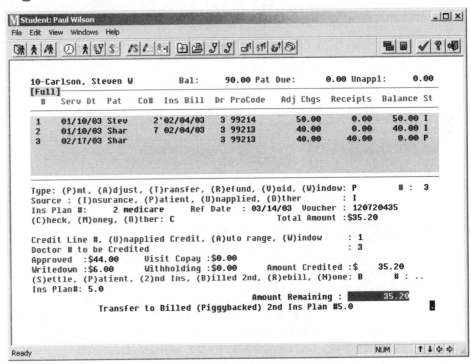

EXERCISE 18: Claire E. League

Posting a Medicare Payment—Patient Deductible

Each year, Medicare patients are expected to pay a certain portion of their own medical expenses before Medicare begins paying. This portion is called the patient deductible and is omitted from Medicare payments until the full deductible has been collected. The Explanation of Medicare Benefits attached to Ms. League's check advises that items one, two, and three of her account have been approved, but payment is being applied to the patient's deductible; therefore, no money is included in the check for these items (Figure 6-36). To ensure accurate records for the practice, the items should be reduced to the amount approved by Medicare and then transferred to patient responsibility.

Figure 6-36 Claire League's Medicare Check—Voucher 120720438

EXPLANATION OF MEDICARE PART I BENEFITS

THIS IS A STATEMENT OF ACTION TAKEN ON YOUR MEDICARE CLAIM

SERVICES WERE PROVIDED FOR NAME/NUMBER	CONTROL NO.	PROCEDURE CODE	MO. OF SERV.	POS	TOS	SERVICE DATES FROM MO. DAY YR.	SERVICE DATES TO MO. DAY YR.	CHARGES AMOUNT BILLED	CHARGES AMOUNT APPROVED	DEDUCTIBLE	NET PAY
League, Claire 738764128D	B013840388082504200	99213	01 0	1	6	01 10 03	01 10 03	40 00	34 00	34 00	
	B01384	85014	01 0	1	6	01 10 03	01 10 03	18 00	12 00	12 00	
	B01384	99213	01 0	1	6	02 03 03	02 03 03	40 00	34 00	29 00	5 00
	B01384	85031	01 0	1	6	02 03 03	02 03 03	15 00	10 00		8 00
PAT. NO. 30		TOTAL FOR THE ABOVE CLAIM						113 00	90 00		13 00

PROVIDER NUMBER	DATE	CHECK NUMBER	CHECK AMOUNT
		120720438	13 00

	CLAIMS PROCESSED	AMOUT PAYABLE	AMOUNT WITHHELD	NET PAYABLE	CREDITS	TOTAL MEDICARE EARNINGS
THIS EOMB•			00		00	
YEAR TO DATE•			00		00	

KEEP THIS NOTICE FOR YOUR RECORDS

STEP 1 From the Main Menu (Menu 1) select option **3**, PAYMENT Posting, then option **1**, PAYMENT Entry. Key '**30.0**' and press **ENTER** to retrieve Ms. League's account.

STEP 2 In the Type field, select (**P**)ayment. At the Source prompt, choose (**I**)nsurance, then Plan **#2** (for Medicare) to invoke the Automated Medicare Payment Handler. Press **ENTER** at the Ref. Date field to accept the default date. Type the check number ('**120720438**') in the Voucher field and press **ENTER**. Choose (**C**)heck and press **ENTER** and key '**13.00**' as the total amount.

STEP 3 Make sure the highlight bar is over line item **1** (the first item for which Medicare is making a payment), then press **ENTER** to select it. The cursor will automatically position itself at the Approved Amount field. If the Medicare profile was correctly set up in Procedure Code Maintenance, the approved amount will appear as a default amount for this field. If it does not, press **F10** to clear the field, then key '**34.00**'. Press **ENTER** and a $6.00 amount should appear in the writedown field. When **ENTER** is pressed again, the Automated Medicare Payment Handler will calculate the amount credited to be 80 percent of the approved amount or the amount of the payment, $13.00. *Because Medicare did not pay on the item, you must OVERWRITE the amount credited.* Enter '**0.00**'; then select '**P**' to transfer the charge to the patient.

STEP 4

Compare your screen with Figure 6-37, then press **F1** or click on the PROCESS button ('√') to process. When the data is processed, **The Medical Manager** software will reduce the $40.00 charge to the Medicare approved amount ($34.00) and decrease the balance to $34.00. The item status will change to 'PT' to show that it was transferred to patient responsibility.

The screen will continue to show an amount remaining that must be allocated.

STEP 5

Repeat the previous procedure for item 2 (procedure code 85014). Make sure the highlight bar is on item **2** and press **ENTER** to select it. The cursor will position itself at the Approved Amount field. If the Medicare profile was correctly set up in Procedure Code Maintenance, the approved amount ($12.00) should appear. Press **ENTER** to accept $12.00 as the Approved Amount and a $6.00 amount should appear in the Writedown field. Press **ENTER** to accept it and the Medicare Automated Payment Handler will calculate the amount credited. However, because Medicare is not providing payment for

Figure 6-37 Payments with Patient Deductible

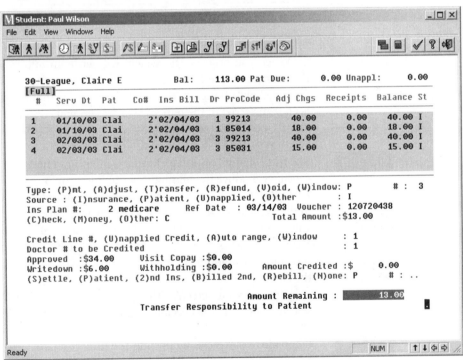

this item, you must overwrite the amount credited as '**0.00**' and press **ENTER**. Select '**P**' to transfer the charge to the patient. Your screen should be similar to Figure 6-38. Press **F1** or click on the PROCESS button ('√') on the top toolbar to process.

Figure 6-38 Payments with Patient Deductible (Continued)

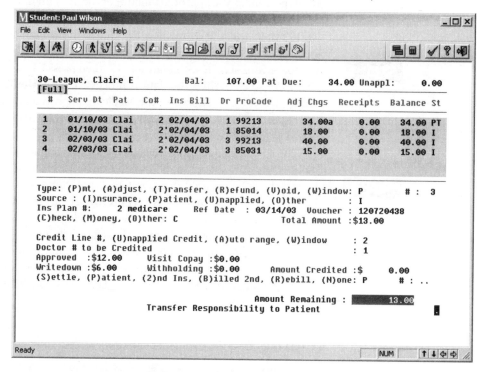

When you process, the system will write an automatic adjusting entry, reducing the charge amount to the Medicare approved amount ($12.00). The balance column for item 2 will change to "12.00 PT" to indicate that the responsibility for this item has been transferred to the patient. The screen will continue to show an amount remaining ($13.00) that must be allocated.

STEP 6

The next item listed on Ms. League's Medicare check is for procedure code 99213 on February 3. Move the highlight bar to line item '**3**' and press **ENTER** to select it. Press **ENTER** to accept '34.00' as the Approved Amount and a $6.00 amount should appear in the Writedown field. Press **ENTER** to accept it and the Medicare Payment Handler will calculate the amount credited. However, if you refer to the Explanation of Medicare Benefits you will see that Medicare withheld a partial deductible on this item; therefore, the amount credited must be overwritten as '**5.00**'. Transfer responsibility to the patient.

Compare your screen with Figure 6-39, then **PROCESS**. After you process your screen, notice that the Receipts column now contains a payment of $5.00 for line item 3.

STEP 7

Complete this exercise by posting the final payment listed on the Medicare check, an $8.00 payment for procedure code 85031, received by Ms. League on her February 2 visit. Move the highlight bar to line item '**4**' and press **ENTER** to select it. Press **ENTER** to accept '10.00' as the Approved Amount and a $5.00 amount should appear in the Writedown field. Press **ENTER** to accept it and the Medicare Payment Handler will calculate the amount to be credited. Press **ENTER** to accept '8.00' as the Amount credited. Choose (**2**)nd to transfer payment responsibility to the secondary insurance and

Figure 6-39 Payment with Partial Deductible

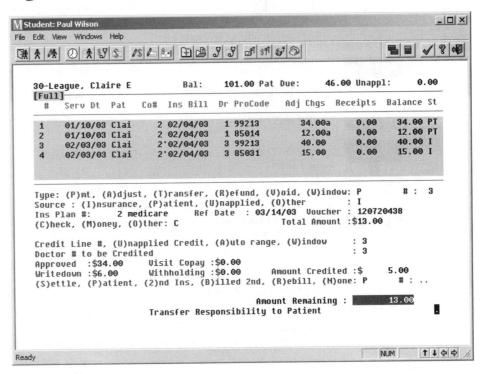

press **ENTER**. Press **ENTER** again to transfer payment responsibility to insurance plan #10.

Compare your screen with Figure 6-40, then **PROCESS**. Press **EXIT** until you reach the Main Menu (Menu 1).

Figure 6-40 Medicare Payment with Transfer to Secondary Carrier

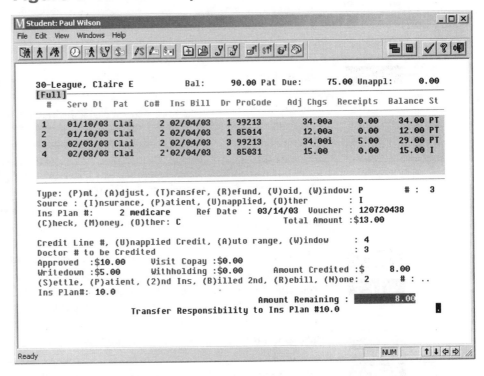

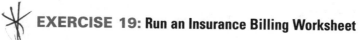

EXERCISE 19: Run an Insurance Billing Worksheet

Because you have now corrected several billing problems, you are ready to print an Insurance Billing Worksheet.

STEP 1 From the Main Menu (Menu 1), select option **6**, BILLING & EDI, then option **3**, INSURANCE Billing Worksheet.

STEP 2 Press **ENTER** to accept 03/14/03, as the Bill-Thru Date.

STEP 3 Press **ENTER** to accept '1' as the default for Physical Form #.

STEP 4 Press **ENTER** to accept 'N' to not print all diagnoses.

STEP 5 Press **ENTER** to accept the default scope of (A)ll outstanding items.
Press **F1** or click on the PROCESS button ('√') on the top toolbar to process. Compare your Insurance Prebilling Worksheet with Figure 6-41.

Figure 6-41 Insurance Prebilling Worksheet

```
03/14/03                          INSURANCE PREBILLING WORKSHEET                                    Page   1
                                        Student: Paul Wilson
                                 Form # 1 - Thru 03/14/03 - All Claims

Ins Plan Dates of Service Diag Code  Proc Code Mod Voucher  POS/TOS   Units  Dr/Al/As  2nd Plan Bill Amt   Receipts      Net
================================================================================================================================
      5 - Epsilon Life & Casualty        Fmt : A:ins0101a.fmt   Bill Amt = Adjusted
     21.2 - Edwards, Andrea
        01/10/03 -          783.0       99214         1057      3/1      1.00   3/ Y/ Y      0      50.00      0.00      50.00
                                                                                                 ---------- ---------- ----------
                                                                                 Totals      :          50.00      0.00      50.00
                                                                                                                      ==========
                                      TOTAL TO BE BILLED FOR INSURANCE PLAN #      5 :                                  50.00
      9 - Worker's Compensation          Fmt : A:ins0101a.fmt   Bill Amt = Adjusted
     21.0 - Edwards, Portia
        02/17/03 -          724.2       99214         1063      3/1      1.00   3/ Y/ Y      0      50.00      0.00      50.00
                                                                                                 ---------- ---------- ----------
                                                                                 Totals      :          50.00      0.00      50.00
                                                                                                                      ==========
                                      TOTAL TO BE BILLED FOR INSURANCE PLAN #      9 :                                  50.00
     10 - Medicare Plus                  Fmt : A:ins0101a.fmt   Bill Amt = Adjusted
     30.0 - League, Claire
      * 02/03/03 -          285.9       85031         1060      3/1      1.00   3/ N/ Y      2      10.00      8.00       2.00
                                                                                                 ---------- ---------- ----------
                                                                                 Totals      :          10.00      8.00       2.00
                                                                                                                      ==========
                                      TOTAL TO BE BILLED FOR INSURANCE PLAN #     10 :                                   2.00
     12 - Fringe Benefit Center          Fmt : A:ins0101a.fmt   Bill Amt = Adjusted
     80.0 - Davis, Timothy
        02/17/03 -          841.2       29705         1062      3/1      1.00   2/ Y/ Y      0      38.00      0.00      38.00
                                                                                                 ---------- ---------- ----------
                                                                                 Totals      :          38.00      0.00      38.00
                                                                                                                      ==========
                                      TOTAL TO BE BILLED FOR INSURANCE PLAN #     12 :                                  38.00
================================================================================================================================
                                      TOTAL TO BE BILLED FOR ALL INSURANCE PLANS :                                    140.00
```

Perform Insurance Billing

Once you have carefully checked the information on the Insurance Prebilling Worksheet, you are ready to perform your actual insurance billing. Load insurance forms or blank paper into your printer and proceed to perform your insurance billing routine

STEP 1 From the Main Menu (Menu 1), choose option **6**, BILLING & EDI. On the Billing & EDI Menu (Menu 4), choose option **5**, INSURANCE Billing.

STEP 2 Press **ENTER** to accept 03/14/03 as the Bill-Thru Date.

STEP 3 Press **ENTER** to accept '1' as the default for Physical Form #.

STEP 4 Press **ENTER** to accept the default scope of (A)ll outstanding items.

STEP 5 Press **F1** or click on the PROCESS button ('√') on the top toolbar to process. Hand in all insurance bills to your instructor.

STEP 6 Enter (**N**)o because a form alignment is not needed.

STEP 7 Enter (**Y**)es to accept insurance billing.

EXERCISE 20: Running a Trial Daily Report for March 14

In Exercise 21, you will perform a Daily Close for March 14, 2003. However, you will first need to run the Trial Daily Report. From the Main Menu (Menu 1), select option 5, REPORT Generation, then option **4**, DAILY Report.

STEP 1 Key '**Y**' to request a Trial Daily Report. Key '**P**' to request a check register by (P)ractice. Press **ENTER** to bypass the prompt "Selective Appointment Location." Key '**A**' for (A)ll.

STEP 2 Press **F1** or click on the PROCESS button ('√') on the top toolbar to process. Press **ENTER** at the prompt '**Daily Close NOT Performed **.'
    Check your work carefully against the financial and other information shown in Figures 6-42 to 6-46, and make any necessary corrections through File Maintenance (Menu 2). When you are sure everything is correct, run the Final Daily Close.

EXERCISE 21: Running a Final Daily Close for March 14

From the Reports Menu (Menu 7), select option **4**, DAILY Report.

STEP 1 Key '**N**' to request a Final Daily Report. Key '**P**' again to request a check register for the practice.

STEP 2 Key '**0**' to not purge appointments.

STEP 3 Press **F1** or click on the PROCESS button ('√') on the top toolbar to process and the report will be generated. Hand in the Final Daily Report to your instructor.

Figure 6-42 Daily Report for 03/14/03—James Monroe, M.D.

```
03/14/03                              DAILY REPORT FOR 03/14/03                              Page   1
                                          James T Monroe MD (1)

                                                                  [to Vchr  Total Ref Date]
Account   Patient Name      Dt Post   Type Dates of Service Dept Voucher Proc Code   Units  Pri/Sec Ail  Loc  Exc  Amount
=========================================================================================================================
30        League,Claire     03/14/03  A03  Medicare Adjustme  0  120720438  [1054       6.00  03/14/03]              -6.00
30        League,Claire     03/14/03  A03  Medicare Adjustme  0  120720438  [1054       6.00  03/14/03]              -6.00

Exception Codes:
overrides: c= charge, p= profile, w= writedown, o= overpay, i= pmt not from resp. ins, e= item edited, x= rebuilt dlyfile.tmp used


                                    Summary for : James T Monroe MD

         -----------------------------------------------------------------------------------
              Item           Today        Period-to-Date          Year-to-Date
           Description      03/14/03    01/01/03 - 03/14/03     01/01/03 - 03/14/03
         -----------------------------------------------------------------------------------
         Total Charges          0.00          182.00                  182.00
         Total Receipts         0.00            4.00                    4.00
         Refunds                0.00            0.00                    0.00
         Cross-Alloc Unapplied  0.00            0.00                    0.00
         Total Adjustments     12.00          132.00                  132.00
         Accounts Receivable   46.00           46.00                   46.00
         Total # Procedures        0               7                       7
         Service Charges        0.00            0.00                    0.00
         Tax Charges            0.00            0.00                    0.00
         Copay Expected         0.00             ---                     ---
         Copay Paid             0.00             ---                     ---
         Deposit Amount         0.00             ---                     ---
                 Checks   0.00
                 Cash     0.00
                 Other    0.00
         -----------------------------------------------------------------------------------
```

Figure 6-43 Daily Report for 03/14/03—Frances Simpson, M.D.

Account	Patient Name	Dt Post	Type	Dates of Service	Dept	Voucher	Proc Code	[to Vchr Units	Total Pri/Sec	Ref Date] Ail	Loc	Exc	Amount
80	Davis,Timothy	03/14/03	A-1	** Void Item **	0	ERROR		[1062	0.00	03/14/03]			0.00
80.0	Davis,Timothy	03/14/03	CHG	02/17/03-	0	1062	99213	-1.00	0/	0	Y		-40.00

Exception Codes:
overrides: c= charge, p= profile, w= writedown, o= overpay, i= pmt not from resp. ins, e= item edited, x= rebuilt dlyfile.tmp used

Summary for : Frances D Simpson M.D.

Item Description	Today 03/14/03	Period-to-Date 01/01/03 - 03/14/03	Year-to-Date 01/01/03 - 03/14/03
Total Charges	0.00	166.00	166.00
Total Receipts	0.00	0.00	0.00
Refunds	0.00	0.00	0.00
Cross-Alloc Unapplied	0.00	0.00	0.00
Total Adjustments	0.00	0.00	0.00
Accounts Receivable	166.00	166.00	166.00
Total # Procedures	0	4	4
Voided Procedures	1	---	---
Voided Charges	40.00	---	---
Service Charges	0.00	0.00	0.00
Tax Charges	0.00	0.00	0.00
Copay Expected	0.00	---	---
Copay Paid	0.00	---	---
Deposit Amount	0.00	---	---
Checks	0.00		
Cash	0.00		
Other	0.00		

Figure 6-44 Daily Report for 03/14/03—Sydney Carrington, M.D.

Account	Patient Name	Dt Post	Type	Dates of Service	Dept	Voucher	Proc Code	[to Vchr Units	Total Pri/Sec	Ref Date] Ail	Loc	Exc	Amount
21	Edwards,Portia	03/14/03	A01	General Adjustmen	0	Dr. C		[1057	-10.00	03/14/03]			10.00
34	Dudley,Wayne	03/14/03	PMT	Check Patient		420		[1053	300.00	03/14/03]			-85.00
34	Dudley,Wayne	03/14/03	PMT	Check Patient		420		[1053	300.00	03/14/03]			-8.00
34	Dudley,Wayne	03/14/03	PMT	Check Patient		420		[1053	300.00	03/14/03]			-150.00
34	Dudley,Wayne	03/14/03	PMT	Check Patient		420		[1053	300.00	03/14/03]			-57.00
10	Carlson,Steven	03/14/03	PMT	Check Medi #2		120720435		[1050	35.20	03/14/03]		p	-35.20
10	Carlson,Steven	03/14/03	A03	Medicare Adjustme	0	120720435		[1050	6.00	03/14/03]		p	-6.00
30	League,Claire	03/14/03	PMT	Check Medi #2		120720438		[1060	13.00	03/14/03]			-5.00
30	League,Claire	03/14/03	A03	Medicare Adjustme	0	120720438		[1060	6.00	03/14/03]			-6.00
30	League,Claire	03/14/03	PMT	Check Medi #2		120720438		[1060	13.00	03/14/03]			-8.00
30	League,Claire	03/14/03	A03	Medicare Adjustme	0	120720438		[1060	5.00	03/14/03]			-5.00

Exception Codes:
overrides: c= charge, p= profile, w= writedown, o= overpay, i= pmt not from resp. ins, e= item edited, x= rebuilt dlyfile.tmp used

Summary for : Sydney J Carrington M.D.

Item Description	Today 03/14/03	Period-to-Date 01/01/03 - 03/14/03	Year-to-Date 01/01/03 - 03/14/03
Total Charges	0.00	1,465.00	1,465.00
Total Receipts	348.20	459.20	459.20
Refunds	0.00	0.00	0.00
Cross-Alloc Unapplied	0.00	0.00	0.00
Total Adjustments	7.00	7.00	7.00
Accounts Receivable	998.80	998.80	998.80
Total # Procedures	0	26	26
Service Charges	0.00	0.00	0.00
Tax Charges	0.00	0.00	0.00
Copay Expected	0.00	---	---
Copay Paid	0.00	---	---
Deposit Amount	348.20	---	---
Checks	348.20		
Cash	0.00		
Other	0.00		

Figure 6-45 Cash Analysis Report for 03/14/03

```
03/14/03                      DAILY REPORT FOR 03/14/03                    Page    4
                               CASH ANALYSIS REPORT
                                Student: Paul Wilson

===================================================================================

       Change in Cash Position                          Daily Deposit
       ----------------------                           -------------

       CHECKS         348.20                    CHECKS         348.20
       CASH             0.00                    CASH             0.00
       OTHER            0.00                    OTHER            0.00
       REFUNDS          0.00                            ==========
                    ==========                              348.20
                        348.20

                          CHECK REGISTER FOR 03/14/03

      Ref #   Voucher    Dr.    Amount    Date Posted    Received From        Account
      =============================================================================
        1     420         3     300.00    03/14/03       Dudley, Wayne          34
        2     120720435   3      35.20    03/14/03       Medicare               10
        3     120720438   3      13.00    03/14/03       Medicare               30
                                ----------
            TOTAL CHECKS :       348.20
```

Figure 6-46 Daily Report Totals for 03/14/03

```
03/14/03                      DAILY REPORT FOR 03/14/03                    Page    5
                                Student: Paul Wilson

===================================================================================
```

                          TOTALS FOR 03/14/03

Doctor	Charges	Receipts	Adjustments	Net A/R	Total A/R	# Proc.	Serv Chg	Tax Chg
1. James T Monroe MD	0.00	0.00	12.00	-12.00	46.00	0	0.00	0.00
2. Frances D Simpson M.D.	-40.00	0.00	0.00	-40.00	166.00	-1	0.00	0.00
3. Sydney J Carrington M.D.	0.00	348.20	7.00	-355.20	998.80	0	0.00	0.00
TOTAL	-40.00	348.20	19.00	-407.20	1,210.80	-1	0.00	0.00

                  PERIOD-TO-DATE TOTALS FOR 01/01/03 - 03/14/03

Doctor	Charges	Receipts	Adjustments	Net A/R	Total A/R	# Proc.	Serv Chg	Tax Chg
1. James T Monroe MD	182.00	4.00	132.00	46.00	46.00	7	0.00	0.00
2. Frances D Simpson M.D.	166.00	0.00	0.00	166.00	166.00	4	0.00	0.00
3. Sydney J Carrington M.D.	1,465.00	459.20	7.00	998.80	998.80	26	0.00	0.00
TOTAL	1,813.00	463.20	139.00	1,210.80	1,210.80	37	0.00	0.00

                  YEAR-TO-DATE TOTALS FOR 01/01/03 - 03/14/03

Doctor	Charges	Receipts	Adjustments	Net A/R	Total A/R	# Proc.	Serv Chg	Tax Chg
1. James T Monroe MD	182.00	4.00	132.00	46.00	46.00	7	0.00	0.00
2. Frances D Simpson M.D.	166.00	0.00	0.00	166.00	166.00	4	0.00	0.00
3. Sydney J Carrington M.D.	1,465.00	459.20	7.00	998.80	998.80	26	0.00	0.00
TOTAL	1,813.00	463.20	139.00	1,210.80	1,210.80	37	0.00	0.00

STEP 4

When the report is complete, accept the Final Daily Close by keying '**Y**' at the prompt "Do You Wish To Accept Daily Close? (Y/N)."

Press **ENTER** at the prompt "Daily Close is Complete. Returning to Log-On," so that you will be able to advance the date in the next exercise.

 EXERCISE 22: Advancing the Date to March 20

STEP 1

Carefully key '**03202003**' and press **ENTER** to change the date. Do not change the date again until instructed to do so again in these lessons.

Note: Your Final Daily close will contain both a GL Daily Distribution Report and a Daily Close Status Report, neither of which is shown in the figures above.

EXERCISE 23: Posting Insurance Payment Split Between Patients

Insurance plan #5, Epsilon Life and Casualty, sends check 52-17118730 for $211.60 (Figure 6-47). The check is to be split between three of Dr. Carrington's patients. Epsilon is paying a percentage (generally 80 percent) of the total amount billed, and you must determine the amount to apply to each individual item. The Explanation of Benefits (EOB) from the insurance plan indicates the payment allocations as shown on the following page:

Figure 6-47 Epsilon Check—Voucher 52-17118730

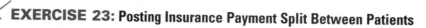

Epsilon Life & Casualty
P.O. Box 189
Macon, GA 31298

EXPLANATION OF PROVIDER PAYMENT

52-17118730

SYDNEY CARRINGTON & ASSOCIATES   E-59-2699965   PAGE 1   03/20/03
34 SYCAMORE STREET SUITE 300
MADISON, CA 95653

ENCLOSED IS A DRAFT (52-17118730) IN THE AMOUNT OF $211.60 IN PAYMENT OF THE FOLLOWING ASSIGNED BENEFITS. IF YOU HAVE ANY QUESTIONS ABOUT THE INDIVIDUAL PAYMENTS LISTED BELOW, PLEASE CONTACT THE APPROPRIATE ISSUING OFFICE.

NOTE: ALL INQUIRIES AND CLAIMS SHOULD REFERENCE THE INSURED ID NUMBER FOR PROMPT RESPONSE.

INSURED NAME	CLAIMANT NAME	PATIENT NUMBER	SERVICE DATES	SUBMITTED EXPENSES	PENDING OR NOT PAYABLE		PAYMENT AMOUNT	EPSILON USE	INSURED ID
EVANS	PATRICIA	110	01/27/03	$180.00		A	144.00	4388295	756575675
EDWARDS	ANDREA	21	01/10/03	76.00		A	60.80	4388295	19FV293D01F
CARLSON	STEVEN	10	02/03/03	8.80		A	6.80	4288293	M5A876587665
						A			
					TOTAL		$211.60		
					AMOUNT		$211.60		

ISSUING CLAIM OFFICE-EPSILON LIFE & CASUALTY, P.O. BOX 189, MACON, GA 31298 – TEL. (800) 555-7654

Patient	Payment Allocation
Patricia Evans	$144.00
Andrea Edwards	$ 60.80
Steven Carlson	$ 6.80
TOTAL	$211.60

The Batch Total line at the bottom of the Payment Entry screen will help you complete the procedure. To clear the batch totals, exit the Payment Entry screen, then choose the screen again. Once this is done you will only exit as far as the Patient Retrieval prompt as you process the Epsilon check. This will permit the payment feature to maintain a running batch total.

Post the amount of payment for each patient separately. *Do not enter the check total in the total amount field.* The first patient is Patricia Evans, whose patient number is given on the check. A $144.00 payment has been made for line 6, her hospital stay.

STEP 1   From the Main Menu (Menu 1), select option **3**, PAYMENT Posting, then option **1**, PAYMENT Entry. Key Ms. Evans's account number, '**110.0**', and press **ENTER** to retrieve her account.

STEP 2   Key '**P**' for (P)ayment, and (**I**)nsurance as the source of the payment. Key '**5**' as the Ins Plan #. Press **ENTER** at the Ref. Date field to accept the current system date of 03/20/03. Key '**17118730**' as the Voucher No. and press **ENTER**. Key '**C**' for (C)heck and press **ENTER**. Key '**144.00**' in the Total Amount field and press **ENTER**. Highlight line item **6** (99232 on 01/28/03 for Patricia), and press **ENTER** to select it. Press **ENTER** again to accept $144.00 as the amount credited. Enter '**P**' to transfer responsibility for any remaining charges to the patient. Compare your screen with Figure 6-48. Press **F1** or click on the PROCESS button ('√') on the top toolbar to process and press **ENTER**.

Figure 6-48 Split Check, First Patient Item 1 of 1

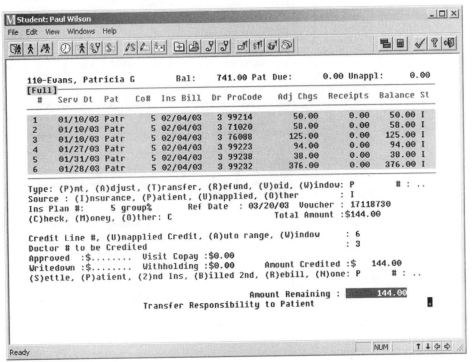

Once the payment information has been processed, the screen will change to reflect the payment. Line 6 will now have a receipt of $144.00. The item balance will be $232.00. Responsibility will be transferred to the patient. The status column will change to PT. Review your screen carefully as no figure is provided.

STEP 3

To continue allocating the check, exit only as far as the Patient Retrieval prompt. Key Mrs. Portia Edwards's account number, '**21.0**', and press **ENTER** to retrieve her account. Notice that the Batch Total line at the bottom of the Payment Entry screen will now reflect the $144.00 posted during Patricia Evans's transaction.

Note: Remember that this insurance plan is paying only a percentage (usually 80 percent) of the amount billed for each item. The amount they are paying you adds up to the first three of Andrea's items. You must calculate what 80 percent of each item is and allocate only that portion of the check to each item. For item 1, 80 percent of $50 is $40. Transfer the remaining portion of each item to patient responsibility.

STEP 4

Key '**P**' for (P)ayment, and (**I**)nsurance as the source of the payment. Key '**5**' as the Ins Plan # and press **ENTER**. Press **ENTER** at the Ref. Date field to accept the current system date of 03/20/03. Key '**17118730**' as the Voucher No. and '**C**' for (C)heck. Enter '**60.80**' in the Total Amount field, press **ENTER**, highlight line item **1** (99214 on 01/10/03 for Andrea) and press **ENTER** again to select it. Press **F10** to clear the field. Carefully key '**40.00**' (80 percent of the original charge) in the Amount Credited field and press **ENTER**. Enter '**P**' to transfer responsibility for the remaining charges to the patient. Compare your screen with Figure 6-49, then press **F1** or click on the PROCESS button ('√') on the top toolbar to process.

Figure 6-49 Split Check, Second Patient, Item 1 of 3

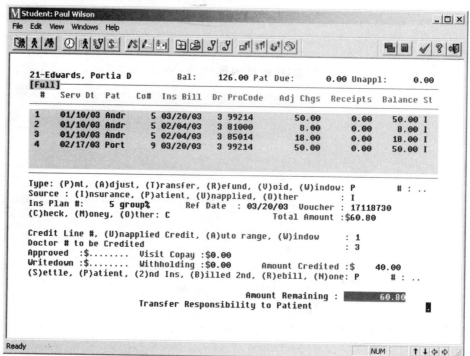

After you process the first of the three lines to be credited for this patient, the receipts column for this item will increase to $40.00, and the balance column will decrease to $10.00. Note that the item status will also change to PT indicating that you transferred the amount to patient responsibility.

Note: Fee profiles are sometimes set incorrectly in the medical practice. However, it is important to credit each item with the exact payment amount intended for the item. As in the example provided above in Step 4, it may be necessary to use the F10 key to clear the field so that the correct payment amount may be written in.

STEP 5

For Andrea Edwards's second charge, make sure the highlight bar is over item **2** (81000) and press **ENTER**. Press **F10** to clear the Amount Credited field. Key '**6.40**' (this is 80 percent of the $8.00 charge that was billed) in the Total Amount field and press **ENTER**. Key '**P**' to transfer responsibility for the remaining charges to the patient. Compare your screen with Figure 6-50, then press **F1** or click on the PROCESS button ('√') on the top toolbar to process.

Figure 6-50 Split Check, Second Patient, Item 2 of 3

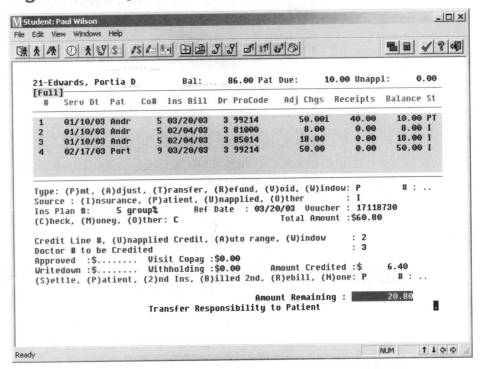

After you process the second of the three lines to be credited for this patient, the receipts column for this item will increase to $6.40 and the balance will be decreased to $1.60.

STEP 6

For Andrea's final charge, highlight line item **3** (85014) and press **ENTER**. Press **ENTER** to accept $14.40 as the Amount Credited. Enter '**P**' to transfer responsibility for the remaining charges to the patient. Compare your screen with Figure 6-51, then press **F1** or click on the PROCESS button ('√') on the top toolbar to process.

Figure 6-51 Split Check, Second Patient, Item 3 of 3

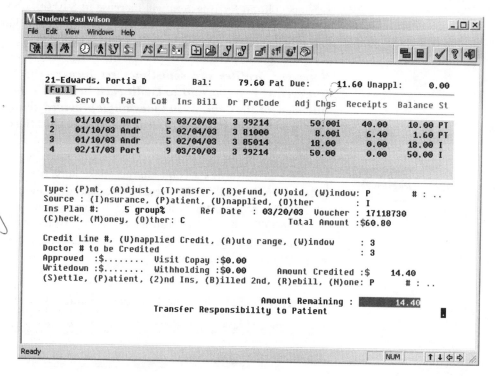

When you process, the receipts column will increase to $14.40, the balance will decrease to $3.60, and the item status PT will indicate that the amount was transferred to patient responsibility. The Batch Total line will now appear, summing both Andrea Edwards's and Patricia Evans's portions of the check. Press **ESCAPE** or click on the EXIT button on the top toolbar to return to the Patient Retrieval screen and begin the next exercise.

EXERCISE 24: Steven W. Carlson

Posting Insurance Payment with Settlement Option

STEP 1 Exit only as far as the Patient Retrieval prompt. Enter the name or number of the third patient on the check by keying '**10.0**' and pressing **ENTER** to retrieve Mr. Carlson's account. The Batch Total line at the bottom of the payment screen will now reflect the receipts from Patricia Evans's transaction and the receipts and adjustments processed for Andrea Edwards. Steven Carlson's portion of the check is a payment of $6.80 for item 1.

STEP 2 Key '**P**' for (P)ayment, '**I**' for (I)nsurance, and enter '**5**' for the plan number. Press **ENTER** at the Ref. Date field to accept the current system date. Enter '**17118730**' for the Voucher number, key '**C**' for (C)heck, and type '**6.80**' for the Total Amount. Make sure line item **1** is highlighted and press **ENTER** to select it. Press **ENTER** to accept $6.80 as the Amount Credited.

STEP 3 Because this patient has no other insurance that can be billed, the practice will accept the payment and write off the remainder using the settlement option. Enter '**S**' for (S)ettle, followed by '**2**' for adjustment type "General Write-Off." Compare your screen with Figure 6-52 and press **F1** or click on the PROCESS button ('√') to process.

Figure 6-52 Split Check, Third Patient, Item 1 of 1 (Before Processing)

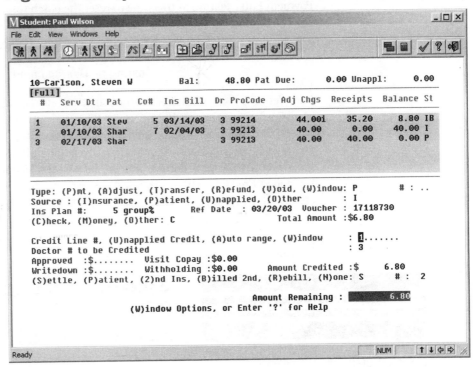

When the allocation is processed, compare your screen with Figure 6-53. The net charges on line 1 will decrease to $42.00, the receipts will increase to $42.00, and the balance column will decrease to $0.00. The Edit Payment screen will show an additional entry of an adjustment for $2.00. The batch total will increase net payments to $211.60 to indicate the total receipts posted among all three patients.

Figure 6-53 Split Check, Third Patient, Item 1 of 1 (After Processing)

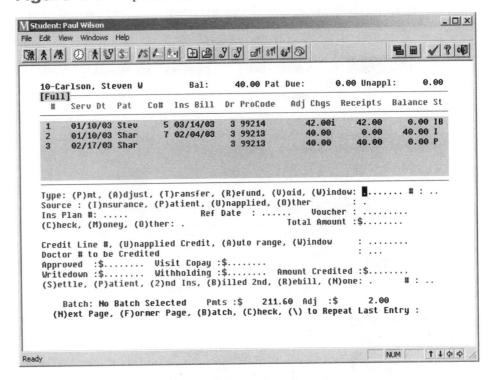

This concludes the split of this check amongst these patients. Completely exit the Payment Entry feature at this time to reset the batch totals to zero.

EXERCISE 25: Alice J. Spivey

Posting an Overpayment

Carrington & Associates, P.A., erroneously billed Alice Spivey's secondary insurance plan, Epsilon Life & Casualty, for $4.00 (Figure 6-54) for an immunization (procedure code 90701) she received during her visit on 01/10/03. However, this procedure was already billed to Alice's primary insurance carrier and was paid on 02/17/03. For adequate record keeping purposes, you should post the payment to the account using the Unapplied Credit function. You will perform a refund for $4.00 to plan 5 for this amount in a subsequent exercise in Unit 7.

Figure 6-54 Epsilon Check—Voucher 52-17181765

Epsilon Life & Casualty
P.O. Box 189
Macon, GA 31298

EXPLANATION OF PROVIDER PAYMENT   52-17181765

SYDNEY CARRINGTON & ASSOCIATES   E-59-2699965   PAGE 1   03/20/03
34 SYCAMORE STREET SUITE 300
MADISON, CA 95653

ENCLOSED IS A DRAFT (52-17181765) IN THE AMOUNT OF $4.00 IN PAYMENT OF THE FOLLOWING ASSIGNED BENEFITS. IF YOU HAVE ANY QUESTIONS ABOUT THE INDIVIDUAL PAYMENTS LISTED BELOW, PLEASE CONTACT THE APPROPRIATE ISSUING OFFICE.

NOTE: ALL INQUIRIES AND CLAIMS SHOULD REFERENCE THE INSURED ID NUMBER FOR PROMPT RESPONSE.

INSURED NAME	CLAIMANT NAME	PATIENT NUMBER	SERVICE DATES	SUBMITTED EXPENSES	PENDING OR NOT PAYABLE		PAYMENT AMOUNT	EPSILON USE	INSURED ID
YOR ID EMPLOYER- POLICY NUMBER		SUB-ID 065000-10-000							
SPIVEY	ALICE	120.4	01/10/03	$ 4.00		A	$ 4.00	4188316	76432079
					TOTAL		$ 4.00		
					AMOUNT		$ 4.00		

ISSUING CLAIM OFFICE-EPSILON LIFE & CASUALTY, P.O. BOX 189, MACON, GA 31298 – TEL. (800) 555-7654

Note: When using Unapplied Credit and subsequent refunds, be sure to enter the doctor number correctly. The system will automatically default to the doctor who performed the original procedure.

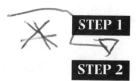

STEP 1   From the Main Menu (Menu 1), choose option 3, PAYMENT Posting, then option **1**, PAYMENT Entry. Key '**120.2**' and press **ENTER** to retrieve Alice Spivey's account.

STEP 2   Choose '**P**' for (P)ayment, '**I**' for (I)nsurance, and choose plan **5**, Epsilon Life & Casualty, as the source of the payment. Press **ENTER** at the Ref. Date field to accept the current system date. Key '**17181765**' (again, the entire voucher number is too large for this field) as the Voucher number, '**C**' for (C)heck, and key '**$4.00**' in the Total Amount field. Finally, choose to apply this amount to (**U**)napplied Credit (Figure 6-55), press **ENTER** to accept the default and credit doctor **#1**, Dr. Monroe, and to accept the default of one. Compare your screen with Figure 6-56 and press **F1** or click on the PROCESS button ('√') on the top toolbar to process.

Figure 6-55 Posting an Overpayment

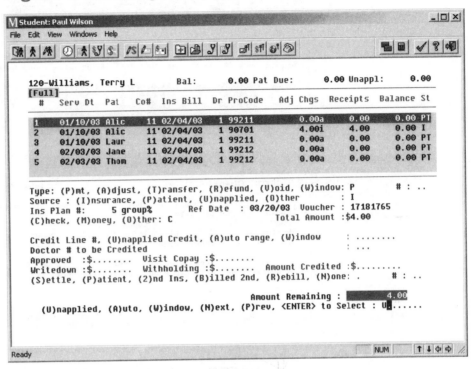

Figure 6-56 Posting an Overpayment (Continued)

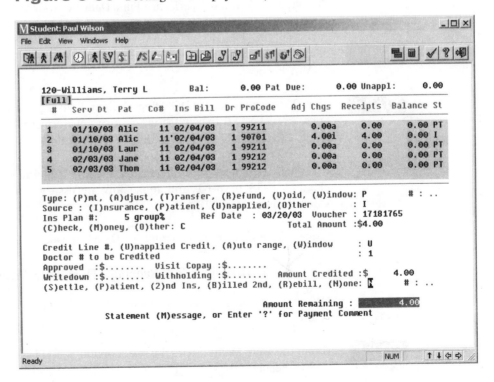

Once the payment information has been processed (Figure 6-57), the line at the top of the screen will show a balance of negative four dollars (-$4.00), a patient due amount of negative four dollars (-$4.00), and an unapplied credit amount of positive $4.00.

Figure 6-57 Payment Screen with Unapplied Credit Balance

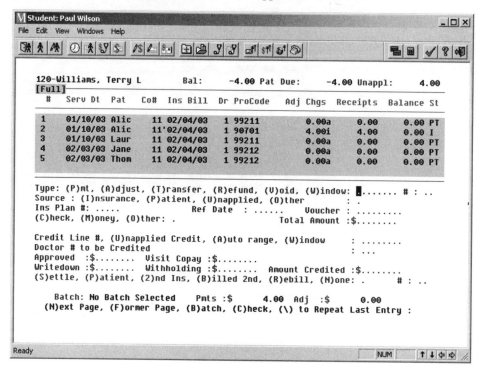

 EXERCISE 26: Running a Trial Daily Report for March 20

In Exercise 27, you will perform a Final Daily Close for March 20, 2003. But you must first run the Trial Daily Report.

STEP 1   From the Main Menu (Menu 1), select option **5**, REPORT Generation, then option **4**, DAILY Report.

STEP 2   Key '**Y**' to request a Trial Daily Report, then '**P**' to request a check register for the practice. Press **ENTER** to bypass the Selective Appointment Location field. Choose '**A**' for (A)ll, then press **F1** or click on the PROCESS button ('√') to process. Press **ENTER** to bypass the prompt "**Daily Close NOT Performed**."

Check your work carefully against the financial and other information shown in Figures 6-58 to 6-61 and make any necessary corrections through the File Maintenance (Menu 2).

Note: There will not be a report for Dr. Simpson.

EXERCISE 27: Running a Final Daily Close for March 20

When you are sure everything in your Trial Daily Report is correct, run the Final Daily Close.

STEP 1   From the Main Menu (Menu 1), select option **5**, REPORT Generation, then option **4**, DAILY Report.

Figure 6-58 Daily Report for 03/20/03—James Monroe, M.D.

```
03/20/03                          DAILY REPORT FOR 03/20/03                                    Page   1
                                    James T Monroe MD (1)

                                                          [to Vchr   Total  Ref Date]
Account   Patient Name    Dt Post  Type Dates of Service Dept Voucher Proc Code  Units  Pri/Sec Ail Loc Exc   Amount
=================================================================================================================
120       Williams,Terry  03/20/03 PMT  Check Ins #5          17181765 [UNAPPL   4.00      03/20/03]          -4.00

Exception Codes:
overrides: c= charge, p= profile, w= writedown, o= overpay, i= pmt not from resp. ins, e= item edited, x= rebuilt dlyfile.tmp used


                                  Summary for : James T Monroe MD
         --------------------------------------------------------------------------
               Item            Today       Period-to-Date          Year-to-Date
            Description       03/20/03    01/01/03 - 03/20/03    01/01/03 - 03/20/03
         --------------------------------------------------------------------------
            Total Charges         0.00           182.00               182.00
            Total Receipts        4.00             8.00                 8.00
            Refunds               0.00             0.00                 0.00
            Cross-Alloc Unapplied 0.00             0.00                 0.00
            Total Adjustments     0.00           132.00               132.00
            Accounts Receivable  42.00            42.00                42.00
            Total # Procedures       0               7                    7
            Service Charges       0.00             0.00                 0.00
            Tax Charges           0.00             0.00                 0.00
            Copay Expected        0.00             ---                  ---
            Copay Paid            0.00             ---                  ---
            Deposit Amount        4.00             ---                  ---
                 Checks      4.00
                 Cash        0.00
                 Other       0.00
         --------------------------------------------------------------------------
```

Figure 6-59 Daily Report for 03/20/03—Sydney Carrington, M.D.

```
03/20/03                          DAILY REPORT FOR 03/20/03                                    Page   2
                                  Sydney J Carrington M.D. (3)

                                                          [to Vchr   Total  Ref Date]
Account   Patient Name    Dt Post  Type Dates of Service Dept Voucher Proc Code  Units  Pri/Sec Ail Loc Exc   Amount
=================================================================================================================
110       Evans,Patricia   03/20/03 PMT  Check Ins #5         17118730 [HOSP    144.00     03/20/03]        -144.00
21        Edwards,Portia   03/20/03 PMT  Check Ins #5         17118730 [1057     60.80      03/20/03]         -40.00
21        Edwards,Portia   03/20/03 PMT  Check Ins #5         17118730 [1057     60.80      03/20/03]          -6.40
21        Edwards,Portia   03/20/03 PMT  Check Ins #5         17118730 [1057     60.80      03/20/03]         -14.40
10        Carlson,Steven   03/20/03 PMT  Check Ins #5         17118730 [1050      6.80      03/20/03]          -6.80
10        Carlson,Steven   03/20/03 A02  General Write-Off  0 17118730 [1050      2.00      03/20/03]          -2.00

Exception Codes:
overrides: c= charge, p= profile, w= writedown, o= overpay, i= pmt not from resp. ins, e= item edited, x= rebuilt dlyfile.tmp used


                                Summary for : Sydney J Carrington M.D.
         --------------------------------------------------------------------------
               Item            Today       Period-to-Date          Year-to-Date
            Description       03/20/03    01/01/03 - 03/20/03    01/01/03 - 03/20/03
         --------------------------------------------------------------------------
            Total Charges         0.00          1,465.00             1,465.00
            Total Receipts      211.60           670.80               670.80
            Refunds               0.00             0.00                 0.00
            Cross-Alloc Unapplied 0.00             0.00                 0.00
            Total Adjustments     2.00             9.00                 9.00
            Accounts Receivable 785.20           785.20               785.20
            Total # Procedures       0              26                   26
            Service Charges       0.00             0.00                 0.00
            Tax Charges           0.00             0.00                 0.00
            Copay Expected        0.00             ---                  ---
            Copay Paid            0.00             ---                  ---
            Deposit Amount      211.60             ---                  ---
                 Checks    211.60
                 Cash        0.00
                 Other       0.00
         --------------------------------------------------------------------------
```

Figure 6-60 Cash Analysis Report for 03/20/03

```
03/20/03                          DAILY REPORT FOR 03/20/03                        Page    3
                                     CASH ANALYSIS REPORT
                                      Student: Paul Wilson

===================================================================================================

        Change in Cash Position                           Daily Deposit
        -----------------------                           -------------

    CHECKS         215.60                          CHECKS         215.60
    CASH             0.00                          CASH             0.00
    OTHER            0.00                          OTHER            0.00
    REFUNDS          0.00
                ==========                                     ==========
                   215.60                                        215.60


                                CHECK REGISTER FOR 03/20/03

        Ref #  Voucher    Dr.     Amount    Date Posted    Received From                 Account
               ======================================================================================
          1   17118730     3      144.00     03/20/03      Epsilon Life & Casualty         110
          2   17118730     3       60.80     03/20/03      Epsilon Life & Casualty          21
          3   17118730     3        6.80     03/20/03      Epsilon Life & Casualty          10
          4   17181765     1        4.00     03/20/03      Epsilon Life & Casualty         120
                                 ----------
              TOTAL CHECKS :       215.60
```

Figure 6-61 Daily Report Totals for 03/20/03

```
03/20/03                          DAILY REPORT FOR 03/20/03                        Page    4
                                      Student: Paul Wilson

===================================================================================================




                            TOTALS FOR 03/20/03

-----------------------------------------------------------------------------------------------------
Doctor                  Charges     Receipts   Adjustments    Net A/R    Total A/R   # Proc.  Serv Chg  Tax Chg
-----------------------------------------------------------------------------------------------------
  1. James T Monroe MD     0.00        4.00        0.00         -4.00       42.00       0       0.00     0.00
  3. Sydney J Carrington M.D.  0.00  211.60        2.00       -213.60      785.20       0       0.00     0.00
-----------------------------------------------------------------------------------------------------
TOTAL                      0.00      215.60        2.00       -217.60      827.20       0       0.00     0.00




                  PERIOD-TO-DATE TOTALS FOR 01/01/03 - 03/20/03

-----------------------------------------------------------------------------------------------------
Doctor                  Charges     Receipts   Adjustments    Net A/R    Total A/R   # Proc.  Serv Chg  Tax Chg
-----------------------------------------------------------------------------------------------------
  1. James T Monroe MD     182.00      8.00      132.00        42.00       42.00       7       0.00     0.00
  2. Frances D Simpson M.D.  166.00    0.00        0.00       166.00      166.00       4       0.00     0.00
  3. Sydney J Carrington M.D. 1,465.00 670.80      9.00       785.20      785.20      26       0.00     0.00
-----------------------------------------------------------------------------------------------------
TOTAL                    1,813.00    678.80      141.00       993.20      993.20      37       0.00     0.00




                  YEAR-TO-DATE TOTALS FOR 01/01/03 - 03/20/03

-----------------------------------------------------------------------------------------------------
Doctor                  Charges     Receipts   Adjustments    Net A/R    Total A/R   # Proc.  Serv Chg  Tax Chg
-----------------------------------------------------------------------------------------------------
  1. James T Monroe MD     182.00      8.00      132.00        42.00       42.00       7       0.00     0.00
  2. Frances D Simpson M.D.  166.00    0.00        0.00       166.00      166.00       4       0.00     0.00
  3. Sydney J Carrington M.D. 1,465.00 670.80      9.00       785.20      785.20      26       0.00     0.00
-----------------------------------------------------------------------------------------------------
TOTAL                    1,813.00    678.80      141.00       993.20      993.20      37       0.00     0.00


          ********** Daily Close Has NOT Been Performed for 03/20/03 **********
```

STEP 2

Key 'N' to request a Final Daily Report, then 'P' to request a check register for the practice. Key '0' to not purge appointments, then press the **F1** key or click the PROCESS button ('√') to process and the Final Daily Report will be generated.

Press 'Y' to accept the Final Daily Close, then press **ENTER** to return to log-on and proceed to the next exercise to advance the date.

stuckby comp.

EXERCISE 28: Advancing the Date to March 31

STEP 1

Carefully key '03312003' and press **ENTER** to advance the date.

STEP 2

Key (Y)es and press **ENTER** to bypass the warning message "184: * WARNING* Skip > 7 days: Continue (Y/N)?" In a real practice situation, you would *never* bypass such a warning. However, for the purposes of the exercises in the Student Edition, you may do so when instructed. Key 'Y' and press **ENTER**.

STEP 3

You will be prompted to reenter your password to verify the date advance. Key 'ICAN' and press **ENTER** and you will return to the Main Menu (Menu 1).

UNIT 6 SUMMARY

Patients with insurance coverage must file a claim with their carrier. Most practices file these claims on behalf of the patient and accept assignment of benefits. This results in the payment being sent directly from the insurance company to the practice. To file these claims, they use the Insurance Billing system.

Insurance billing begins by generating a Prebilling Worksheet. The Insurance Prebilling Worksheet allows you to verify that the charges and information previously posted is correct. You should be able to verify the charges by the procedure codes, and verify that they have the proper diagnosis codes and ailment. You should be able to determine if they were assigned to the proper primary and secondary companies. By eliminating mistakes at this point in the billing process, you can expect faster payment from the insurance plan.

When the Prebilling Worksheet has been checked, the final insurance billing is run. When the billing is completed, you are given a final opportunity to confirm that the information that has been printed is correct. Once you accept the insurance billing, each item is marked as having been billed with a date and a claim number. The item status changes to prevent the editing of certain additional fields in the charge record.

Complete and correct claims submitted to the insurance company will result in faster payments from the insurance company. Typically payments from the insurance company are accompanied by a document called an Explanation of Benefits (EOB). The EOB includes information about the patient and procedures for which payment is being made as well as any financial adjustments that the practice is contractually obligated to make. In most cases, the insurance will not pay the entire cost of the patient's procedures. This can be due to the patient's benefit coverage, a copay due from the patient, or a contractual agreement between the practice and the insurance company. Insurance policies may also have a deductible which makes the patient responsible for the first $75 or $100 of health care charges each year.

Patient payments may be collected at the time of the patient's visit or after the insurance company has paid. Payments from either patients or insurance may be entered into the system through the Payment Entry module. Alternatively, patient payments made at the time of the visit can be entered in the system when the charge is posted through the Patient Pay module (automatically accessible at the end of each charge posting session).

Certain managed care and HMO plans prepay the physician at the beginning of each month for most routine patient visits. Therefore, when HMO patients are seen, typically the physician will collect only the patient's copay; the rest of the usual and customary charge for that visit will be automatically adjusted off.

Some patients have multiple insurance policies, such as a patient who has two working parents or a Medicare patient with a supplemental policy. In these cases, when an insurance payment is posted, responsibility for the remaining portion of the balance can be transferred to the secondary company. The transfer will cause the system to produce a new claim form for the second company the next time insurance billing is run. If the patient does not have a secondary plan, responsibility for any remaining balance on the item should be transferred to the patient. Once an item is paid by insurance, responsibility should always be transferred either to a secondary plan, if one exists, or to the patient.

If a payment posting error is made, the incorrect payment and adjustment records may be deleted before daily close through the Edit Payment/Adjustments option in File Maintenance. Once payments and adjustments have been daily closed, no further deletion of the items is possible. Therefore, the trial daily close should be checked carefully for any errors in posting payments or adjustments, as well as charges.

Chapter 6 → p. 289-290

1) Why's insurance billing imp. to the med. office? Why'd e an office prefer to submit forms for pts. instead of having pts. submit their claim form directly 2 the Ins. carrier.

2) Explain why an ins. billing wksheet should be run in advance of billing.

3) How is the sys. date changed in Med. Manager.sys? Why should this date be changed only when ur specifically instructed 2 do so?

4) What does it mean when the Ins. co. makes a full pymt ⊖ (minus) a pt. deductible. How can the pt. due amount of the pts. account change as a result of this situation?

5) What's meant by primary & secondary Ins. coverage? What portion of a claim is generally pd. by each plan?

6) Discuss diff. btwn. the amount charged for a procedure & the "Medicare approval" amount.

7) What's it mean 4 a pt. 2 have dual Ins. coverage? Provide an ex. of how billing would be handled 4 a pt. w/ this type of coverage.

[Answers]

The reason 2 to 2 screen.
1) Transfer account liability.
2) Post pymt. at a later date.
3) To make any type of adjustments

① For the dr. to get pd. + a way to produce revenues for the practice. Rather have office for unaccuracey. make sure we're entering

② B/c it allows u to see previous pymts

Shatterfly.

(continued).

im a fail this class!

② procedures correctly.

after final close.

③ You backclick it & put the date you are told B/C if you change it on ur own, you ~~will lose all your work~~ match all work done in

④ that one particular day.

④ → ~~it means~~ Pt. 2 → that amount has been added.

⑤ Primary is 1st ins. 2nd is 2nd insurance. Liable is pd. by ↑ Non-coverage is pd by ↑. Primary means who gets billed first.

⑥ The diff. btwn the amt. charged 4 a procedure is that they sent the procedure to the insurance. Medicare approved is when the office sends A paper stating if a certain procedure if medicare would approve it.

7) Dual coverage - 2. Primary + Secondary.
Did already.

↑ Primary 1st Secondary 2nd.
A pt. is insured by more than 1 ins. plan.

#4) The pt. is liable for the amount ~~the~~ Insurance. didn't pay. It will increase the pts. account.

#3) The date changes on Medical Manager every time you do a final daily close. The reason that the date show & change only when u do a final day close & you tell the program that u are ready for the next day.

2) b/c it helps double check if the proper primary + secondary Ins. co. Also, if the procedure codes match the ailment info.
At the same time u can check all related info. 2 make sure its correct. It eliminates mistakes at this point, 4 can expect faster pymt. from the Insurance.

1) It's how the $ comes 2 the business. The reason that office submits the claim form for the pt. is b/c there would be less errors. Pt. won't come back 2 fill out claim forms or w/ Questions.

TESTING YOUR KNOWLEDGE

1. Why is insurance billing important to the medical office? Why would an office prefer to submit forms for patients instead of having the patients submit their claim forms directly to the insurance carrier?

2. Explain why an insurance billing worksheet should be run in advance of billing.

3. How is the system date changed in **The Medical Manager** system? Why should this date be changed only when you are specifically instructed to do so?

4. What does it mean when the insurance company makes a full payment minus a patient deductible? How can the patient due amount of the patient's account change as a result of this situation?

(continues)

5. What is meant by primary and secondary insurance coverage? What portion of a claim is generally paid by each plan?

6. Discuss the difference between the amount charged for a procedure and the "Medicare approved" amount.

7. What does it mean for a patient to have dual insurance coverage? Provide an example of how billing would be handled for a patient with this type of coverage.

Report Generation

LEARNING OUTCOMES

After completing this unit, you should be able to:

◆ Describe the functions of the Guarantor's Financial Summary Report.

◆ Describe the function of the Current Period Report.

◆ Describe the function of the System Summary Report.

◆ Print the Guarantor, Current Period and System Summary Reports.

◆ Explain several methods for billing patients on a regular basis.

◆ Print patient statements.

One of the most important responsibilities in a medical office is to generate daily, weekly, or monthly lists and reports. Many types of reports can be generated that can supply financial information, trace the activities of patient accounts, develop an audit trail for insurance payments, and monitor the procedure and treatment activities of the physician.

Reports can be generated any time you wish to recall data. Many of them will display on the console screen; all of them can be printed. Reports are useful for error checking and analysis of data. Printed reports are an essential form of data backup.

TYPES OF REPORTS

The five basic types of reports available in **The Medical Manager** software are (1) guarantor reports, (2) financial activity reports, (3) support reports, (4) daily reports, and (5) special reports.

Guarantor reports provide patient personal information, extended information, and insurance information from the guarantor's file.

Financial activity reports provide item-by-item summaries on patients, insurance companies, and accounts receivable. From this file, you can analyze insurance plan payments or request an insurance plan payment review.

Support reports give information on procedure and diagnosis codes, insurance plans, service facilities, doctors, insured parties, referring doctors, and ailment history.

The Daily Report lists the day's activity in both detailed and summary formats and includes the Daily Close function.

Special reports include the referring doctor analysis, patient and dependent name and number cross-references, and special notices such as referring doctor thank-you notes, new patient introductory letters, and patient birthday greetings.

The guarantor report provides information about an account.

Financial Reports

To generate a Guarantors' Financial Summary Report, complete the following steps:

STEP 1

Select option **5**, REPORT Generation, at the Main Menu (Menu 1). Select option **2**, FINANCIAL Activity Reports, at the Reports Menu (Menu 7). The screen shown in Figure 7-1 will appear.

Figure 7-1 Financial Activity Reports Menu (Menu 8) Screen

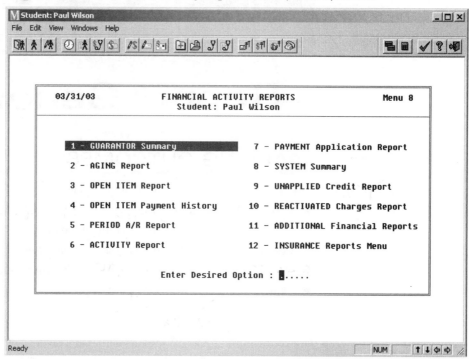

```
03/31/03              FINANCIAL ACTIVITY REPORTS          Menu 8
                          Student: Paul Wilson


          1 - GUARANTOR Summary        7 - PAYMENT Application Report

          2 - AGING Report             8 - SYSTEM Summary

          3 - OPEN ITEM Report         9 - UNAPPLIED Credit Report

          4 - OPEN ITEM Payment History   10 - REACTIVATED Charges Report

          5 - PERIOD A/R Report        11 - ADDITIONAL Financial Reports

          6 - ACTIVITY Report          12 - INSURANCE Reports Menu


                     Enter Desired Option : ▌.....
```

STEP 2 Select option **1**, GUARANTOR Summary, at the Financial Activity Reports menu (Menu 8). The Guarantors' Financial Summary Report screen shown in Figure 7-2 will appear.

The Guarantors' Financial Summary Report permits you to select a report based on (1) printer or console; (2) account number, name, or doctor number; and (3) a single account, a selective range of accounts, or all accounts. Note that you have additional options within each category from which you may select.

Figure 7-2 Blank Guarantors' Financial Summary Report Screen

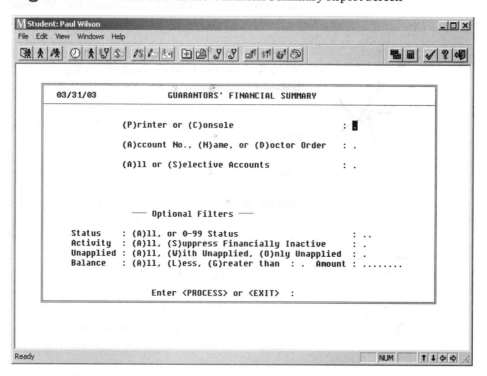

```
03/31/03              GUARANTORS' FINANCIAL SUMMARY

              (P)rinter or (C)onsole              : ▌

              (A)ccount No., (N)ame, or (D)octor Order  : .

              (A)ll or (S)elective Accounts        : .



                    —— Optional Filters ——
   Status   : (A)ll, or 0-99 Status               : ..
   Activity : (A)ll, (S)uppress Financially Inactive  : .
   Unapplied : (A)ll, (W)ith Unapplied, (O)nly Unapplied  : .
   Balance  : (A)ll, (L)ess, (G)reater than : .  Amount : ........

                  Enter <PROCESS> or <EXIT>  :
```

Although there are a number of options and filters you can use to run the Guarantors' Financial Summary Report, for this exercise, choose the following options:

(**P**)rinter
(**A**)ccount Number Order
(**A**)ll Accounts

Status:	(**A**)ll		
Activity:	(**A**)ll		
Unapplied:	(**O**)nly unapplied		
Balance:	(**A**)ll	Amount:	**0.00**

STEP 3

After the selections have been made, make sure your printer is on, has paper in it, and is online. Press **F1** or click on the PROCESS button ('√') on the top toolbar to process, and the requested Guarantors' Financial Summary Report will be generated.

REFERENCE LIST OF OPTIONS AVAILABLE #1
FOR GUARANTORS' FINANCIAL SUMMARY

◆ a. Status: (A)ll, or 0–9 Status: You may enter 'A' for all account statuses or 1–9 for a specific account status listed below:
- 0   Inactive Account
- 1   Active Account
- 2   Account Referred to Collection Agency
- 3   Temporary Account
- 4–9   User-Defined

◆ b. Activity: (A)ll, (S)uppress Financially Inactive: Enter 'A' for all accounts or 'S' to suppress accounts that are not financially active. Financially active accounts are those that have a balance due and/or have unapplied credit.

◆ c. Unapplied: (A)ll, (W)ith Unapplied, (O)nly Unapplied: Enter 'A' for all accounts, 'W' for all accounts with unapplied credit, or 'O' for those accounts with only unapplied credit.

◆ d. Balance: (A)ll, (L)ess, (G)reater than Amount: Enter 'A' for all accounts, 'L' for accounts with balances less than an amount you specify, or 'G' for accounts with a balance greater than an amount you specify. If A, L, or G is selected, the cursor will appear at the Amount field to permit entry of a dollar value.

◆ e. Default option: To default to (C)onsole, (A)ccount No. order, (A)ll accounts, (A)ll statuses, (A)ll activity levels, (A)ll unapplied levels, and (A)ll balances, press ENTER at each of the respective fields.

APPLYING YOUR KNOWLEDGE

EXERCISE 1: Running the Guarantors' Financial Summary Report

STEP 1

Using the previous instructions as a guide, select and run the Guarantors' Financial Summary Report again.

At the Main Menu (Menu 1), select option **5**, REPORT Generation. At the Reports Menu (Menu 7), select option **2**, FINANCIAL Activity Reports. At the Financial Activity Reports Menu (Menu 8), select option **1**, GUARANTOR Summary.

Choose (**P**)rinter, then accept default responses through the next four fields on the screen.

STEP 2 Select (**O**)nly at the Unapplied option, then default for the remaining fields.

Compare your screen with the completed screen shown in Figure 7-3. When you are sure it is accurate, press **F1** or click on the PROCESS button ('√') on the top toolbar to process the report. Your report should be similar to Figure 7-4. Hand in your report to your instructor.

Figure 7-3 Completed Guarantors' Financial Summary Report Screen

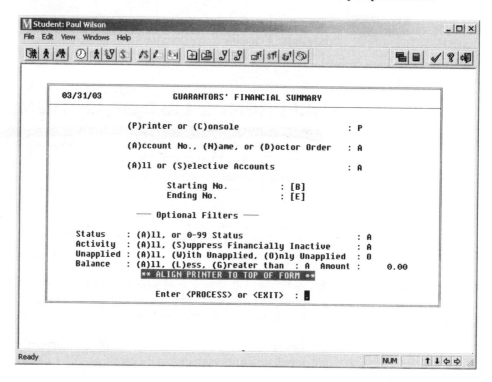

Figure 7-4 Guarantors' Financial Summary Report

```
03/31/03                    GUARANTORS' FINANCIAL SUMMARY BY ACCOUNT                    Page   1
                                   Student: Paul Wilson
                                      All Accounts
                              Status : All / Only Unapplied

Accnt #  Last Name       -Last Statement Data-   --Last Payment Data--   YTD Chgs   Unappl Cr  Pat Due AR      Balance
================================================================================================================
120      Williams,Terry                  0.00   03/20/03         4.00       4.00        4.00       -4.00        -4.00
================================================================================================================

            TOTALS :                                                        4.00        4.00       -4.00        -4.00


                            ****  Number Printed : 1  ****
                            ****  Number Active  : 8  ****
```

The current period is usually one month.

The purpose of the Current Period Report is to show the changes in a guarantor's financial status during the present period. The report begins with this period's beginning balance; itemizes all charges, adjustments, payments, write-offs, and refunds for the period; and shows the ending balance. It differs from other financial activity reports for the patient since it details only financial information for the current period.

The Current Period Report can be used any time you want to look at the current financial activity within a guarantor's account, either in summary or in detail. Follow the instructions below to see how a Current Period Report may be generated.

 From the Main Menu (Menu 1), select option **5**, REPORT Generation, then option **2**, FINANCIAL Activity Reports. From the Financial Activity Reports Menu (Menu 8), select option **5**, PERIOD A/R Report, and the Current Period Report screen shown in Figure 7-5 appears.

Figure 7-5 Blank Current Period Report Screen

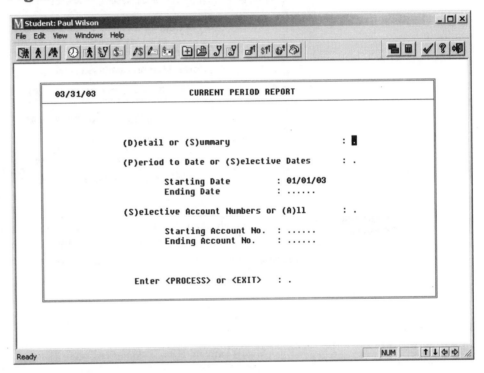

Current Period Report presents a standard selection screen for you to select a report based on (1) detail or summary information; (2) period-to-date or selective dates; and (3) a single account number, a selective range of account numbers, or all account numbers.

EXERCISE 2: Running the Summary Current Period Report

STEP 1

To run the Summary Current Period Report, carefully key in the options shown on the Completed Current Period Report Screen, shown in Figure 7-6.

Figure 7-6 Completed Current Period Report Screen

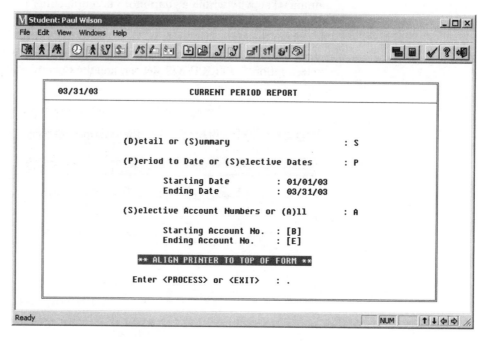

STEP 2

When you have checked that all your selections match those in the computer screen shown in Figure 7-6, press **F1** or click on the PROCESS button ('√') on the top toolbar to process and generate your report. Compare your report with Figure 7-7 and hand in the report to your instructor.

Figure 7-7 Summary Current Period Report

Acct No	Name	Phone No.	Bal Fwd	Charges	Receipts	Adjust	Balance
10	Carlson, Steven W	(916) 988-3293		130.00	82.00	8.00	40.00
14	Evans, Deborah A	(916) 678-5674		123.00	71.00		52.00
21	Edwards, Portia D	(916) 899-7800		116.00	60.80	-10.00	65.20
30	League, Claire E	(408) 907-4352		113.00	13.00	23.00	77.00
34	Dudley, Wayne R	(408) 789-6654		300.00	300.00		0.00
80	Davis, Timothy R	(916) 908-7657		166.00			166.00
110	Evans, Patricia G	(916) 544-8275		741.00	144.00		597.00
120	Williams, Terry L	(916) 875-3256		124.00	8.00	120.00	-4.00

```
03/31/03                    SUMMARY CURRENT PERIOD REPORT FOR 01/01/03 - 03/31/03                    Page    1
                                           Student: Paul Wilson
                                              All Accounts


                             TOTALS                    0.00    1813.00    678.80    141.00    993.20

                             UNAPPLIED CREDIT ONLY OMITTED                                      0.00
                               ( included      4.00 )
                             SYSTEM TOTAL A/R                                                 993.20

              ** Report Does Not Include Guarantors with ONLY Unapplied Credit Balances **
```

System Summary Report #3

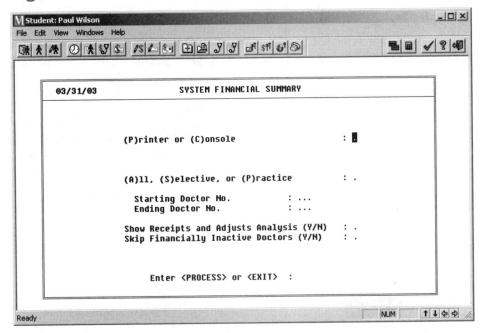

The System Summary Report provides totals.

The System Summary Report provides a quick look at the practice's accounts receivable and practice totals for the period-to-date and the year-to-date. The summary can be printed for the practice as a whole or for all or selective doctors. The System Summary Report shows total charges, receipts, adjustments, accounts receivable, net accounts receivable, total number of procedures performed, and the percentage of net charges that have been collected. Follow the instructions below to see how a System Summary Report may be generated

From the Main Menu (Menu 1), select option **5**, REPORT Generation, then option **2**, FINANCIAL Activity Reports. Then, select option **8**, SYSTEM Summary from the Financial Activity Reports Menu (Menu 8). The System Financial Summary screen shown in Figure 7-8 appears.

Figure 7-8 Blank System Financial Summary Screen

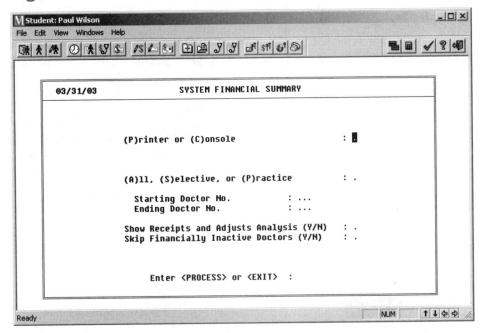

The System Financial Summary presents a standard selection screen for you to select a report based on (1) printer or console; and (2) all doctors, selective doctors, or the practice as a whole. Another selection, (3) Receipts and adjustments analysis, is optionally available with this report.

EXERCISE 3: Running the System Financial Summary Report

STEP 1

To run the System Financial Summary Report, carefully key in the options shown on the Completed System Financial Summary Report Screen, shown in Figure 7-9.

Figure 7-9 Completed System Financial Summary Report Screen

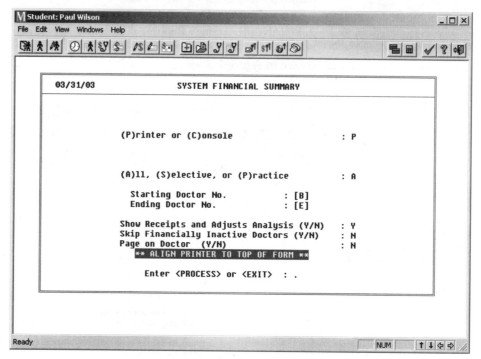

STEP 2

When you have checked that all your selections match those in the completed screen shown in Figure 7-9, press **F1** or click on the PROCESS button ('√') on the top toolbar to process and generate your report. Compare your report with Figures 7-10 through 7-15, then hand in your System Financial Summary Report to your instructor.

Figure 7-10   System Financial Summary Report, Page 1 of 6

```
03/31/03                    SYSTEM FINANCIAL SUMMARY - DETAIL                    Page    1
                                  Student: Paul Wilson
                                    All Entries

                        Totals For : James T Monroe MD (1)

-------------------------------------------------------------------------------------------
Dates                      Charges    Receipts   Adjustments    Net A/R    Total A/R  # Proc.   Col %
-------------------------------------------------------------------------------------------
01/01/03 - 03/20/03         182.00       8.00       132.00       42.00       42.00      7      16.0%
01/01/03 - 03/20/03         182.00       8.00       132.00       42.00       42.00      7      16.0%
-------------------------------------------------------------------------------------------



                        Receipts Analysis for : James T Monroe MD (1)
-------------------------------------------------------------------------------------------
             Net Receipts                     PTD             YTD
-------------------------------------------------------------------------------------------
                 Medicare                     0.00            0.00
                 Insurance                    8.00            8.00
                 Capitation Payments         60.00          180.00
                 Patient                      0.00            0.00
                 Other                        0.00            0.00
                                         -----------     -----------
                 Total Receipts              68.00          188.00
                 Refunds                      0.00            0.00
                                         ============    ============
                 Gross Receipts             68.00          188.00


                        Adjustments for : James T Monroe MD (1)
-------------------------------------------------------------------------------------------
Adjustments              PTD            YTD      Adjustments                PTD           YTD
-------------------------------------------------------------------------------------------
1) General Adjustment     0.00           0.00    2) General Write-Off       0.00          0.00
3) Medicare Adjustment   12.00          12.00    4) Medicare Write-Off      0.00          0.00
5) HMO Adj & Write-Off  120.00         120.00
                      ==============  ==============
Total Adjustments       132.00         132.00


                        Refunds for : James T Monroe MD (1)
-------------------------------------------------------------------------------------------
Refunds                  PTD            YTD      Refunds                    PTD           YTD
-------------------------------------------------------------------------------------------
0) Unspecified Refund     0.00           0.00    1) Incorrect Data Entry    0.00          0.00
2) Overpayment Refund     0.00           0.00    3) Returned Check          0.00          0.00
96) Acct Transfer To      0.00           0.00    97) Acct Transfer From     0.00          0.00
98) Cross-Alloc To        0.00           0.00    99) Cross-Alloc From       0.00          0.00
                      ==============  ==============
Total Refunds             0.00           0.00
```

Figure 7-11 System Financial Summary Report, Page 2 of 6

```
                           SYSTEM FINANCIAL SUMMARY - DETAIL                    Page   2
                                Student: Paul Wilson
                                   All Entries

                          Totals For : Frances D Simpson M.D. (2)

--------------------------------------------------------------------------------------------
Dates                        Charges    Receipts   Adjustments    Net A/R    Total A/R  # Proc.   Col %
--------------------------------------------------------------------------------------------
01/01/03 - 03/20/03           166.00      0.00        0.00        166.00      166.00      4       0.0%
01/01/03 - 03/20/03           166.00      0.00        0.00        166.00      166.00      4       0.0%
--------------------------------------------------------------------------------------------



                      Receipts Analysis for : Frances D Simpson M.D. (2)
--------------------------------------------------------------------------------------------
               Net Receipts              PTD                YTD
--------------------------------------------------------------------------------------------
               Medicare                  0.00               0.00
               Insurance                 0.00               0.00
               Capitation Payments       0.00               0.00
               Patient                   0.00               0.00
               Other                     0.00               0.00
                                       ----------         ----------
               Total Receipts            0.00               0.00
               Refunds                   0.00               0.00
                                       ============       ============
               Gross Receipts            0.00               0.00


                        Adjustments for : Frances D Simpson M.D. (2)
--------------------------------------------------------------------------------------------
Adjustments          PTD          YTD        Adjustments               PTD          YTD
--------------------------------------------------------------------------------------------
1) General Adjustment   0.00      0.00       2) General Write-Off       0.00         0.00
3) Medicare Adjustment  0.00      0.00       4) Medicare Write-Off      0.00         0.00
5) HMO Adj & Write-Off  0.00      0.00
                   ==============  ==============
Total Adjustments       0.00      0.00


                         Refunds for : Frances D Simpson M.D. (2)
--------------------------------------------------------------------------------------------
Refunds              PTD          YTD        Refunds                   PTD          YTD
--------------------------------------------------------------------------------------------
0) Unspecified Refund   0.00      0.00       1) Incorrect Data Entry    0.00         0.00
2) Overpayment Refund   0.00      0.00       3) Returned Check          0.00         0.00
96) Acct Transfer To    0.00      0.00       97) Acct Transfer From     0.00         0.00
98) Cross-Alloc To      0.00      0.00       99) Cross-Alloc From       0.00         0.00
                   ==============  ==============
Total Refunds           0.00      0.00
```

Figure 7-12 System Financial Summary Report, Page 3 of 6

```
03/31/03                        SYSTEM FINANCIAL SUMMARY - DETAIL                     Page   3
                                    Student: Paul Wilson
                                       All Entries
                          Totals For : Sydney J Carrington M.D. (3)

------------------------------------------------------------------------------------------------
Dates                    Charges    Receipts   Adjustments    Net A/R    Total A/R   # Proc.   Col %
------------------------------------------------------------------------------------------------
01/01/03 - 03/20/03      1,465.00    670.80        9.00        785.20     785.20       26     46.1%
01/01/03 - 03/20/03      1,465.00    670.80        9.00        785.20     785.20       26     46.1%
------------------------------------------------------------------------------------------------


                       Receipts Analysis for : Sydney J Carrington M.D. (3)
------------------------------------------------------------------------------------------------
          Net Receipts                          PTD          YTD
------------------------------------------------------------------------------------------------
          Medicare                              48.20        48.20
          Insurance                            211.60       211.60
          Capitation Payments                  235.00       625.00
          Patient                              411.00       828.00
          Other                                  0.00         0.00
                                            -----------  -----------
          Total Receipts                       905.80     1,712.80
          Refunds                                0.00         0.00
                                            ===========  ===========
          Gross Receipts                       905.80     1,712.80


                         Adjustments for : Sydney J Carrington M.D. (3)
------------------------------------------------------------------------------------------------
Adjustments            PTD          YTD      Adjustments                 PTD          YTD
------------------------------------------------------------------------------------------------
1) General Adjustment  -10.00      -10.00    2) General Write-Off        2.00         2.00
3) Medicare Adjustment  17.00       17.00    4) Medicare Write-Off       0.00         0.00
5) HMO Adj & Write-Off   0.00        0.00
                     ==============  ==============
Total Adjustments        9.00        9.00


                          Refunds for : Sydney J Carrington M.D. (3)
------------------------------------------------------------------------------------------------
Refunds                PTD          YTD      Refunds                     PTD          YTD
------------------------------------------------------------------------------------------------
0) Unspecified Refund    0.00        0.00    1) Incorrect Data Entry     0.00         0.00
2) Overpayment Refund    0.00        0.00    3) Returned Check           0.00         0.00
96) Acct Transfer To     0.00        0.00    97) Acct Transfer From      0.00         0.00
98) Cross-Alloc To       0.00        0.00    99) Cross-Alloc From        0.00         0.00
                     ==============  ==============
Total Refunds            0.00        0.00
```

Figure 7-13 System Financial Summary Report, Page 4 of 6

```
03/31/03                    SYSTEM FINANCIAL SUMMARY - DETAIL                      Page    4
                                   Student: Paul Wilson
                                      All Entries

                          Totals For : Sandra A Shiller, RPT (4)

--------------------------------------------------------------------------------------------
Dates                  Charges    Receipts   Adjustments    Net A/R    Total A/R   # Proc.   Col %
--------------------------------------------------------------------------------------------
01/01/03 - 03/20/03       0.00       0.00         0.00         0.00        0.00       0      0.0%
01/01/03 - 03/20/03       0.00       0.00         0.00         0.00        0.00       0      0.0%
--------------------------------------------------------------------------------------------



                     Receipts Analysis for : Sandra A Shiller, RPT (4)
--------------------------------------------------------------------------------------------
        Net Receipts                        PTD              YTD
--------------------------------------------------------------------------------------------
        Medicare                            0.00             0.00
        Insurance                           0.00             0.00
        Capitation Payments                 0.00             0.00
        Patient                             0.00             0.00
        Other                               0.00             0.00
                                        -----------      -----------
        Total Receipts                      0.00             0.00
        Refunds                             0.00             0.00
                                        ===========      ===========
        Gross Receipts                      0.00             0.00


                       Adjustments for : Sandra A Shiller, RPT (4)
--------------------------------------------------------------------------------------------
Adjustments            PTD          YTD       Adjustments            PTD          YTD
--------------------------------------------------------------------------------------------
1) General Adjustment    0.00       0.00      2) General Write-Off     0.00        0.00
3) Medicare Adjustment   0.00       0.00      4) Medicare Write-Off    0.00        0.00
5) HMO Adj & Write-Off   0.00       0.00
                     ============ ============
Total Adjustments        0.00       0.00


                         Refunds for : Sandra A Shiller, RPT (4)
--------------------------------------------------------------------------------------------
Refunds                PTD          YTD       Refunds                PTD          YTD
--------------------------------------------------------------------------------------------
0) Unspecified Refund    0.00       0.00      1) Incorrect Data Entry  0.00        0.00
2) Overpayment Refund    0.00       0.00      3) Returned Check        0.00        0.00
96) Acct Transfer To     0.00       0.00      97) Acct Transfer From   0.00        0.00
98) Cross-Alloc To       0.00       0.00      99) Cross-Alloc From     0.00        0.00
                     ============ ============
Total Refunds            0.00       0.00
```

Figure 7-14 System Financial Summary Report, Page 5 of 6

PERIOD-TO-DATE TOTALS FOR 01/01/03 - 03/20/03

Doctor	Charges	Receipts	Adjustments	Net A/R	Total A/R	# Proc.	Col %
1. James T Monroe MD	182.00	8.00	132.00	42.00	42.00	7	16.0%
2. Frances D Simpson M.D.	166.00	0.00	0.00	166.00	166.00	4	0.0%
3. Sydney J Carrington M.D.	1,465.00 541	670.80	9.00	785.20	785.20	26	46.1%
4. Sandra A Shiller, RPT	0.00	0.00	0.00	0.00	0.00	0	0.0%
TOTALS	1,813.00	678.80	141.00	993.20	993.20	37	40.6%
Practice Totals :	1,813.00	678.80	141.00	993.20	993.20	37	40.6%

YEAR-TO-DATE TOTALS FOR 01/01/03 - 03/20/03

Doctor	Charges	Receipts	Adjustments	Net A/R	Total A/R	# Proc.	Col %
1. James T Monroe MD	182.00	8.00	132.00	42.00	42.00	7	16.0%
2. Frances D Simpson M.D.	166.00	0.00	0.00	166.00	166.00	4	0.0%
3. Sydney J Carrington M.D.	1,465.00	670.80	9.00	785.20	785.20	26	46.1%
4. Sandra A Shiller, RPT	0.00	0.00	0.00	0.00	0.00	0	0.0%
TOTALS	1,813.00	678.80	141.00	993.20	993.20	37	40.6%
Practice Totals :	1,813.00	678.80	141.00	993.20	993.20	37	40.6%

1,0490

Receipts Analysis for Practice

Net Receipts	PTD	YTD
Medicare	48.20	48.20
Insurance	219.60	219.60
Capitation Payments	295.00	805.00
Patient	411.00	828.00
Other	0.00	0.00
Total Receipts	973.80	1,900.80
Refunds	0.00	0.00
Gross Receipts	973.80	1,900.80

.80   .80

Figure 7-15 System Financial Summary Report, Page 6 of 6

Adjustments	PTD	YTD	Adjustments	PTD	YTD
1) General Adjustment	-10.00	-10.00	2) General Write-Off	2.00	2.00
3) Medicare Adjustment	29.00	29.00	4) Medicare Write-Off	0.00	0.00
5) HMO Adj & Write-Off	120.00	120.00			
Total Adjustments	141.00	141.00			

Refunds	PTD	YTD	Refunds	PTD	YTD
0) Unspecified Refund	0.00	0.00	1) Incorrect Data Entry	0.00	0.00
2) Overpayment Refund	0.00	0.00	3) Returned Check	0.00	0.00
96) Acct Transfer To	0.00	0.00	97) Acct Transfer From	0.00	0.00
98) Cross-Alloc To	0.00	0.00	99) Cross-Alloc From	0.00	0.00
Total Refunds	0.00	0.00			

EXERCISE 4: Performing a Final Daily Close for March 31

You will perform a Final Daily Close for March 31, even though no additional entries have been made into the system. This is done only for the purposes of an upcoming exercise; therefore, you do not need to turn your report in to your instructor. Because no additional entries have been made, it is *not* necessary to run a Trial Daily Report first.

STEP 1 From the Main Menu (Menu 1), select option **5**, REPORT Generation, then option **4**, DAILY Report.

STEP 2 Press '**N**' to request a Final Daily Close, '**P**' to request a check register for the practice, and '**0**' to not purge appointments.

STEP 3 Press **F1** or click on the PROCESS button ('√') to process and the Final Daily Close will be generated.

Press '**Y**' to accept the Final Daily Close, then press **ENTER** to return to log-on and advance the date.

EXERCISE 5: Advancing the Date to April 3

Carefully key '**04032003**' and press **ENTER** to advance the date and return to the Main Menu (Menu 1).

PATIENT BILLING

Patients often receive their first bill at the time of their visit. This statement may be as simple as a copy of the encounter form marked by the physician, or it may be a computerized listing of services performed. The best opportunity for collection of an account is at the time of service; therefore, it is becoming increasingly common for practices to require payment at the time of service. When a patient bill is printed after posting a patient payment, it is also sometimes used as a payment receipt.

Patient Statement

The patient statement feature of **The Medical Manager** system produces a list of outstanding charges in a patient's account. The patient statement is generally sent to the guarantor at the end of the month before the period close, but it may be sent as many times as desired.

You may wish to bill all patients at the end of each month, or you may bill in batches according to an alphabetical formula or by some other batch method. For example, using an alphabetical formula, you might bill A through F during the first week of the month, G through L during the second week, M through R during the third week, and S through Z during the fourth week. Statements may also be done in a batch, or they may be batched by account number, name, primarily responsible doctor, zip code, or bill type. Batch statements can be mailed or electronically processed in small groups.

Two types of patient statements may be used: the Open Item Statement and the Current Period Activity Statement. The Open Item Statement generates an up-to-date list of each outstanding charge. This statement includes all outstanding charges from the beginning of the account through the billing date, and the remaining balance. This statement has the ability to separate charges awaiting insurance payment from charges to be paid by the patient.

The Current Period Activity Statement is a *balance forward* statement. It begins with a balance forward amount, which is the total balance due from the previous period. Then it lists the current period's charges, payments, and adjustments in detail to arrive at the patient's current balance. This type of statement must be run only at the end of the month. As with the Open Item Statement, the Current Period Activity Statement with balance forward information shows the amount due from insurance companies and amount due from the patient.

The Open Item Statement and the Current Period Activity Statement both generate the same balances, but one shows more detail of each outstanding item, and the other shows more detail of the current period activities. An Open Item type of statement provides more detail and can be billed in small batches or for separate doctors.

Account Aging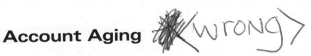

Account aging identifies how long a balance is overdue.

A process called *account aging* establishes how long an account has been unpaid. Statements mailed to the patient show the age of an account, including a breakdown of the amount overdue: 30 days, more than 60 days, more than 90 days, or more than 120 days.

The aging on patient statements may be set up to age all items or to age patient-due items only. In addition to proper aging, **The Medical Manager** system permits you to print running notices of outstanding balances.

The following procedures will be completed using the Patient Statement feature:

STEP 1

Select option **6**, BILLING & EDI, from the Main Menu (Menu 1), then select option **2**, PATIENT Statement. The screen shown in Figure 7-16 appears.

Before attempting data entry, study the following list of available options for Patient Statement Routines. After you study the list, follow the instructions provided in the *Applying Your Knowledge exercise*.

Figure 7-16 Patient Statements Routine Screen

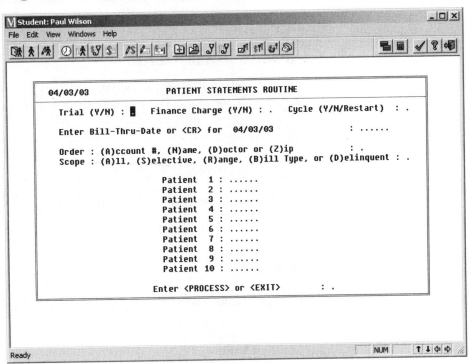

REFERENCE LIST OF AVAILABLE OPTIONS
FOR PATIENT STATEMENT ROUTINES

◆   a.   Trial Bill? (Y/N): (Press ENTER to default)

This field asks whether you want a trial billing, or if a regular billing routine is desired. The default value is (N)o.

◆   b.   Enter Bill-Thru Date or press ENTER for the current system date

This field requires that you enter a bill-thru date or that you press ENTER to default to the current system date. This date represents the last posting date on which charges will be listed on the patient statement.

◆   c.   Order: (A)ccount #, (N)ame, (D)octor, or (Z)ip:

Select the order by which you want patient statements to be printed. When used with "Range," which is discussed next, the order option provides various means of dividing the patient statements into manageably sized mailings. Your options for order include:

1. Account number: Statements are printed in account number order, permitting the practice to limit each printing to a range of statements by account number.

2. Name: Statements are printed in alphabetical order by the guarantor's last name, permitting the practice to limit each printing to only a portion of the alphabet.

3. Doctor: Statements are printed based on the doctor primarily responsible for the account, permitting the practice to print statements for a given doctor or doctors.

4. Zip: Statements are printed in zip code order, enabling the practice to take advantage of presorted mail discounts. When used with the range option, below, this will also permit the practice to batch statements by sectors of the city or state.

◆   d.   Scope: (A)ll, (S)elective, (R)ange, (B)ill Type, or (D)elinquent

Enter whether all accounts, individually selected accounts, a range of accounts, accounts with a specific bill type, or delinquent accounts are to be billed. If (S)elective is chosen, you may enter up to ten patient account numbers. Since (R)ange, (B)ill Type, and (D)elinquent bring up different prompts, these prompts are explained below.

(R)ange can be used for batch billing.

If (A)ccount # order is selected, you are prompted to enter the range of account numbers:

Start Account #:
End Account #:

If (N)ame order is selected, you are prompted to enter the range of account names:

Start Last Name:
End Last Name:

If (D)octor order is selected, you are prompted to enter the range of doctor numbers for the account's primarily responsible doctor:

Start Doctor #:
End Doctor #:

If (Z)ip Code order is selected, you are prompted to enter the range of zip codes:

Start Zip Code:
End Zip Code:

If (B)ill Type is chosen, the numbers you assigned to Bill Type when you opened the account for the guarantor will be used:

Start Bill Type (1–9):
End Bill Type (1–9):

If (D)elinquent is chosen, you will be permitted to limit the range of delinquency notices to the oldest unpaid items.

After information is entered in the fields, the Patient Statement Monitor screen shown in Figure 7-17 appears.

Figure 7-17 Patient Statement Monitor Screen

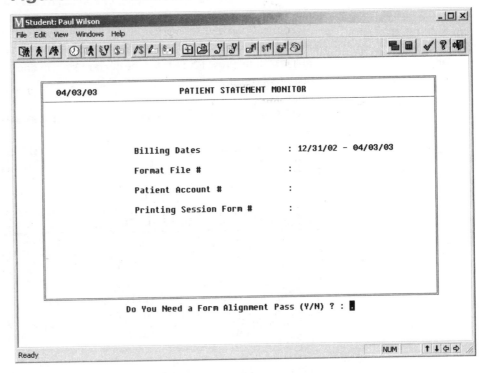

◆ e. Before printing begins, you are given the opportunity to align the billing form in the printer. The following prompt appears:

Do You Need a Form Alignment Pass (Y/N)?

If a form alignment pass is requested, you will have to key a format file number that was created earlier to identify different formats. Choose any of the items monitored during the billing process, shown below:

1. Billing Dates: Two dates are displayed: the date of the last period close and the bill-thru date.

2. Format File #: The format file that is currently being used to generate the statement for this account.

3. Patient Account #: The patient presently being processed in the statement routine.

4. Printing Session Form #: A counter for the number of forms generated during this billing session.

APPLYING YOUR KNOWLEDGE

✓EXERCISE 6: Printing Patient Statements

Although **The Medical Manager** software can print statements on any type of form, the formats provided will create statements on plain paper so that no special forms are required.

Generate statements for all of your accounts. From the Main Menu (Menu 1), choose option **6**, BILLING & EDI, then option **2**, PATIENT Statement. Then, choose the following options:

Trial: **N**
Bill-Thru Date: Press **ENTER** for the current system date
Order: (**A**)ccount
Scope: (**A**)ll
Press **F1** or click on the PROCESS button ('√') to generate your patient statements.

After patient statements are finished, press **ENTER** and the system will return to the Billing & EDI Menu (Menu 4). Hand in your statements to your instructor.

SYSTEM UTILITIES

As part of our month end routine, we would normally perform two of the functions on the System Utility Menu (Menu 3) shown in Figure 7-18; option 1, PERIOD Close with Purge, and option 8, GL Transfer/Distribution Report. In the next exercise, *you will perform only the GL Report.* The Period Close will not be performed in the Student Edition course. The purge is omitted at this point only for the purposes of the student exercises but should always be performed in a timely fashion in an actual medical office.

General Ledger Transfer/Distribution Report

The General Ledger (GL) Transfer Distribution Report summarizes how accounts and departments were affected financially by each Daily Close. The Trial Distribution Report can be used any time during the billing period when you wish to see a summary of General Ledger activities.

Figure 7-18 System Utility Menu (Menu 3) Screen

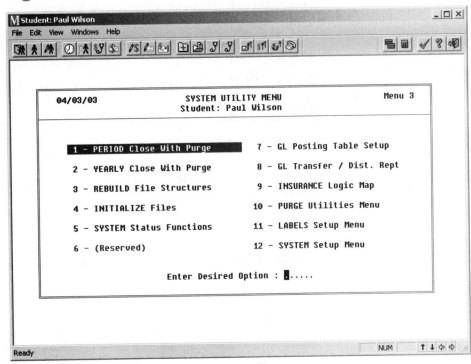

From the Main Menu (Menu 1), select option **9**, SYSTEM Utilities. At the System Utility Menu (Menu 3), select option **8**, GL Transfer / Dist. Rept. This refers to the General Ledger/Transfer Distribution Report. The screen shown in Figure 7-19 will appear.

Figure 7-19 GL Transfer with Distribution Report Screen

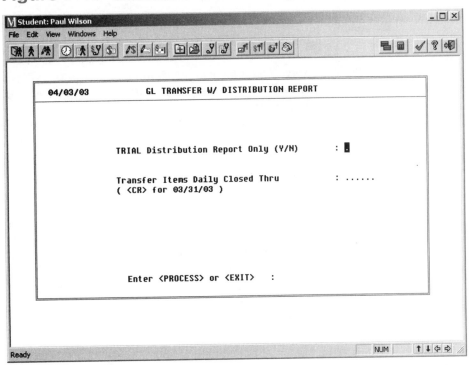

Before attempting any data entry, study the following list of options available. Then, proceed to the *Applying Your Knowledge* section.

REFERENCE LIST OF AVAILABLE OPTIONS FOR THE GENERAL LEDGER/DISTRIBUTION REPORT

1. TRIAL Distribution Report Only (Y/N):

Enter (Y)es only if a Trial Distribution Report is desired. This will not carry out the actual transfer.

2. Transfer Items Daily Closed Thru:

This function will signify which items should be transferred to the general ledger at this time.

APPLYING YOUR KNOWLEDGE

 EXERCISE 7: Running the GL Transfer Report

STEP 1 From the Main Menu (Menu 1), select option **9**, SYSTEM Utilities. From the System Utility menu (Menu 3), select option **8**, GL Transfer Dist. Rept.

STEP 2 Because we do *not* want to run a Trial Report, enter '**N**' for the first selection on the screen. Press **ENTER** to accept the date of 03/31/03 (this is the date of the last Final Daily Close). Hand this report in to your instructor. It should be similar to Figures 7-20 and 7-21.

STEP 3 Press **ENTER** at the prompt "Transfer Processed Successfully" to return to the System Utility Menu (Menu 3).

Note: If you have made financial edits to correct your Daily Reports, your GL Transfer Report may differ slightly. Check with your instructor if you have any questions.

Figure 7-20 GL Transfer with Distribution Report, Page 1 of 2

```
04/03/03               GL DISTRIBUTION REPORT - TRANSFER          Page    1
                             Student: Paul Wilson
                        For Items Daily Closed Thru 03/31/03

GL Account        Daily Close Date    Debit        Credit         Net
==============================================================================
10001.00
                   02/17/03            4.00          0.00          4.00
                   03/20/03            4.00          0.00          4.00
                                    ------------  ------------  ------------
                  [10001.00]           8.00          0.00          8.00


10003.00
                   02/17/03          111.00          0.00        111.00
                   03/14/03          348.20          0.00        348.20
                   03/20/03          211.60          0.00        211.60
                                    ------------  ------------  ------------
                  [10003.00]         670.80          0.00        670.80


15001.00
                   01/10/03          122.00         60.00         62.00
                   02/03/03           60.00         60.00          0.00
                   02/17/03            0.00          4.00         -4.00
                   03/14/03            0.00         12.00        -12.00
                   03/20/03            0.00          4.00         -4.00
                                    ------------  ------------  ------------
                  [15001.00]         182.00        140.00         42.00


15002.00
                   01/10/03          128.00          0.00        128.00
                   02/17/03           78.00          0.00         78.00
                   03/14/03            0.00         40.00        -40.00
                                    ------------  ------------  ------------
                  [15002.00]         206.00         40.00        166.00


15003.00
                   01/10/03          689.00          0.00        689.00
                   02/03/03          615.00          0.00        615.00
                   02/17/03          161.00        111.00         50.00
                   03/14/03           10.00        365.20       -355.20
                   03/20/03            0.00        213.60       -213.60
                                    ------------  ------------  ------------
                  [15003.00]       1,475.00        689.80        785.20


60001.00
                   01/10/03            0.00        122.00       -122.00
                   02/03/03            0.00         60.00        -60.00
                                    ------------  ------------  ------------
                  [60001.00]           0.00        182.00       -182.00


60002.00
                   01/10/03            0.00        128.00       -128.00
                   02/17/03            0.00         78.00        -78.00
                   03/14/03           40.00          0.00         40.00
                                    ------------  ------------  ------------
                  [60002.00]          40.00        206.00       -166.00


60003.00
                   01/10/03            0.00        689.00       -689.00
                   02/03/03            0.00        615.00       -615.00
```

Figure 7-21 GL Transfer with Distribution Report, Page 2 of 2

```
04/03/03                 GL DISTRIBUTION REPORT - TRANSFER              Page    2

GL Account         Daily Close Date   Debit          Credit          Net
=============================================================================
                      02/17/03          0.00          161.00         -161.00
                                     ------------   ------------    ------------
                      [60003.00]        0.00        1,465.00       -1,465.00

60023.00
                      03/14/03          0.00           10.00          -10.00
                                     ------------   ------------    ------------
                      [60023.00]        0.00           10.00          -10.00

60033.00
                      03/20/03          2.00            0.00            2.00
                                     ------------   ------------    ------------
                      [60033.00]        2.00            0.00            2.00

60041.00
                      03/14/03         12.00            0.00           12.00
                                     ------------   ------------    ------------
                      [60041.00]       12.00            0.00           12.00

60043.00
                      03/14/03         17.00            0.00           17.00
                                     ------------   ------------    ------------
                      [60043.00]       17.00            0.00           17.00

60061.00
                      01/10/03         60.00            0.00           60.00
                      02/03/03         60.00            0.00           60.00
                                     ------------   ------------    ------------
                      [60061.00]      120.00            0.00          120.00

                                     ============   ============    ============
TOTAL TRANSFERRED THRU 03/31/03      2,732.80       2,732.80           0.00


          ********** GL Transfer WAS Performed Thru 03/31/03 **********
```

UNIT 7 SUMMARY

One of the most important uses of a modern computer system is to report data that has been previously entered into the system. These reports can assist in managing the practice in several different ways. Financial reports allow the practice to look at the same data from various points of view. Some ways of looking at open items, for instance, include organizing them by guarantor responsible, insurance responsible, or by the physician who performed the service. Reports can also list the balance on each patient's account, or summarize physician financial totals. Comparing totals from some of these different reports helps verify that the system is in financial balance. Reports are also helpful in being able to identify and analyze mistakes, duplicates, or erroneous entries.

Special reports can be useful in maintaining good relationships. These include referring doctor analysis, referring doctor thank you notices, patient introductory letters, and even reminders of patient birthday greetings.

Another important function of the office is to generate bills and statements to patient accounts. Patient statements report to the guarantor charges to the account, payments by the insurance company, and balances expected from the guarantor. Clear and easy-to-read patient statements can eliminate or reduce phone calls from patients about their account balances. Patient statements can also include reminder information such as upcoming appointments.

TESTING YOUR KNOWLEDGE

1. What type of information does the Guarantors' Financial Summary Report contain? How may this information be used by the medical practice?

293.

2. How is the Current Period Report used by the medical practice?

295

3. Describe the function and importance of the System Summary Report.

p.297

4. What are several different methods that can be used to bill patients? Explain each method you list.

Advanced Functions

LEARNING OUTCOMES

After completing this unit, you should be able to:

◆ Discuss three unique payment situations and describe how each situation should be handled.
◆ Post a variety of unique payments.
◆ Discuss the account aging process.
◆ Name and discuss several types of patient data that can be retrieved and displayed.
◆ Display and print patient data.
◆ Explain the purpose and importance of period close and purge.

The Medical Manager software is a sophisticated, comprehensive practice management system that allows you to develop advanced procedures for working with accounts and financial reports. A few advanced functions plus unique payment methods are covered in this unit.

UNIQUE PAYMENTS

A variety of unusual situations may occur that test your knowledge of posting accounts. Four of the more common examples are: (1) refunding an overpayment, (2) removing the credit for a bad check, (3) automatic payment from insurance, and (4) rebilling lost insurance claims.

Refunding an Overpayment

A refund is provided when a patient or insurance carrier overpays an account. An overpayment may be the result of the patient's or carrier's mistake when preparing a check, a mistake by the medical office during the posting procedure, or an incorrect treatment indicated by the physician.

Removing the Credit for a Bad Check

When an account is paid by check, the amount of the check is applied to any outstanding balance. If the check is returned for insufficient funds, the credit originally applied to the account must be removed.

Automatic Payment from Insurance Company

The Automatic Payment feature (referred to as *Auto Pay*) of **The Medical Manager** software can be used when an insurance plan pays an account in full.

Rebilling Lost Insurance Claims

Lost claim forms are not uncommon among insurance carriers. The easiest method of replacing a lost form is to photocopy the file version and send it to the carrier. In the event that a file version does not exist, you may use the Rebill feature by entering an adjustment for zero dollars.

APPLYING YOUR KNOWLEDGE

In the following exercises, you will be given clear directions as to which screens are used. If you need to refresh your memory, refer to the appropriate unit in the text. Figures are also provided for use in comparison.

EXERCISE 1: Terry L. Williams

Refunding an Overpayment

When Ms. Terry Williams brought her daughter, Alice Spivey, into the office on January 10, 2003, Alice was given an immunization for which her insurance company, Health Maintenance Org., was correctly billed an additional $4.00. Accordingly, Dr. Carrington's office received payment for this amount on February 17, 2003. However, Alice's secondary policy (through her father's employer), Epsilon Life & Casualty, was *ALSO billed and subsequently paid the $4.00 amount*. Because this amount was rightfully the responsibility of Alice's primary insurance company, it is necessary that a refund be issued to Epsilon Life & Casualty for their overpayment.

After you write the refund check (Figure 8-1), you must update the account. Carefully follow the instructions shown below to complete the refund for the insurance company.

STEP 1   From the Main Menu (Menu 1), choose option **3**, PAYMENT Posting, then option **1**, PAYMENT Entry. Key '**120.0**' and press **ENTER** to retrieve Ms. Williams's account.

Figure 8-1   Refund Check for Epsilon Life & Casualty

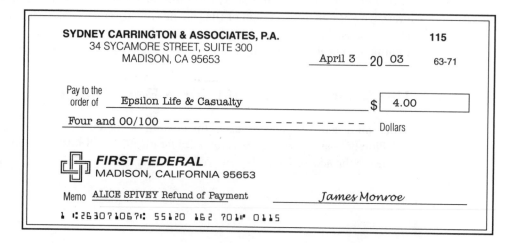

STEP 2 Enter (**R**)efund as the Payment Type and notice that a new screen appears showing $4.00 as "Unapplied Available" (this is the amount of money you have available to refund). Press **ENTER** to mark (with an asterisk) $4.00 as the amount you want to refund to Epsilon Life & Casualty. Press **F1** or click on the PROCESS button ('√') on the top toolbar to process this request for a refund of Unapplied Credit monies.

STEP 3 Key '?' in the # field or click on the Help button ('?') on the top toolbar to view a help window for Refund Reason Codes. Move the highlight bar to '**02 Overpayment Refund**' and press **ENTER** to select it. Press **ENTER** at the Ref. Date field to accept the current system date of 04/03/03. Key '**115**' as the voucher number (this is the number of the check you will send the insurance company). Press **ENTER** to accept $4.00 as the Total Amount of the refund. Key '**N**' for 'None' because the account balance will be $0.00. Your screen should be similar to Figure 8-2. Press **F1** or click on the PROCESS button ('√').

Note that once the payment information has been processed, the amount of unapplied credit will decrease to $0.00 and the account balance will increase by $4.00 (i.e., it will increase from -$4.00 to $0.00).

Figure 8-2 Refunding an Overpayment by Epsilon Life & Casualty

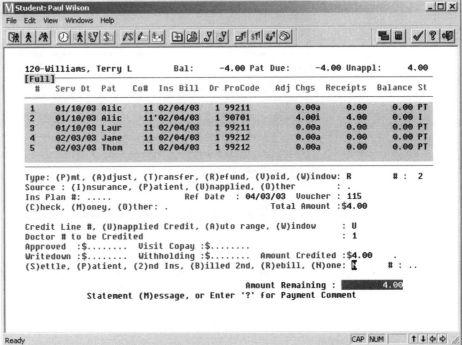

EXERCISE 2: Wayne R. Dudley

First Step—Removing the Credit for a Bad Check

The bank has returned Mr. Wayne Dudley's check, a payment of $300.00, to you marked "NSF" (nonsufficient funds; Figure 8-3).

The check was originally credited to items 1–4 according to the patient's current Payment Report. Normally, two steps are required to make the correction: (1) a negative payment to restore the item balance to unpaid, and (2) a refund to remove the credit from the doctor's receipts. To understand fully the effect of this, notice the patient's balance shown in Figures 8-4 and 8-7 before you begin any entries. Follow the instructions shown below to remove the credit originally posted for Mr. Dudley's check.

Figure 8-3 Wayne Dudley's Check—Voucher 420

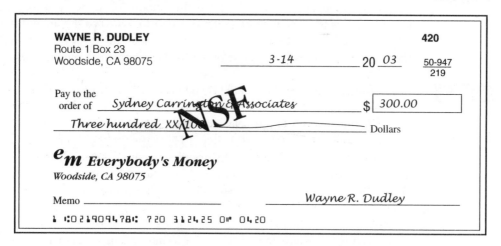

Figure 8-4 Removing Credit for a Bad Check, First Step

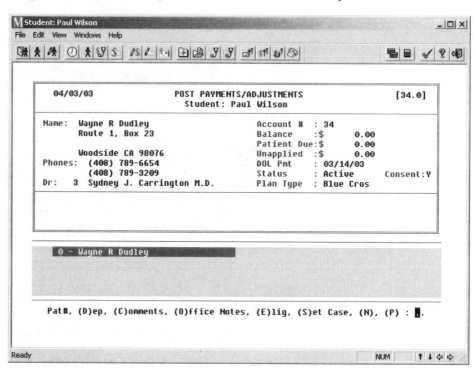

STEP 1 From the Main Menu (Menu 1), choose option **3**, PAYMENT Posting, then option **1**, PAYMENT Entry. Key '**34**' and press **ENTER** to retrieve Mr. Dudley's account.

STEP 2 Choose (**P**)ayment, (**P**)atient, and press **ENTER** at the Ref. Date field to accept the current system date of 04/03/03. Key '**420**' in the Voucher # field (remember, this is the number of the original check from Mr. Dudley). Key (**C**)heck and enter negative $300.00 ('**-300.00**') for the Total Amount of the payment. Because Mr. Dudley's original payment was for all four of the items shown in the current window (i.e., they add up to $300.00), you can use the Automatic Payment feature to once again credit these items. Key '**A**' for (A)uto Pay and '**P**' to transfer the items to (**P**)atient Responsibility. Compare your screen with Figure 8-5.

Notice that when you press **F1** twice or click twice on the PROCESS button ('√') to process, the Receipts column of payments made on each item is changed to '0.00'.

Figure 8-5 Using Auto Pay to Make Negative Payment to Line Items 1–4

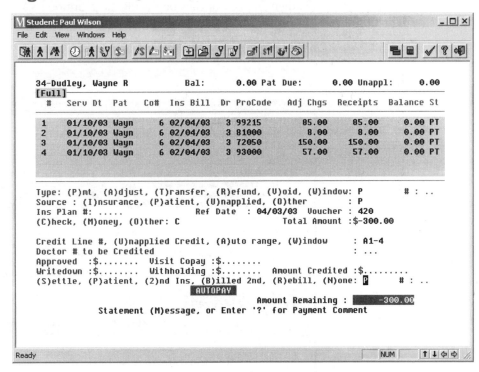

Accordingly, the amounts have been moved to the Balance column and now show as 'PT' (patient) responsibility for each item.

When the negative payment has been allocated, the receipts will have been moved into Unapplied Credit, but still remain on the patient's account. A refund will now be performed to remove the amount from the doctor's receipts. The net effect of the two entries will be to increase the patient's account balance and lower the doctor's period-to-date and year-to-date receipts. Be sure to use the correct doctor number for the refund.

Note: The screen will not show open items if the period has been closed.

EXERCISE 3: Wayne R. Dudley

Second Step—Refund

Once the items on Mr. Dudley's account are reversed, a refund should be performed. This will increase the amount due from the patient and reduce the doctor's receipts. Follow the instructions shown below to perform the refund and reduce the doctor's receipts.

STEP 1 From the Main Menu (Menu 1), choose option **3**, PAYMENT Posting, then option **1**, PAYMENT Entry. Key account number '**34.0**' and press **ENTER** to retrieve Mr. Dudley's account. Key '**R**' for (R)efund, '**A**' to mark (A)ll, and press **ENTER**. Press **F1** or click on the PROCESS button ('√') on the top toolbar to process and request a refund of the Unapplied Credit monies to Dr. Carrington.

STEP 2 Key '?' at the # field or click on the Help button ('?') on the top toolbar to view a help window of Refund Reason Codes. Move the highlight bar to '**03 Returned Check**' and press **ENTER** to select it. Press **ENTER** at the Ref. Date field to accept the current system date of 04/03/03. Enter '**420**' (Mr. Dudley's original check number) as the Voucher No., and press **ENTER** to accept $300.00 as the total amount. Key '**N**' for

'None' because the account balance will be $0.00. Compare your screen with Figure 8-6, then press **F1** or click on the PROCESS button ('√').

Figure 8-6 Removing Credit for a Bad Check, Second Step

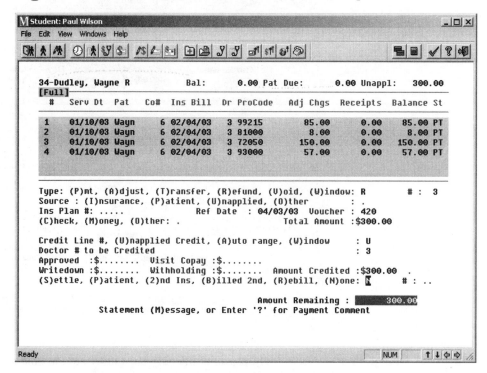

Press **ESCAPE** or click on the EXIT button on the top toolbar to return to the Patient Retrieval screen for Payment Entry. Key '**34**' to reenter Mr. Dudley's account. Compare your screen with Figure 8-7 and notice that the balance due has been restored and the

Figure 8-7 Adjusted Account for Wayne Dudley

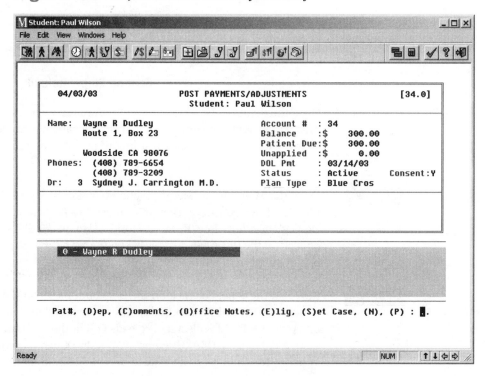

unapplied credit amount now reads $0.00. Dr. Carrington's period-to-date and year-to-date receipts have also been adjusted to account for Mr. Dudley's returned check.

EXERCISE 4: Gene S. Evans

Auto Pay Insurance Mode

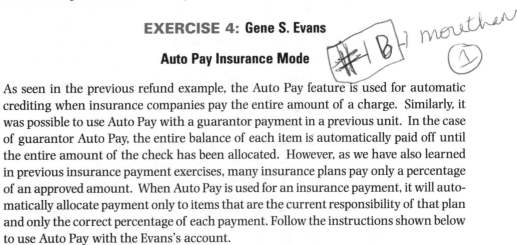

As seen in the previous refund example, the Auto Pay feature is used for automatic crediting when insurance companies pay the entire amount of a charge. Similarly, it was possible to use Auto Pay with a guarantor payment in a previous unit. In the case of guarantor Auto Pay, the entire balance of each item is automatically paid off until the entire amount of the check has been allocated. However, as we have also learned in previous insurance payment exercises, many insurance plans pay only a percentage of an approved amount. When Auto Pay is used for an insurance payment, it will automatically allocate payment only to items that are the current responsibility of that plan and only the correct percentage of each payment. Follow the instructions shown below to use Auto Pay with the Evans's account.

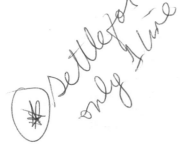

Insurance Plan 7 has paid all charges for Gene Evans as shown on the check in Figure 8-8. Because the first two items shown for the Evans's account match exactly what the plan has paid, it is appropriate to use the Auto Pay feature to post this payment. As in previous exercises, rather than select each item separately, you can use the Auto Pay feature by keying 'A' in the Credit Line # field. Automatic allocation will be used for the remaining balance of each item.

Figure 8-8 Pan American Check—Voucher 97977

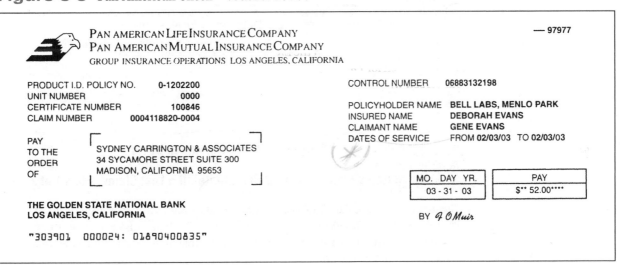

| STEP 1 | From the Main Menu (Menu 1), choose option **3**, PAYMENT Posting, then option **1**, PAYMENT Entry. Key Mr. Evans's patient number, '**14.1**' and press **ENTER** to retrieve his account. Because Gene is a dependent on his wife's account, the screen will display the name of the guarantor '**Evans, Deborah**' in the upper left corner. Gene's name will be displayed in the first two items under the patient column. Choose (**P**)ayment, (**I**)nsurance as the source of the payment, and '**7**' at the Ins Plan # field. *Remember that if you did not know Mr. Evans's plan number, you could enter '?' at this field or click on the Help button ('?') on the top toolbar to choose from a help window.* Press **ENTER** at the Ref. Date field to accept the current system date. |

STEP 2   Key '**97977**' in the voucher field, choose '**C**' for (C)heck, and enter '**52.00**' as the Total Amount of the payment.

Enter '**A**' for (A)uto Pay and press **ENTER**. Press **ENTER** to default to pay on items 'A1-4'. Press **ENTER** to default to (N)one because the item balance will be $0.00. Compare your screen with Figure 8–9, then press **F1** or click on the PROCESS button ('√') on the top toolbar to process to invoke the Auto Pay feature. Notice that the receipts for line 1 increase to $40.00 and the balance decreases to $0.00. Similarly, the receipts for line 2 increase to $12.00 and the balance decreases to $0.00.

This completes posting this insurance check for Mr. Evans.

Figure 8-9 Payment Using Auto Pay

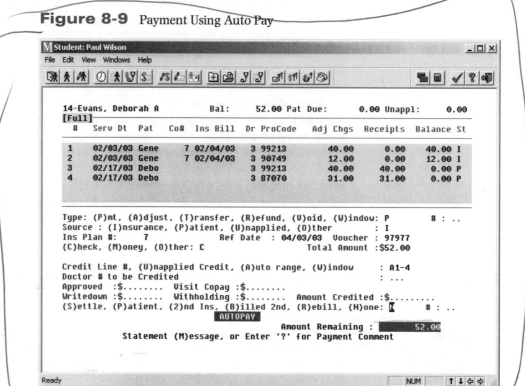

EXERCISE 5: Timothy R. Davis

Using Adjustment for Zero Dollars to Rebill a Lost Claim—Item 1 of 2

The insurance plan, Pan American, reports that a claim has never been received for Mr. Timothy Davis for services rendered on 01/10/03. You must generate a new claim because you cannot locate a file copy. Follow the instructions shown below to make an Adjustment for Zero Dollars.

STEP 1

From the Main Menu (Menu 1), select option **3**, PAYMENT Posting, then option **1**, PAYMENT Entry. Key Mr. Davis's account number ('**80.0**') and press **ENTER** to retrieve his account. Key '**A**' for (A)djustment, '**I**' for (I)nsurance, and plan '**12**' for the carrier to rebill. Press **ENTER** at the Ref. Date field to accept the current system date of 04/03/03. Press **ENTER** to leave the Voucher No. field blank. Type '**0.00**' in the Total Amount field, then highlight line item 1 (99213 for Timothy) and press **ENTER** to select it. Choose to (**R**)ebill, then choose '**N**' at the Review prompt, and press **ENTER** twice. Make sure a '**1**' is in the credit line # field, then press **F1** or click on the PROCESS button. Your screen should be similar to Figure 8-10. Notice that the balance on line item 1 is now shown as $40.00 IR. Remember that the 'I' status stands for insurance billed. Adding an "R" to this status (i.e., "IR") means that the insurance company has been rebilled for this item.

Note: Be sure to repeat the process for item 2, below.

Figure 8-10 Rebilling a Lost Claim—Adjustment to Line Item 1

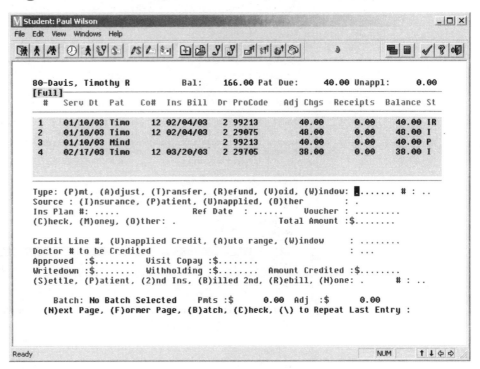

```
┌M Student: Paul Wilson                                              _□×│
File  Edit  View  Windows  Help

  ┌──┬──┬───┬───┬──┬──┬──┬───┬───┬──┬───┬───┬──┬──┬──┬──┐           ┌──┬──┬──┬──┬──┐
  │                                                    │     ∂     │                │

  ┌──────────────────────────────────────────────────────────────────────┐
  │  80-Davis, Timothy R          Bal:    166.00 Pat Due:    40.00 Unappl:    0.00  │
  │  [Full]                                                                          │
  │   #   Serv Dt  Pat   Co#  Ins Bill  Dr ProCode  Adj Chgs  Receipts  Balance St  │
  │                                                                                  │
  │   1   01/10/03 Timo   12  02/04/03   2 99213       40.00     0.00     40.00 IR   │
  │   2   01/10/03 Timo   12  02/04/03   2 29075       48.00     0.00     48.00 I    │
  │   3   01/10/03 Mind                  2 99213       40.00     0.00     40.00 P    │
  │   4   02/17/03 Timo   12  03/20/03   2 29705       38.00     0.00     38.00 I    │
  │                                                                                  │
  └──────────────────────────────────────────────────────────────────────┘

  Type: (P)mt, (A)djust, (T)ransfer, (R)efund, (U)oid, (W)indow: ▮....... # : ..
  Source : (I)nsurance, (P)atient, (U)napplied, (O)ther       : .
  Ins Plan #: .....              Ref Date : ......   Voucher : .........
  (C)heck, (M)oney, (O)ther: .                      Total Amount :$........

  Credit Line #, (U)napplied Credit, (A)uto range, (W)indow    : ........
  Doctor # to be Credited                                      : ...
  Approved  :$........  Visit Copay :$.......
  Writedown :$........  Withholding :$........  Amount Credited :$........
  (S)ettle, (P)atient, (2)nd Ins, (B)illed 2nd, (R)ebill, (N)one: .    # : ..

      Batch: No Batch Selected     Pmts :$   0.00 Adj :$   0.00
      (N)ext Page, (F)ormer Page, (B)atch, (C)heck, (\) to Repeat Last Entry :


Ready                                                  NUM    ↑ ↓ ⇦ ⇨
```

Using Adjustment for Zero Dollars to Rebill a Lost Claim—Item 2 of 2

STEP 2

Because you should already be at the Payment Entry screen for Mr. Davis's account, rebilling item 2 is simply a repeat of the process you completed for line item 1. Key '**A**' for (A)djustment, '**I**' for (I)nsurance, and plan '**12**' for the carrier you want to rebill. Press **ENTER** at the Ref. Date field to accept the current system date of 04/03/03. Press **ENTER** to leave the Voucher No. field blank. Type '**0.00**' in the Total Amount field, then highlight line item **2** (procedure code 29075) and press **ENTER** to select it. Choose to (**R**)ebill, then choose '**N**' at the Review prompt, and press **ENTER** twice. Make sure a 2 is in the credit line # field, then press **F1** or click on the PROCESS button. Notice that the balance on line item 2 is now shown as $48.00 IR, indicating that the item has been successfully rebilled.

Neither the item balances, nor patient or receipts balances, will be affected. Another bill to insurance plan 12 will be generated for this item on the next billing run. Because line item 3, a service also received on 1/10/03, is patient responsibility, you will not need to make any adjustment to this item.

Note: Payment for zero dollars may also be used to rebill items. To do so, follow the above example exactly, except enter 'P' for (P)ayment in the Type field.

EXERCISE 6: Portia D. Edwards

Adding a Patient to Hospital Rounds

Follow the instructions shown below to make an entry to add Mrs. Portia Edwards to hospital rounds. Review Unit 5 if you need further assistance with this procedure. You will use the information shown in Figure 8-11 to complete this exercise.

STEP 1

From the Main Menu (Menu 1), select option **8**, OFFICE Management, then option **6**, HOSPITAL Tracking, then option **1**, Hospital Rounds Entry. Key Mrs. Edwards's account number ('**21.0**') and press **ENTER** to retrieve her account.

Figure 8-11 Hospital Rounds Screen

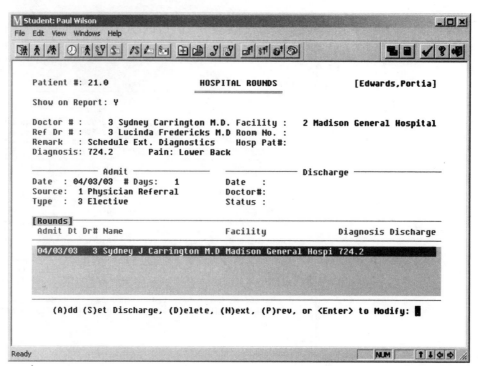

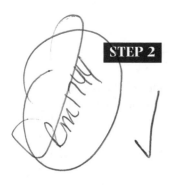

STEP 2 Choose (A)dd. Key '**Y**' (yes, to show on the Hospital Rounds Report). Choose Doctor No. **3.** Her referring physician is doctor **3,** Lucinda Fredericks, M.D. Dr. Carrington's remark for the reason for Mrs. Edwards's admission is **Schedule Ext. Diagnostics** and her initial diagnosis was '**724.2**', Lower Back Pain. Key in the Service Facility No. **2**, and press **ENTER** at the Room No. and Hosp. Pat. # to leave it blank. Enter '**04032003**' as Mrs. Edwards's Admit Date. Mrs. Edwards is expected to be in the hospital for '**1**' day, the Source: **1** physician referral and Type: **3** elective. Press **F1** or click on the PROCESS button ('√') on the top toolbar to process and Mrs. Edwards will be added to Hospital Rounds as shown in Figure 8-11.

EXERCISE 7: Running A Trial Daily Report for April 3

STEP 1 From the Main Menu (Menu 1), select option **5**, REPORT Generation, then option **4**, DAILY Report.

STEP 2 Key '**Y**' to request a Trial Daily Report and '**P**' to request a check register for the practice. Press **ENTER** at the Selective Appointment Location prompt to leave it blank.

STEP 3 Choose '**A**' for (A)ll and press **F1** or click on the PROCESS button ('√'). Compare your report to Figures 8-12 through 8-16. Press **ENTER** at the "Daily close not performed" prompt.

now 2 print from Rm1744

Figure 8-12 Trial Daily Report for 04/03/03—James Monroe, M.D.

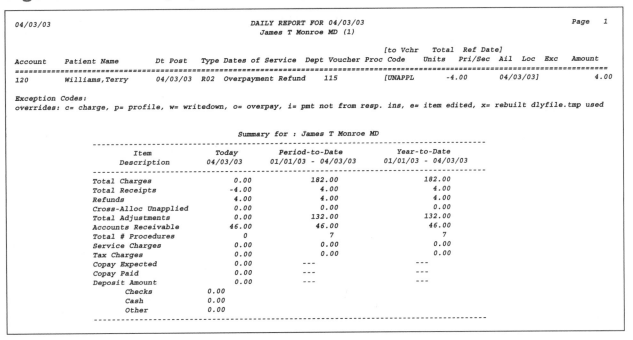

```
04/03/03                          DAILY REPORT FOR 04/03/03                                    Page    1
                                    James T Monroe MD (1)

                                                            [to Vchr   Total   Ref Date]
Account    Patient Name      Dt Post   Type Dates of Service Dept Voucher Proc Code   Units   Pri/Sec Ail  Loc  Exc   Amount
=====================================================================================================================
120        Williams,Terry    04/03/03  R02  Overpayment Refund   115    [UNAPPL       -4.00   04/03/03]              4.00

Exception Codes:
overrides: c= charge, p= profile, w= writedown, o= overpay, i= pmt not from resp. ins, e= item edited, x= rebuilt dlyfile.tmp used


                                   Summary for : James T Monroe MD
         -------------------------------------------------------------------
            Item            Today       Period-to-Date         Year-to-Date
          Description      04/03/03   01/01/03 - 04/03/03    01/01/03 - 04/03/03
         -------------------------------------------------------------------
         Total Charges       0.00          182.00                182.00
         Total Receipts     -4.00            4.00                  4.00
         Refunds             4.00            4.00                  4.00
         Cross-Alloc Unapplied 0.00          0.00                  0.00
         Total Adjustments   0.00          132.00                132.00
         Accounts Receivable 46.00          46.00                 46.00
         Total # Procedures     0              7                     7
         Service Charges     0.00            0.00                  0.00
         Tax Charges         0.00            0.00                  0.00
         Copay Expected      0.00            ---                   ---
         Copay Paid          0.00            ---                   ---
         Deposit Amount      0.00            ---                   ---
             Checks    0.00
             Cash      0.00
             Other     0.00
         -------------------------------------------------------------------
```

Figure 8-13 Trial Daily Report for 04/03/03—Frances Simpson, M.D.

```
04/03/03                          DAILY REPORT FOR 04/03/03                                    Page    2
                                   Frances D Simpson M.D. (2)

                                                            [to Vchr   Total   Ref Date]
Account    Patient Name      Dt Post   Type Dates of Service Dept Voucher Proc Code   Units   Pri/Sec Ail  Loc  Exc   Amount
=====================================================================================================================

Exception Codes:
overrides: c= charge, p= profile, w= writedown, o= overpay, i= pmt not from resp. ins, e= item edited, x= rebuilt dlyfile.tmp used


                                  Summary for : Frances D Simpson M.D.
         -------------------------------------------------------------------
            Item            Today       Period-to-Date         Year-to-Date
          Description      04/03/03   01/01/03 - 04/03/03    01/01/03 - 04/03/03
         -------------------------------------------------------------------
         Total Charges       0.00          166.00                166.00
         Total Receipts      0.00            0.00                  0.00
         Refunds             0.00            0.00                  0.00
         Cross-Alloc Unapplied 0.00          0.00                  0.00
         Total Adjustments   0.00            0.00                  0.00
         Accounts Receivable 166.00        166.00                166.00
         Total # Procedures     0              4                     4
         Service Charges     0.00            0.00                  0.00
         Tax Charges         0.00            0.00                  0.00
         Copay Expected      0.00            ---                   ---
         Copay Paid          0.00            ---                   ---
         Deposit Amount      0.00            ---                   ---
             Checks    0.00
             Cash      0.00
             Other     0.00
         -------------------------------------------------------------------
```

Figure 8-14 Trial Daily Report for 04/03/03—Sydney Carrington, M.D.

```
04/03/03                            DAILY REPORT FOR 04/03/03                                    Page    3
                                    Sydney J Carrington M.D. (3)

                                                        [to Vchr   Total   Ref Date]
Account   Patient Name    Dt Post   Type Dates of Service  Dept Voucher Proc Code  Units  Pri/Sec Ail Loc Exc  Amount
==================================================================================================================
34        Dudley,Wayne    04/03/03  PMT  Patient              420         [1053    -300.00        04/03/03]      85.00
34        Dudley,Wayne    04/03/03  PMT  Patient              420         [1053    -300.00        04/03/03]       8.00
34        Dudley,Wayne    04/03/03  PMT  Patient              420         [1053    -300.00        04/03/03]     150.00
34        Dudley,Wayne    04/03/03  PMT  Patient              420         [1053    -300.00        04/03/03]      57.00
34        Dudley,Wayne    04/03/03  R03  Returned Check       420         [UNAPPL  -300.00        04/03/03]      85.00
34        Dudley,Wayne    04/03/03  R03  Returned Check       420         [UNAPPL  -300.00        04/03/03]       8.00
34        Dudley,Wayne    04/03/03  R03  Returned Check       420         [UNAPPL  -300.00        04/03/03]     150.00
34        Dudley,Wayne    04/03/03  R03  Returned Check       420         [UNAPPL  -300.00        04/03/03]      57.00
14        Evans,Deborah   04/03/03  PMT  Check Ins #7        97977        [1061      52.00        04/03/03]     -40.00
14        Evans,Deborah   04/03/03  PMT  Check Ins #7        97977        [1061      52.00        04/03/03]     -12.00

Exception Codes:
overrides: c= charge, p= profile, w= writedown, o= overpay, i= pmt not from resp. ins, e= item edited, x= rebuilt dlyfile.tmp used


                               Summary for : Sydney J Carrington M.D.
               --------------------------------------------------------------------
                   Item           Today        Period-to-Date         Year-to-Date
                Description      04/03/03     01/01/03 - 04/03/03    01/01/03 - 04/03/03
               --------------------------------------------------------------------
               Total Charges         0.00           1,465.00              1,465.00
               Total Receipts     -248.00             422.80                422.80
               Refunds             300.00             300.00                300.00
               Cross-Alloc Unapplied  0.00              0.00                  0.00
               Total Adjustments     0.00               9.00                  9.00
               Accounts Receivable 1,033.20          1,033.20              1,033.20
               Total # Procedures       0                 26                    26
               Service Charges       0.00               0.00                  0.00
               Tax Charges           0.00               0.00                  0.00
               Copay Expected        0.00                ---                   ---
               Copay Paid            0.00                ---                   ---
               Deposit Amount       52.00                ---                   ---
                   Checks       52.00
                   Cash          0.00
                   Other         0.00
               --------------------------------------------------------------------
```

(handwritten: 1089)

Figure 8-15 Cash Analysis Report for 04/03/03

```
04/03/03                            DAILY REPORT FOR 04/03/03                                    Page    4
                                    CASH ANALYSIS REPORT
                                    Student: Paul Wilson
==================================================================================================================

        Change in Cash Position                              Daily Deposit
        -----------------------                              -------------

        CHECKS        52.00                          CHECKS        52.00
        CASH           0.00                          CASH           0.00
        OTHER          0.00                          OTHER          0.00
        REFUNDS     -304.00                                     ==========
                  ==========                                        52.00
                    -252.00


                               CHECK REGISTER FOR 04/03/03

        Ref #  Voucher   Dr.      Amount    Date Posted   Received From              Account
        ==========================================================================================
          1    97977      3       52.00     04/03/03      Pan American Health Ins.      14
                                 ----------
             TOTAL CHECKS :        52.00
```

EXERCISE 8: Running A Final Daily Close for April 3

Now, you will run a Final Daily Close, then advance the date to April 4, 2003 in Exercise 9.

STEP 1   From the Main Menu (Menu 1), choose option **5**, REPORT Generation, then option **4**, DAILY Report.

Figure 8-16 Trial Daily Report Totals for 04/03/03

```
04/03/03                        DAILY REPORT FOR 04/03/03                    Page   5
                                   Student: Paul Wilson

========================================================================================


                              TOTALS FOR 04/03/03

-----------------------------------------------------------------------------------------
Doctor              Charges    Receipts   Adjustments   Net A/R   Total A/R   # Proc.  Serv Chg   Tax Chg
-----------------------------------------------------------------------------------------
 1. James T Monroe MD      0.00       -4.00        0.00       4.00       46.00       0      0.00      0.00
 2. Frances D Simpson M.D. 0.00        0.00        0.00       0.00      166.00       0      0.00      0.00
 3. Sydney J Carrington M.D. 0.00    -248.00       0.00     248.00    1,033.20       0      0.00      0.00
-----------------------------------------------------------------------------------------
TOTAL                      0.00     -252.00        0.00     252.00    1,245.20       0      0.00      0.00
```

1301

```
                     PERIOD-TO-DATE TOTALS FOR 01/01/03 - 04/03/03

-----------------------------------------------------------------------------------------
Doctor              Charges    Receipts   Adjustments   Net A/R   Total A/R   # Proc.  Serv Chg   Tax Chg
-----------------------------------------------------------------------------------------
 1. James T Monroe MD    182.00       4.00      132.00      46.00       46.00       7      0.00      0.00
 2. Frances D Simpson M.D. 166.00     0.00        0.00     166.00      166.00       4      0.00      0.00
 3. Sydney J Carrington M.D. 1,465.00 422.80      9.00   1,033.20    1,033.20      26      0.00      0.00
-----------------------------------------------------------------------------------------
TOTAL                   1,813.00     426.80      141.00   1,245.20    1,245.20      37      0.00      0.00
```

1520   1520

```
                     YEAR-TO-DATE TOTALS FOR 01/01/03 - 04/03/03

-----------------------------------------------------------------------------------------
Doctor              Charges    Receipts   Adjustments   Net A/R   Total A/R   # Proc.  Serv Chg   Tax Chg
-----------------------------------------------------------------------------------------
 1. James T Monroe MD    182.00       4.00      132.00      46.00       46.00       7      0.00      0.00
 2. Frances D Simpson M.D. 166.00     0.00        0.00     166.00      166.00       4      0.00      0.00
 3. Sydney J Carrington M.D. 1,465.00 422.80      9.00   1,033.20    1,033.20      26      0.00      0.00
-----------------------------------------------------------------------------------------
TOTAL                   1,813.00     426.80      141.00   1,245.20    1,245.20      37      0.00      0.00
```
39

```
            ********** Daily Close Has NOT Been Performed for 04/03/03 **********
```

STEP 2 Key '**N**' to request a Final Daily Close and '**P**' to request a check register for the practice. Make sure to key '**0**' to not purge appointments.

STEP 3 Finally, press **F1** or click on the PROCESS button ('√') and the report will be generated. Hand in the Final Daily Close Report to your instructor.

Once your report has been generated, press **ENTER** to return to the log-on screen so you will be able to advance the date in the next exercise.

EXERCISE 9: Advancing the Date to April 4

Key '**04042003**' at the prompt and press **ENTER** to advance the date. Note that because you chose to advance the date by less than 7 days (i.e., 03/31/2003 to 04/04/2003), you did not receive a warning message.

AGING REPORT

Dunning letters are based on the Aging Report.

Aging Reports provide information that aid in collections of accounts. Both patients and insurance companies are sometimes slow in paying outstanding balances. To maintain cash flow and financial viability for the practice, dunning notices or follow-up letters must be sent. These notices and reminders become more demanding the longer the account remains unpaid.

The Aging Report categorizes an account's outstanding balance by the length of time it has been due. The guarantor's or insurance plan's current balance is "aged" to show which charges have been outstanding the longest; therefore, the Aging Report shows which accounts need the most attention for collection.

Accounts are aged in six categories:

1—Current
2—31–60 days
3—61–90 days
4—91–120 days
5—121–150 days
6—151 + days – End

The Aging Report can be printed at any time to aid in payment collection. You may generate a report by account, doctor, or by insurance plan, and you can also print the report in summary or in detail. At the summary level, all of the items aged are added together by account or by insurance plan, and only the Aging Summary is printed. At the detail level, each outstanding open item is aged and printed.

The first step in analyzing the accounts outstanding for a medical practice is to determine which portion is to be paid by the insurance plan and which portion is the patient's responsibility. This is done by running the Aging Report using the (A)nalysis option. The report will provide an aged analysis comparing the patient and insurance due portions of the accounts. The analysis may be generated either by doctor or practice.

Review these directions for printing an Aging Report. After the directions are complete, you will be asked to print an Aging Report.

To get to the Aging Report Screen, from the Main Menu (Menu 1), select option **5**, REPORT Generation. From the Report Menu, select option **2**, FINANCIAL Activity Report followed by option **2**, AGING Report. The Aging Report screen in Figure 8-17

Figure 8-17 Aging Report Screen

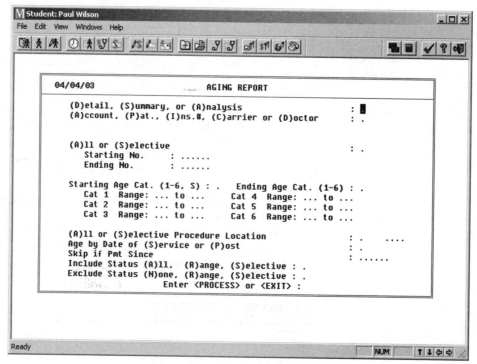

appears. A description of the meaning of each section of the screen is given in the following paragraphs. After you have studied the descriptions, proceed to *Applying Your Knowledge* and follow the instructions to run the Aging Reports listed.

(D)etail, (S)ummary, or (A)nalysis

The Aging Report may be selected in (D)etail, (S)ummary, or (A)nalysis level. Summary level ages all open items into one line providing totals in each category. (D)etail level provides a detail of each open item plus the summary totals. If (A)nalysis is selected, the report compares an analysis of patient and insurance due portions of accounts. The report is automatically generated in (D)octor order, and each item associated with a doctor is aged exclusively for that doctor. The aging is based upon the original date of service, and all aging categories are included. A (P)ractice option, a summary analysis of the aged accounts of all physicians in the practice, provides only a single page practice analysis. If the (P)ractice option is *not* selected, the analysis will generate a separate analysis page for each doctor and the summary analysis page for the practice.

(A)ccount, (P)at., (I)ns. #, (C)arrier, or (D)octor

If the Aging Report is retrieved by (A)ccount, aging is based on the original date of services. If the report is retrieved by (P)atient due, only the items currently the patient's responsibility are aged, and they are aged based upon the date of patient responsibility. If the report is called up by (I)nsurance plan, only the items currently shown as insurance responsibility are aged, based upon the insurance billing date. If the report is called up by (C)arrier, the items shown as that carrier's responsibility will be aged. If the report is called up by (D)octor, aging is based on the original date of service, and only the items that are associated with that doctor are aged.

Separate by Doctor? (Y/N)

If the report is called by insurance plan, the user will have the option to generate separate Insurance Aging reports for all or selective doctors. Insurance aging will be based on insurance billing date.

Display by Claim? (N)one, (F)orced, (A)ll

To view the items by claim, choose (A)ll. Choosing (N)one will not display the items by claim. (F)orced refers to an item that is billed as a "forced claim," a special condition used when billing Medicare, part A. You will probably not encounter this in most physicians' offices. However, it is used in some outpatient clinics.

(A)ll, (S)elective, (P)ractice

If the Analysis Report is selected, the above prompt will display. If (A)ll or (S)elective is chosen, the Aging Analysis Report will be generated for all or selective doctors. If (P)ractice is chosen, a single page report will analyze the practice's accounts receivable as a whole.

Starting Aging Cat. (1–6, S)—Ending Aging Cat. (1–6)

Enter the aging categories from which to begin and end the report. If 'S' is chosen, categories 1–3 remain the same but the user is allowed to enter the number of days for categories 4–6. The age category options are:

1—0–30 days

2—31–60 days

3—61–90 days

4—91–120 days

5—121–150 days

6—151+ days–End

Skip if Payment Since

All accounts showing payment since the entered date will be skipped and not shown in the report.

Include Status? (Y/N)

In New Patient Entry (See Unit 3), you assigned a status to each account (e.g., Active or Inactive). The information you originally entered into this field can be used as a filter for specific account statuses. You can choose to include all status codes, a range of statuses, or up to five selective status codes. For example, you can choose to run an Aging Report for only patients with an account status of "Active."

Exclude Status? (Y/N)

You can choose not to exclude any status code or a range of statuses, or up to five selective status codes.

Default Options

To default through all categories, press **ENTER** six times. An explanatory list of items included on an Aging Report is shown in Figure 8-18.

You then press **F1** or click on the PROCESS button ('√') on the top toolbar to process and the requested Aging Report would be generated. Generate the reports requested in the *Applying Your Knowledge* section.

APPLYING YOUR KNOWLEDGE

EXERCISE 10: Running Aging Reports

Run each of the following Aging Reports using the instructions provided below. Note that all of the Aging Reports are requested from the same screen. For clarity, the procedure for each Aging Report is listed as a separate step. Remember to press ENTER to

Figure 8-18 Items Included on an Aging Report

Aging Report	Items
Account	The guarantor's account number.
Date of Service	The dates when procedures were performed. If a service was performed over a period of time, the beginning and ending dates will be printed.
Patient	The first name of the patient treated.
Dr #	The number representing the physician who performed the procedure.
Voucher	The number assigned to the procedure for identification purposes.
Proc Code	The code number representing the procedure performed.
Diag Code	The code number representing the doctor's diagnosis.
Pat Resp	The date of patient responsibility for the procedure. (This will be either the serviced date or the transfer date.)
Units	The number of times this procedure was performed on the given date(s) of service.
Stat	The financial status of the procedure.
Ins 1—Billed	The date on which the primary insurance plan was billed for the procedure. This date is preceded by the insurance plan number, and followed by an "E" if this claim has been filed via EMC.
Ins 2—Billed	The date on which a secondary insurance plan was billed for the procedure.
Current	Aging of accounts receivable; account is up-to-date.
31–60	Aging of accounts receivable; account is 31–60 days outstanding.
61–90	Aging of accounts receivable; account is 61–90 days outstanding.
91–120	Aging of accounts receivable; account is 91–120 days outstanding.
121–150	Aging of accounts receivable; account is 121–150 days outstanding.
151+	Aging of accounts receivable; account is over 151 days outstanding.

accept default information at fields for which no information is provided. If you need to, take a few moments to go back and review the steps for printing an Aging Report. Be sure your printer is ready before you begin printing. For comparison purposes, the reports are illustrated in Figures 8-19 through 8-22. Hand in the reports to your instructor.

STEP 1

Aging Analysis by Practice. From the Main Menu (Menu 1), select option **5**, REPORT Generation, option **2**, FINANCIAL Activity Report, then option **2**, AGING Report. Choose 'A' for (A)nalysis and 'P' for (P)ractice. Press **ENTER** two more times to accept the defaults of All Procedure Locations and Age by Date of Source. Press the **F1** key or click on the PROCESS button ('√') and the Analysis By Practice Aging Report will be generated.

Figure 8-19 Aging Analysis Summary for Practice

```
04/04/03                        SYSTEM AGING ANALYSIS BY DOCTOR                        Page    1
                                      Student: Paul Wilson
                                     SUMMARY FOR PRACTICE
                                    All Procedure Locations


                    -------------------------------------------------------------------------------
                        0 - 30        31 - 60       61 - 90       91 -120       121 -150      151 +
                    -------------------------------------------------------------------------------
         Patient  :     622.20          0.00         40.00          0.00          0.00         0.00
            %     :      94.0%          0.0%          6.0%          0.0%          0.0%         0.0%
         Insurance :     90.00        493.00          0.00          0.00          0.00         0.00
            %     :      15.4%         84.6%          0.0%          0.0%          0.0%         0.0%
                    -------------------------------------------------------------------------------
         Totals   :     712.20        493.00         40.00          0.00          0.00         0.00
            %     :      57.2%         39.6%          3.2%          0.0%          0.0%         0.0%
                    -------------------------------------------------------------------------------


         Total Patient Receivables        :     662.20        53.2%    (Date-Patient-Responsible)
         Total Insurance Receivables      :     583.00        46.8%    (Date-Company-Billed)
         Total Open Items                 :    1245.20       100.0%    (Summation-of-Above)
         Unapplied Credits & Overpaid     :       0.00
         Total Accounts Receivable        :    1245.20
```

STEP 2

Summary Aging Report by Patient Due (All Accounts). At the Aging Report screen, choose 'S' for (S)ummary, 'P' for (P)atient, and 'A' for (A)ll. Press **ENTER** twice to bypass the Starting Aging Category and Ending Aging Category fields. Choose 'A' for (A)ll Procedure Location and 'S' for Age By Date of (S)ervice. Press **ENTER** to accept the current system date at the Skip If Pmt Since field. Choose 'A' for (All) and 'N' for (None). Press **F1** or click on the PROCESS button ('√') and the Summary Aging Report by Patient Due will be generated (Figure 8-20).

Figure 8-20 Summary Aging Report by Patient Due

```
04/04/03          SUMMARY AGING REPORT BY ACCOUNT BASED ON DATE PATIENT BILLED (Pat. Only)       Page    1
                                       Student: Paul Wilson
                                          All Accounts
                            Aging Category: 1 - 6 / DOL Pay <= 04/04/03
                                      All Procedure Locations

                                       Overpd &                                                      Total
Acct #  Name          Phone No.    DOL Pay  Unapplied  0 - 30   31 - 60  61 - 90  91 -120  121 -150  151 +   Balance
======================================================================================================================
21    Edwards,Portia (916) 899-7800 03/20/03            15.20                                                 15.20
30    League,Claire  (408) 907-4352 03/14/03            75.00                                                 75.00
34    Dudley,Wayne R (408) 789-6654 03/14/03           300.00                                                300.00
80    Davis,Timothy  (916) 908-7657                                       40.00                               40.00
110   Evans,Patricia (916) 544-8275 03/20/03           232.00                                               232.00
                                               ======== ========= ======== ======== ======== ======== ======== =========
      REPORT TOTALS              :     0.00            622.20     0.00    40.00     0.00     0.00     0.00    662.20

      PERCENT OF TOTAL AGED      :                     94.0%     0.0%     6.0%     0.0%     0.0%     0.0%
```

STEP 3

Summary Aging Report by Insurance Billed Date (Not Separated by Doctor). At the Aging Report screen, choose '**S**' for (S)ummary, '**I**' for (I)nsurance, and '**N**' to not separate the report by doctor. Key '**A**' for (A)ll. Press **ENTER** twice to bypass the Starting Aging Category and Ending Aging Category fields. Choose '**A**' for (A)ll Procedure Location and '**S**' for Age by Date of (S)ervice. Press **ENTER** to accept the current system date at the Skip If Pmt Since field. Choose '**A**' for (All) and '**N**' for (None). Press **F1** or click on the PROCESS button ('√') and the Summary Aging Report by Insurance Billed Date will be generated (Figure 8-21).

Figure 8-21 Summary Aging Report by Insurance Billed Date

```
04/04/03                  SUMMARY AGING REPORT BY INS PLAN BASED ON DATE INSURANCE BILLED               Page   1
                                         Student: Paul Wilson
                                            All Ins Plans
                               Aging Category: 1 - 6 / DOL Pay <= 04/04/03
                                         All Procedure Locations

                                                                                                          Total
Plan#  Name            Carrier   Phone No.     Overpd    0 - 30   31 - 60   61 - 90   91 -120  121 -150   151 +   Balance
=======================================================================================================================
5      Epsilon Life &  EPSLON   (800) 908-7654                    365.00                                         365.00
7      Pan American H  PANAMC   (213) 456-7654                     40.00                                          40.00
9      Worker's Compe  BENIND   (800) 654-2323           50.00                                                    50.00
10     Medicare Plus   MEDIP    (800) 675-4354            2.00                                                     2.00
12     Fringe Benefit  FRGBEN   (800) 999-1234           38.00     88.00                                         126.00
                                              ======== ========== ========== ========== ========== ========== ========== ==========
       REPORT TOTALS              :            0.00     90.00    493.00      0.00      0.00      0.00      0.00   583.00

       PERCENT OF TOTAL AGED      :                     15.4%     84.6%      0.0%      0.0%      0.0%      0.0%
```

STEP 4

Detailed Aging Report by Insurance Billed Date (Not Separated by Doctor). Choose '**D**' for (D)etail at the Aging Report screen. Then key '**I**' for (I)nsurance, '**N**' to not separate the report by doctor, '**F**' for (F)orced Claim, and '**A**' for (A)ll. Press **ENTER** twice to bypass the Starting Aging Category and Ending Aging Category fields. Choose '**A**' for (A)ll Procedure Location, '**S**' for Age by Date of (S)ervice. Press **ENTER** to accept the current system date at the Skip If Pmt Since field. Choose '**A**' for (All) and '**N**' for (None). Press **F1** or click on the PROCESS button ('√') and the Detailed Aging Report by Insurance Billed Date will be generated (Figure 8-22).

Figure 8-22 Detailed Aging Report by Insurance Billed Date

```
04/04/03                 DETAILED AGING REPORT BY INS PLAN BASED ON DATE INSURANCE BILLED                    Page    1
                                          Student: Paul Wilson
                                             All Ins Plans
                              Aging Category: 1 - 6 / DOL Pay <= 04/04/03
                                        All Procedure Locations

          Dates of  Patient              Proc Code    Ins 1-Billed
Plan# Acc Service   Dr#/Voucher Units/Stat Diag        Ins 2-Billed    0 - 30   31 - 60   61 - 90   91 -120   121 -150   151 +
=================================================================================================================================
5        Epsilon Life & Casualty            (800)  908-7654      EPSLON Epsilon Life & Casualty
   110    01/10/03 Evans,Patricia G  99214            5-02/04/03           50.00
                   3/1056    1/2      174.9           0-
   110    01/10/03 Evans,Patricia G  71020            5-02/04/03           58.00
                   3/1056    1/2      174.9           0-
   110    01/10/03 Evans,Patricia G  76088            5-02/04/03          125.00
                   3/1056    1/2      174.9           0-
   110    01/27/03 Evans,Patricia G  99223            5-02/04/03           94.00
                   3/HOSP    1/2      174.9           0-
   110    01/31/03 Evans,Patricia G  99238            5-02/04/03           38.00
                   3/HOSP    1/2      174.9           0-

      BALANCE FOR PLAN 5    :      365.00   OVERPD:    0.00          365.00

7        Pan American Health Ins.           (213)  456-7654     PANAMC Pan American Health Ins.
   10     01/10/03 Carlson,Sharon A  99213            7-02/04/03           40.00
                   3/1051    1/2      461.9           0-

      BALANCE FOR PLAN 7    :       40.00   OVERPD:    0.00           40.00

9        Worker's Compensation              (800)  654-2323     BENIND Beneficial Industrial Co.
   21     02/17/03 Edwards,Portia D  99214            9-03/20/03           50.00
                   3/1063    1/2      724.2           0-

      BALANCE FOR PLAN 9    :       50.00   OVERPD:    0.00           50.00

10       Medicare Plus                      (800)  675-4354      MEDIP Medicare Plus
   30     02/03/03 League,Claire E   85031           10-03/20/03            2.00
                   3/1060    1/5      285.9            2-02/04/03

      BALANCE FOR PLAN 10   :        2.00   OVERPD:    0.00            2.00

12       Fringe Benefit Center              (800)  999-1234     FRGBEN Fringe Benefit Center
   80     02/17/03 Davis,Timothy R   29705           12-03/20/03           38.00
                   2/1062    1/2      841.2           0-
   80     01/10/03 Davis,Timothy R   99213           12-02/04/03 r         40.00
                   2/1055    1/2      841.2           0-
   80     01/10/03 Davis,Timothy R   29075           12-02/04/03 r         48.00
                   2/1055    1/2      841.2           0-

      BALANCE FOR PLAN 12   :      126.00   OVERPD:    0.00           38.00     88.00
=================================================================================================================================
TOTALS:  BAL:      583.00              OVERPD:    0.00      90.00    493.00      0.00      0.00      0.00      0.00

PERCENT OF TOTAL AGED  :                                   15.4%     84.6%      0.0%      0.0%      0.0%      0.0%
```

(handwritten annotations: "638." above 583.00; "584." above 493.00; "14.1 85.9" below the 15.4% 84.6% line)

DISPLAY PATIENT DATA

Display Patient Data is among the most powerful of **The Medical Manager** software's features. Through this one menu item, you have access to every existing piece of account data found in the Guarantor reports, the Financial Activity reports, the Ailment File report, and the Office Management reports. You can have an immediate full screen look at an account's activities. You have options available that focus on dependents, insurance companies, charges, payments, appointments, hospital confinements, estimates, patient-extended information, word processing records, recall information, selected historical data, or open item aging summary. Display Patient Data allows you to look at the details of a specific item within an account without printing a long report. Every screen also provides a hard copy option.

Display Patient Data first presents an account's demographic and summary financial information. You may select options for additional information on dependents, insurance plans, open items, current period payments, appointments, hospital confinements, procedure history, clinical history, financial history, open item aging summary, patient-extended information, recall, estimates, or patient's word processing file. Each individual charge or payment can be analyzed in further detail. Any ailment information that is linked to a charge is also available when charges are reviewed.

Display Patient Data is an invaluable tool for easily tapping the entire scope of data stored by **The Medical Manager** system. It is an excellent tool for reviewing a patient's account or for tracing detailed information on an account.

Follow the instructions below to display patient data.

Select option 4. DISPLAY Patient Data, at the Main Menu (Menu 1). Key '21' and press **ENTER** to retrieve Portia Edwards's account. The patient number you entered here will act as the default patient number on all the selection screens accessed via Display Patient Data. If a full patient number with decimal extension is entered, only that patient's data will be displayed for Procedure and Clinical History. If the account number is entered without decimal extension, history will be shown for all dependents of the account. The screen in Figure 8-23 will appear providing demographic, account status, and financial summary information. Whenever you desire to return to any preceding screen in the Display Patient Data process, you may press ESCAPE or click on the EXIT button on the top toolbar.

The Display Patient Data screen is divided into three portions. The upper portion provides demographic information about the account, the middle portion provides a financial summary of the account, and the lower portion provides 14 options for detailed information. You may select the option (1–14) desired and press ENTER. Detailed processing instructions for each of the available options may be found in the following sections.

Figure 8-23 Display Patient Data Screen

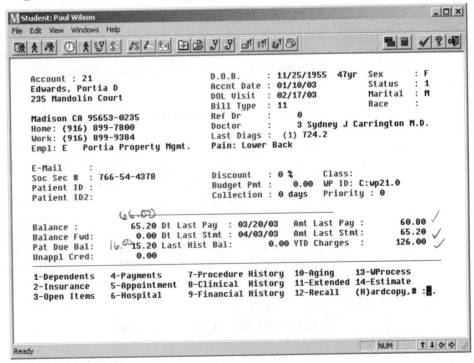

Option 1: Dependents

At the Display Patient Data screen, key **1**, Dependents, and press **ENTER**. The Dependents display, shown in Figure 8-24, includes the dependent's number, name, date of birth, sex, relationship to the guarantor, and Social Security number. Use the

Figure 8-24 Dependents on Portia Edwards' Account

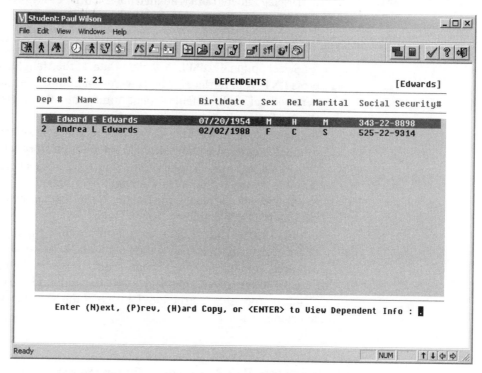

highlight bar to select a dependent and press **ENTER** to see more detailed information. From this screen, choose '**E**' to view this dependent's extended information. Press **ESCAPE** or click on the EXIT button on the top toolbar until you return to the Display Patient Data screen, shown in Figure 8-23, page 335.

Option 2: Insurance Coverage

At the Display Patient Data screen, key '**2**' and press **ENTER** to view insurance information for this account. A screen similar to Figure 8-25 will appear. The Insurance Coverage display presents a summary list of the guarantor's insurance plan, including insurance plan number, insurance plan name, effective dates, assignment, and notes. You can use the highlight bar to view more about each plan. In addition, you can choose (**A**)ll Plans to see information on all plans on the account. At the prompt, select whether a hard copy is desired. If you key (H)ard copy, the information will be printed. Press **ESCAPE** or click on the EXIT button on the top toolbar until you return to the Display Patient Data screen for Mrs. Edwards.

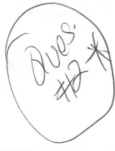

Option 3: Open Items

Key option '**3**', Open Items, at the Display Patient Data screen and press **ENTER**. The Open Items display presents an open item list of a patient's charges. Only enough information is given to identify a charge. A screen similar to Figure 8-26 will appear. Full

Figure 8-25 Insurance Coverage for Edward Edwards

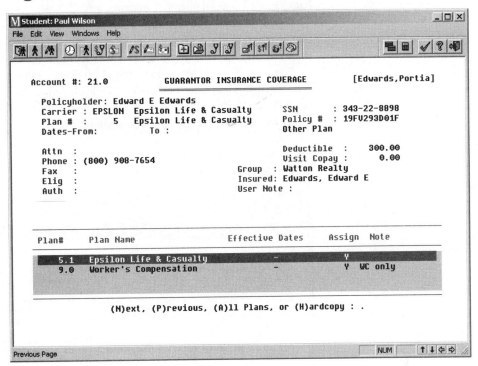

```
M Student: Paul Wilson                                              _ □ X
File  Edit  View  Windows  Help

[toolbar icons]                                              [toolbar icons]

   Account #: 21.0           GUARANTOR INSURANCE COVERAGE      [Edwards,Portia]

    Policyholder: Edward E Edwards
    Carrier : EPSLON   Epsilon Life & Casualty      SSN     : 343-22-8898
    Plan #  :     5    Epsilon Life & Casualty      Policy # : 19FU293D01F
    Dates-From:         To :                        Other Plan

    Attn  :                                         Deductible  :     300.00
    Phone : (800) 908-7654                          Visit Copay :       0.00
    Fax   :                               Group   : Watton Realty
    Elig  :                               Insured : Edwards, Edward E
    Auth  :                               User Note :


    Plan#    Plan Name                  Effective Dates    Assign  Note

     5.1   Epsilon Life & Casualty          -              Y
     9.0   Worker's Compensation            -              Y   WC only


           (N)ext, (P)revious, (A)ll Plans, or (H)ardcopy : .


Previous Page                                              NUM      ↑↓⇦⇨
```

detail on a charge may be viewed by keying the reference number and pressing ENTER. You can also see full detail by moving the highlight bar to an item and pressing ENTER *#2B* or by using the mouse to double-click on an item. Highlighting and pressing ENTER after the reference number of a charge has been entered will result in full detail on that charge. If the account has more charges than can be displayed on one screen, use (N)ext or (P)revious to page forward and backward to see charges not displayed on the

Figure 8-26 Open Items Display for the Edwards Account

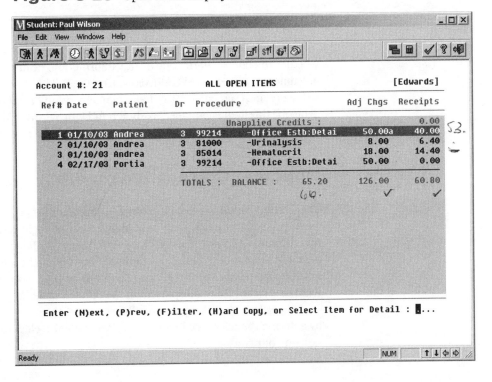

```
M Student: Paul Wilson                                              _ □ X
File  Edit  View  Windows  Help

[toolbar icons]                                              [toolbar icons]

   Account #: 21               ALL OPEN ITEMS                   [Edwards]

   Ref# Date      Patient   Dr  Procedure              Adj Chgs  Receipts
                              Unapplied Credits :                   0.00
      1 01/10/03 Andrea    3  99214    -Office Estb:Detai  50.00a  40.00   S3.
      2 01/10/03 Andrea    3  81000    -Urinalysis          8.00   6.40
      3 01/10/03 Andrea    3  85014    -Hematocrit         18.00  14.40
      4 02/17/03 Portia    3  99214    -Office Estb:Detai  50.00   0.00

                    TOTALS : BALANCE :      65.20    126.00     60.80
                                             66.             ✓        ✓


   Enter (N)ext, (P)rev, (F)ilter, (H)ard Copy, or Select Item for Detail : ▌...


Ready                                                      NUM      ↑↓⇦⇨
```

current page. Remember that you can also use the arrow buttons on the bottom toolbar to move between pages of information.

Select whether a hard copy of the display is desired or if further detailed information is necessary for a particular charge by entering its reference line number. For example, highlight line item '**1**', and press **ENTER** to select it to view Open Item Detail.

Figure 8-27 provides an example of an Open Item Detail screen for one procedure, code 99214. The upper portion of the display gives full detail of the charge as it was entered. The bottom portion of the display gives full detail of all payments and adjustments that have been posted to the system.

Figure 8-27 Open Item Detail

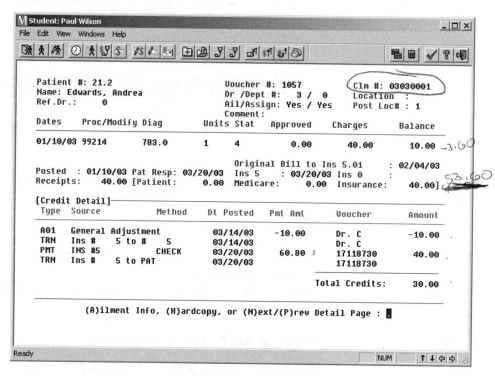

To view Ailment information linked to this charge, key '**A**' and press **ENTER**. Decide whether to obtain a hard copy of this information, or just view it on your console. At any time you may press ESCAPE or click on the EXIT button on the top toolbar to return to the previous screen. Notice that when ailment information is requested, the ailment detail for this item is provided as shown in Figure 8-28. Press **ESCAPE** or click on the EXIT button on the top toolbar until you return to the Display Patient Data screen.

Option 4: Current Payments

The Current Payments display presents a summary list of a patient's current payments, as shown in Figure 8-29. Only enough information is given to identify a payment. From Mrs. Edwards's Display Patient Data screen, key '**4**', Payments, and press **ENTER**. If payment application detail is required, highlight the desired payment and press **ENTER**. Remember that you can use (**N**)ext or (**P**)revious to page forward and backward to see charges not displayed on the current page.

Now, select whether you want a hard copy of the display or a payment's application by entering the reference line number. You can also elect to simply view this information on your console.

Figure 8-28 Ailment Information Screen

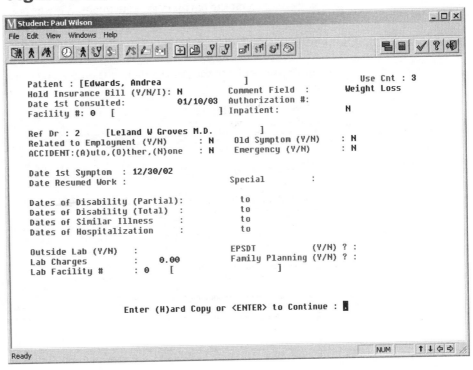

Figure 8-29 Current Payments for Portia Edwards's Account

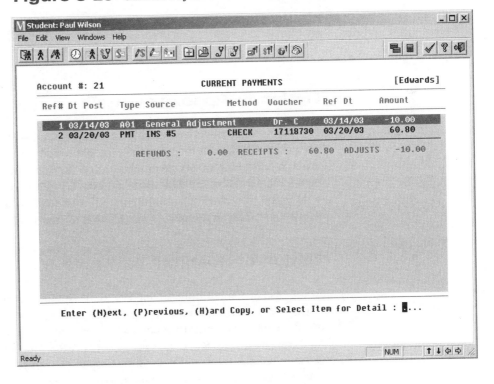

Figure 8-30 shows a Payment Detail screen. The upper portion of the display gives full detail about the payment or adjustment as it was posted. The bottom portion gives detail about which charges were credited during allocation of the payment or adjustment. The charges are identified by date of service and procedure code number and by charge voucher number. Press **ESCAPE** or click on the EXIT button on the top toolbar until you return to the Display Patient Data screen.

Figure 8-30 Payment Detail for Portia Edwards's Account

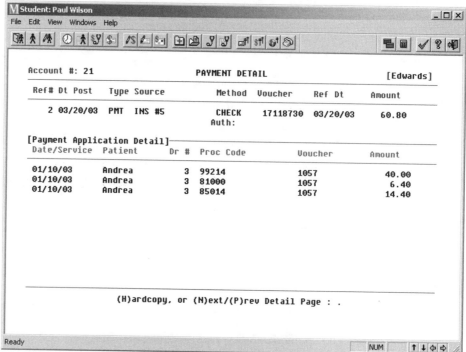

Option 5: Appointments

The Appointment display provides a list of appointments by account number as shown in Figure 8-31. Details include date, time, dependents, reasons, doctor, room number, length of visit, and two phone numbers. Key '**5**', Appointments, at the Display Patient Data screen and press **ENTER**. When option 5 is selected, the "(H)ardcopy ?" prompt is displayed. Enter '**H**' for a hard copy, or press **ENTER** for a console display. Enter (**C**)urrent or (**H**)istory Report. Press **ENTER** to return to the main patient display.

Option 6: Hospital

At the Display Patient Data screen, key '**6**', Hospital, and press **ENTER**. The Hospital display gives current hospital confinement by patient with information on room number, date, diagnosis, referring physician, and remark. You may choose to request a hard copy by keying '**H**', or you can press **ENTER** for a console display. If a hard copy is requested, the number of days in the hospital, referring doctor's phone number, and diagnosis code will be listed in addition to the information shown in Figure 8-32. Press **ESCAPE** or click on the EXIT button until you return to the Display Patient Data screen for Mrs. Edwards.

Figure 8-31 Appointment Report Screen for Portia Edwards's Account

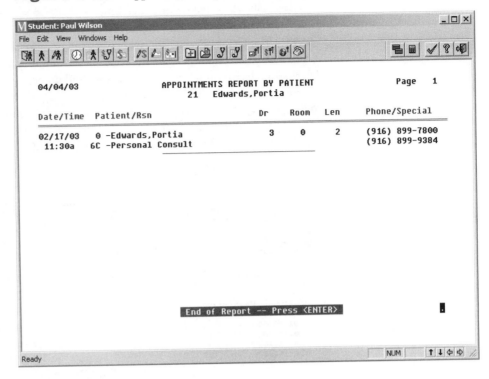

Figure 8-32 Hospital Rounds Report Screen

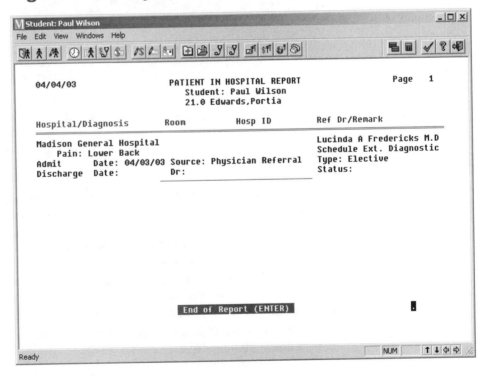

Option 7: Procedure History

From Mrs. Edwards's Display Patient Data screen, key '**7**', Procedure History, and press **ENTER**. The Patient Procedure History display presents a summary of the treatments received by the requested patients. Detail on treatment date, procedure code and description, doctor number, patient number and name, and patient diagnosis is provided. You may choose to request a hard copy by keying '**H**', or you can press **ENTER** for a console display. If a hard copy is requested, department number, units, and charges will be listed in addition to the information shown in Figure 8-33. Press **ESCAPE** or click on the EXIT button until you return to the Display Patient Data screen.

Figure 8-33 Patient Procedure History Screen for Portia Edwards's Account

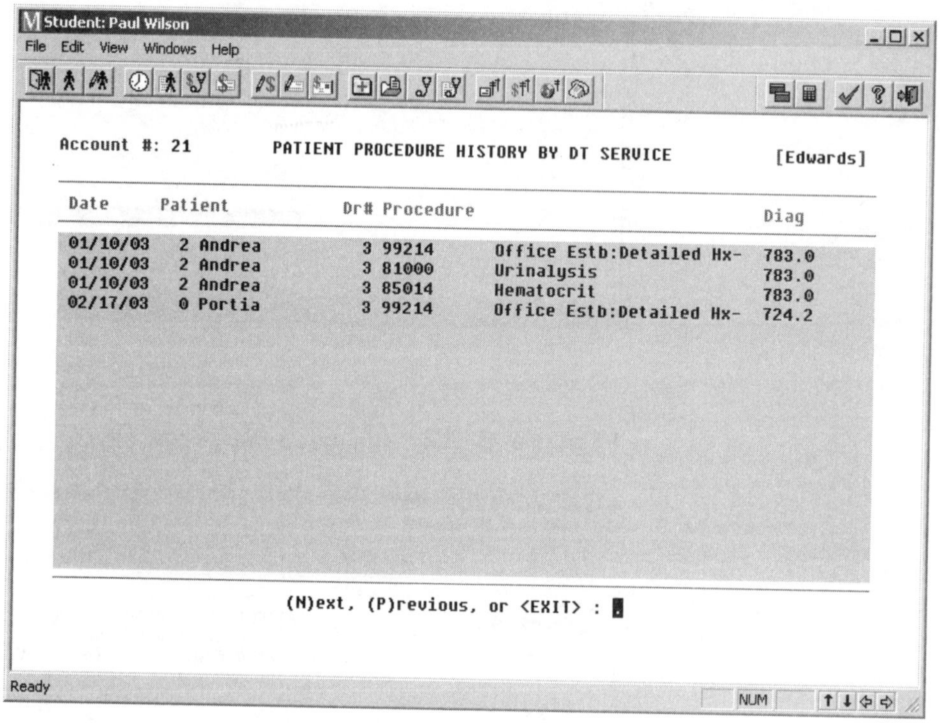

Option 8: Clinical History

The Clinical History Report provides full detail on up to nine different types of patient history data for each patient selected. The possible (optional) types of data are user defined. They could include such data as drug history, allergy history, or other information. Clinical History Detail may be kept online for as long as desired (1 year, 2 years, or indefinitely). From Mrs. Edwards's Display Patient Data screen, key '**8**', Clinical History, and press **ENTER**. You can choose either (I)tem or (F)orm mode. Press **ENTER** to accept the default response for this item. The screen shown in Figure 8-34 appears. Complete the following steps to see how a Clinical History Report is generated.

1. You can enter 'C' for a console display of the data, or 'P' for a hard copy of the Clinical History Report. Press **ENTER** to accept the default response of a (C)onsole display.

2. Enter the type of clinical history data (1–999) you want to be displayed or printed. Press **ENTER** to default to (A)ll types.

Figure 8-34 Clinical History Reports Selection Screen

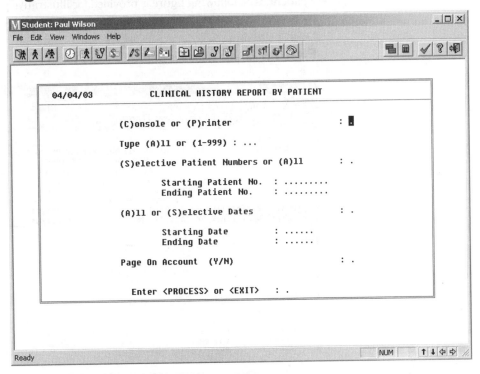

3. You can enter 'S' if you want to select requested patients by number, or 'A' to review data for all patients. Press **ENTER** to default to (S)elective Patient Numbers.

4. You can enter patient number(s) of patient(s) to be displayed or listed. Your entry to these fields is bypassed if (A)ll patients are selected. If the (S)elective Patients Numbers option was requested, press **ENTER** twice to see the number of the patient whose data are currently being reviewed.

5. You can enter 'A' if all dates are to be displayed, or 'S' for (S)elective if you only want to display the requested range of dates. Press **ENTER** to default to (A)ll dates.

6. You can enter beginning and ending dates. Your entry to these fields is bypassed if (A)ll dates are selected. If (S)elective dates are requested, you can press **ENTER** to default to a starting date of 01011800 and then press **ENTER** again to default to an ending date of 12319999.

7. You can enter 'Y' if you want each account to be listed on its own page. Your entry to this field is bypassed if (A)ll dates are selected. Press **ENTER** to default to not paging an account. Then, you can press **F1** or click on the PROCESS button ('√') to process and view the requested data, or press ESCAPE or click on the EXIT button on the top toolbar to return to the Display Patient Data screen.

Figure 8-35 shows an example of an Allergy History Report that might be kept for a patient. The following figure is provided for illustrative purposes only. Press **ENTER** twice to return to the Display Patient Data screen.

Figure 8-35 Sample Clinical History Report

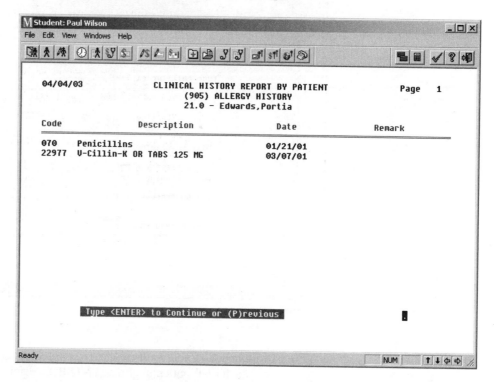

Option 9: Financial History

The Patient Financial History display provides chronological detail on charge and payment information for the account being reviewed. It includes account totals for units of service, charges, payments, adjustments, refunds, and current balance. The doctor number, procedure, description, date of service, and patient name and number are shown. All charges and all patient and insurance payment information are also displayed.

Note that an **OUT OF BALANCE** message will display if the account is out of balance with this report.

At the Display Patient Data screen, key '**9**', Financial History, and press **ENTER**. You can enter '**H**' for a hard copy, or press **ENTER** for a console display without hard copy. If a hard copy is requested, procedure and diagnosis codes will be listed in addition to the information shown in Figure 8-36. Press **ESCAPE** or click on the EXIT button on the top toolbar until you to return to the Display Patient Data screen.

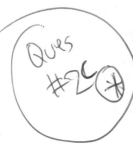

Option 10: Aging Analysis

The Aging Analysis ages all open items for the account into five aging categories by patient and insurance. Aging categories include: current, 31–60 days, 61–90 days, 91–120 days, and over 120 days. Percentages of the total charges to the patient and to the patient's insurance companies are calculated within each of the five categories. The overall balance is also calculated for both patient and carrier. At the Display Patient Data screen, key '**10**', Aging Analysis, and press **ENTER**. The screen shown in Figure 8-37 will appear. If you want to print a hard copy of the display, you can press '**H**'. Press **ENTER** to return to the Display Patient Data screen.

Figure 8-36 Patient Financial History for Portia Edwards' Account

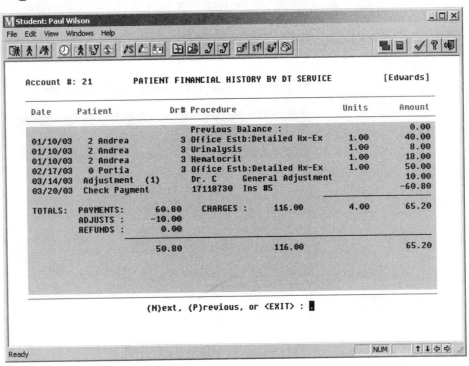

Figure 8-37 Aging Analysis for Portia Edwards's Account

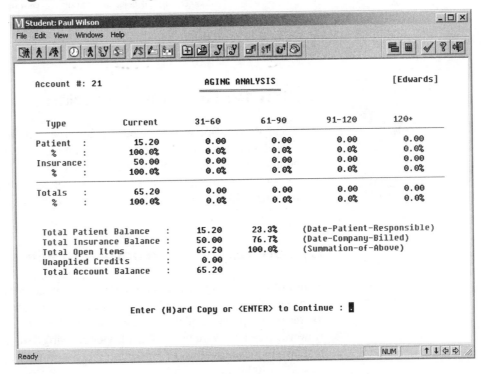

Option 11: Extended Information

Patient Extended Information holds the additional information that was entered during patient entry. It is also possible to label additional fields through the Extended Information Labels routine in System Utilities. Some examples of user-defined fields are "Service Branch", "Retired", "Hobbies", or "Service Organizations". These fields can also be relabeled for legal representative information or other types of information that would be useful for your practice. From Mrs. Edwards's Display Patient Data screen, key '11', Extended, and press **ENTER**. The screen shown in Figure 8-38 will appear. If you want to print a hard copy of the display, you can press 'H'. Press **ENTER** to return to the Display Patient Data screen.

Figure 8-38 Extended Information Screen

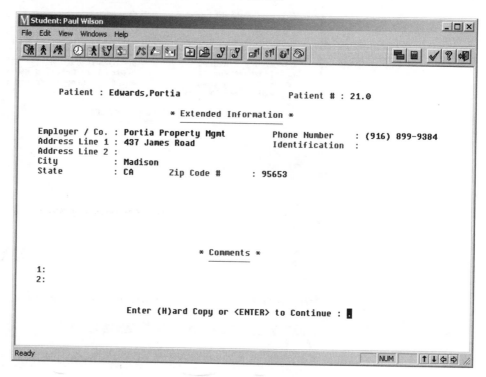

Option 12: Recall Information

The Recall Report, Option 12, provides a convenient method of reviewing all appointment recall information, including patient name, date of contact, reason code, doctor #, and patient's phone numbers. The requested information may be displayed on the console, or a hard copy may be printed. This option will not be addressed in the Student Edition course. However, a sample Recall Report is shown in Figure 8-39.

Option 13: Word Processing File

If the practice is using a word processor to create documents about patients, a particular patient's word processing file (set up during guarantor and dependent entry) may be viewed using option 13. This option will not be addressed in the Student Edition course. However, a sample word processing file viewed using **The Medical Manager** software is shown in Figure 8-40.

Option 14: Estimate

The Estimate Report, Option 14, provides the user with a convenient method of reviewing all online estimate information. The requested information may be displayed on the console or a hard copy may be printed. However, because you have not entered any estimates, none are available for viewing.

Figure 8-39 Sample Recall Report on Console

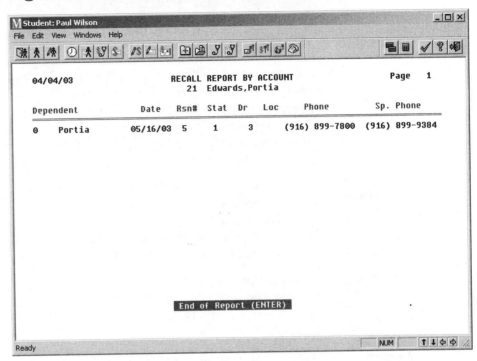

Figure 8-40 Sample Word Processing File

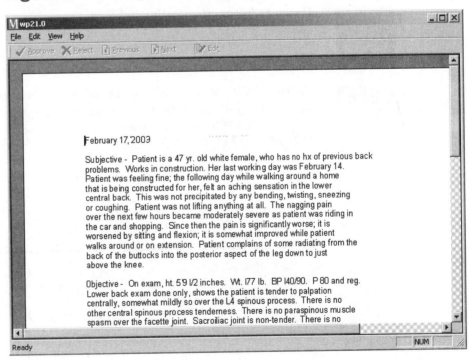

EXERCISE 11: Printing Patient Data

The purpose of this section is to reinforce what you have learned in the preceding section on the Display Patient Data feature of **The Medical Manager** software. For clarity, the procedure for printing each patient data option is listed as a separate step. Practice using this feature again by viewing the options you will *not* be printing (options 1, 4, 7, 11, and 13). Then, using the instructions provided below, as well as the information provided in the preceding section, print hard copies of the options listed below. *Make sure your printer is ready before you begin.* Hand in the reports to your instructor.

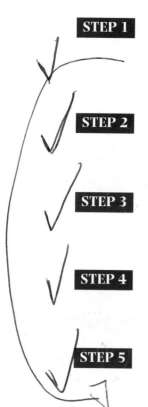

STEP 1

Option 2: Insurance Plan and Insured Party Information. From the Main Menu (Menu 1), select option **4**, DISPLAY Patient Data. Key '**21.0**' and press **ENTER** to retrieve Portia Edwards's account. Key '**2**', Insurance, and press **ENTER**. Key '**A**' for (A)ll, '**H**' for hard copy, press **ENTER** and the Insurance Plan and Insured Party Information will be printed. **EXIT** to return to the Display Patient Data screen.

STEP 2

Option 3: Open Items. From the Display Patient Data screen, key option '**3**', Open Items, and press **ENTER**. Highlight line item **1** and press **ENTER** to select it. Key '**H**' for hard copy, press **ENTER**, and the Open Items list will be printed. **EXIT** to return to the Display Patient Data screen.

STEP 3

Option 5: All Scheduled Appointments. From the Display Patient Data screen, key option '**5**', Appointment, and press **ENTER**. Key '**H**' for hard copy and press **ENTER**. Key '**C**' for current and press **ENTER**; the list of all scheduled appointments for this account will be printed. **EXIT** to return to the Display Patient Data screen.

STEP 4

Option 6: Information on Hospital Stay. From the Display Patient Data screen, key option '**6**', Hospital, and press **ENTER**. Key '**H**' for hard copy, press **ENTER**, and the Information on Hospital Stay will be printed. Press **ENTER** to return to the Display Patient Data screen.

STEP 5

Option 9: Information on All Charges and Payments Posted. From the Display Patient Data screen, key option '**9**', Financial History, and press **ENTER**. Key '**H**' for hard copy, press **ENTER**, and the Financial History for this account will be printed. Press **ESCAPE** or click on the EXIT button on the top toolbar until you return to the Main Menu (Menu 1).

PERIOD CLOSE AND PERIOD CLOSE WITH PURGE

At the end of each billing period, usually once a month, medical offices complete a Period Close. This activity is option 1 on the System Utility Menu (Menu 3).

During the closing activity, all paid-off items are purged from outstanding accounts. This allows you to start the new billing period with accounts up to date.

In the Student Edition, the Period Close and Period Close with Purge will not be performed. However, it is important to note that both of these activities reset the financial figures for each doctor in the practice. These figures represent the doctors' financial totals for the current billing period. These are the same numbers included on the summary page of each Daily Close. The Period Close and Period Close with Purge reset each doctor's financial totals to zero ($0.00) in order to start the new period over.

UNIT 8 SUMMARY

Occasionally, an account or an item on an account is overpaid. This sometimes occurs because duplicate payments are received from both the patient and primary or secondary insurance plans. When this occurs, one or more of the parties who have made the payments will request a refund. **The Medical Manager's** payment module allows you to record the refund of the overpayment.

It is also unfortunately true that patient checks are sometimes returned for nonsufficient funds (NSF). In these instances, the items have usually been daily closed, and therefore, it is necessary to reinstate the balances on the account using a multistep process. The first step is to reverse the credits on each line item that was paid by the NSF check. Once this is completed, the total of the reversed credits will be shown as "unapplied credit". In the next step, the total unapplied credit is refunded into a special category that indicates a bad check. No refund check is sent to the patient as NSF is a special category used to indicate a bad check.

When insurance plans or patients pay off a large number of items on an account, a high-speed, automatic payment feature, referred to as 'Auto Pay', can be used to distribute automatically the check amount across a series of items beginning with the oldest item first. The Auto Pay feature saves the medical office assistant the time it would take to apply these amounts to each line item individually on the account.

Lost claim forms are not uncommon among insurance carriers. The payment module also has a Rebill feature that allows the system to generate a new copy of the insurance claim the next time insurance bills are printed. This is done by posting a zero dollar adjustment for payment and, at the transfer option, choosing 'R' for rebill.

An important part of the medical office assistant's job is to answer queries from patients who call for information about their health or their account. The Display Patient Information module allows you to retrieve and view on screen many different types of information about the patient. Information includes the ability to view insurance coverage, open items, payments made on those items, total check payments received and how they have been applied, as well as appointments, recalls, and many clinical results of the system.

Aging reports span multiple accounts and provide a special view of the system by organizing data according to how long unpaid items have been the responsibility of the guarantor or insurance. Aging reports are useful in allowing the practice to determine how long unpaid or partially paid items have been on the books.

At the end of each month, the practice performs a period financial close of the system. This serves the function of totaling the doctor's revenue receipts and adjustments for the calendar month and allows the doctor's totals for the next month to begin anew.

This comprehensive exercise will enable you and your instructor to evaluate your understanding of **The Medical Manager** software. Complete each procedure using the instructions and other information provided. For clarity, each procedure in this section is listed as a separate step. Refer to previous units for any other supporting material you may need. When you have completed the exercises, give your completed Daily Close Reports, System Financial Summary Report, and Summary Aging Report by Patient to your instructor.

Note: It may take more than one class session to complete the Comprehensive Evaluation. Do not begin an exercise if you will not have enough time to complete it. If you make an error, go to the appropriate File Maintenance program and correct it, before moving on to the next exercise.

STEP 1 Advancing the Date

Before you begin the Comprehensive Evaluation, you must advance the system date to April 7, 2003. This must be done when you log onto **The Medical Manager**. If you are already logged on, you must exit **The Medical Manager**, and reenter your name and password. When the prompt that begins "Enter Today's Date..." appears, key '**04072003**' and press **ENTER**. Press '**Y**' to continue when you see the warning message that the Daily Close has not been done. Under normal office conditions, you would *never* advance the date without first performing a Daily Close. However, for the purposes of this exercise, you may do so.

STEP 2 Adding an Account

The next account for you to enter is for Mr. Joseph Hughes, patient '200'. At New Patient Entry, enter '**?Hughes**' in the field labeled Enter Guarantor Last Name, and press **ENTER** to make sure Mr. Hughes is not already in the system. Since he is not, press **ESCAPE** to continue entering Joseph Hughes's account. The account information is shown In Figure 8-41. You will also add his wife, Sarah. Her patient information is shown in Figure 8-42. Add both family members in this step.

up to mrs. hughes info

Figure 8-41 Joseph Hughes—Patient Registration Form

Patient Registration Form

Sydney Carrington & Associates
34 Sycamore Street ● Madison, CA 95653

FOR OFFICE USE ONLY	
ACCOUNT NO.:	**200**
DOCTOR:	**#1**
BILL TYPE:	**11**
EXTENDED INFO.:	**2**

TODAY'S DATE: _04/07/2003_

PATIENT INFORMATION

Hughes   _Joseph_   _P._
PATIENT LAST NAME   FIRST NAME   MI

Self
RELATIONSHIP TO GUARANTOR

_M_ | _03/09/1974_ | _Married_ | _809-32-7546_
SEX (M/F)   DATE OF BIRTH   MARITAL STATUS   SOC. SEC. #

Current Manufacturing Co.
EMPLOYER OR SCHOOL NAME

9560 Albian Road
ADDRESS OF EMPLOYER OR SCHOOL

Madison | _CA_ | _95653_
CITY   STATE   ZIP CODE

_(916) 544-5639_   _Leland Groves, M.D._
EMPLOYER OR SCHOOL PHONE   REFERRED BY

E-MAIL

GUARANTOR INFORMATION

Hughes   _Joseph_   _P._ | _M_
RESPONSIBLE PARTY LAST NAME   FIRST NAME   MI   SEX (M/F)

1916 Willow Court
MAILING ADDRESS   STREET ADDRESS (IF DIFFERENT)

Madison   _CA_ | _95653_
CITY   STATE   ZIP CODE

_(916) 678-8205_   _(916) 544-5639_
(AREA CODE) HOME PHONE   (AREA CODE) WORK PHONE

_03/09/1974_ | _Married_ | _809-32-7546_
DATE OF BIRTH   MARITAL STATUS   SOC. SEC. #

Current Manufacturing Co.
EMPLOYER NAME

9560 Albian Road
EMPLOYER ADDRESS

Madison | _CA_ | _95653_
CITY   STATE   ZIP CODE

PRIMARY INSURANCE

Cross and Shield Ins. Plan
NAME OF PRIMARY INSURANCE COMPANY

435 Embarcadero
ADDRESS

Madison | _CA_ | _95653_
CITY   STATE   ZIP CODE

_5787653434_   _Current Manufacturing Co._
IDENTIFICATION #   GROUP NAME AND/OR #

Same
INSURED PERSON'S NAME (IF DIFFERENT FROM THE RESPONSIBLE PARTY)

Same
ADDRESS (IF DIFFERENT)

Same |
CITY   STATE   ZIP CODE

_(800) 345-7689_   _809-32-7546_
PRIMARY INSURANCE PHONE NUMBER   SOC. SEC. #

Self
WHAT IS THE RESPONSIBLE PARTY'S RELATIONSHIP TO THE INSURED?

SECONDARY INSURANCE

NAME OF SECONDARY INSURANCE COMPANY

ADDRESS

CITY   STATE   ZIP CODE

IDENTIFICATION #   GROUP NAME AND/OR #

INSURED PERSON'S NAME (IF DIFFERENT FROM THE RESPONSIBLE PARTY)

ADDRESS (IF DIFFERENT)

CITY   STATE   ZIP CODE

SECONDARY INSURANCE PHONE NUMBER   SOC. SEC. #

WHAT IS THE RESPONSIBLE PARTY'S RELATIONSHIP TO THE INSURED?

I hereby consent for Sydney Carrington & Associates, P.A. to use or disclose my health information to carry out treatment, payment, and health care operations. I authorize the use of this signature on all insurance submissions. I understand that I am financially responsible for all charges whether or not paid by the insurance. I acknowledge receipt of the practice's privacy policy.

Joseph P. Hughes   _04/07/2003_
PATIENT SIGNATURE   DATE

Figure 8-42 Sarah Hughes—Patient Registration Form

Pt. Id #?

Patient Registration Form

Sydney Carrington & Associates
34 Sycamore Street ● Madison, CA 95653

TODAY'S DATE: ___04/07/2003___

FOR OFFICE USE ONLY	
ACCOUNT NO.:	**200**
DOCTOR:	**#1**
BILL TYPE:	**11**
EXTENDED INFO.:	**2**

PATIENT INFORMATION

Hughes	Sarah	
PATIENT LAST NAME	FIRST NAME	MI

Wife
RELATIONSHIP TO GUARANTOR

F	05/29/1975	Married	256-78-6314
SEX (M/F)	DATE OF BIRTH	MARITAL STATUS	SOC. SEC. #

Elias Boutique
EMPLOYER OR SCHOOL NAME

7532 Welton Street
ADDRESS OF EMPLOYER OR SCHOOL

Madison	CA	95653
CITY	STATE	ZIP CODE

(916) 233-1490	Leland Groves, M.D.
EMPLOYER OR SCHOOL PHONE	REFERRED BY

E-MAIL

GUARANTOR INFORMATION

Hughes	Joseph	P.	M
RESPONSIBLE PARTY LAST NAME	FIRST NAME	MI	SEX (M/F)

1916 Willow Court
| MAILING ADDRESS | STREET ADDRESS (IF DIFFERENT) |

Madison	CA	95653
CITY	STATE	ZIP CODE

(916) 678-8205	(916) 544-5639
(AREA CODE) HOME PHONE	(AREA CODE) WORK PHONE

03/09/1974	Married	809-32-7546
DATE OF BIRTH	MARITAL STATUS	SOC. SEC. #

Current Manufacturing Co.
EMPLOYER NAME

9560 Albian Road
EMPLOYER ADDRESS

Madison	CA	95653
CITY	STATE	ZIP CODE

PRIMARY INSURANCE

Cross and Shield Ins. Plan
NAME OF PRIMARY INSURANCE COMPANY

435 Embarcadero
ADDRESS

Madison	CA	95653
CITY	STATE	ZIP CODE

5787653434	Current Manufacturing Co.
IDENTIFICATION #	GROUP NAME AND/OR #

Joseph P. Hughes
INSURED PERSON'S NAME (IF DIFFERENT FROM THE RESPONSIBLE PARTY)

1916 Willow Court
ADDRESS (IF DIFFERENT)

Madison	CA	95653
CITY	STATE	ZIP CODE

(800) 345-7689	809-32-7546
PRIMARY INSURANCE PHONE NUMBER	SOC. SEC. #

Self
WHAT IS THE RESPONSIBLE PARTY'S RELATIONSHIP TO THE INSURED?

SECONDARY INSURANCE

NAME OF SECONDARY INSURANCE COMPANY

ADDRESS

CITY	STATE	ZIP CODE

IDENTIFICATION #	GROUP NAME AND/OR #

INSURED PERSON'S NAME (IF DIFFERENT FROM THE RESPONSIBLE PARTY)

ADDRESS (IF DIFFERENT)

CITY	STATE	ZIP CODE

SECONDARY INSURANCE PHONE NUMBER	SOC. SEC. #

WHAT IS THE RESPONSIBLE PARTY'S RELATIONSHIP TO THE INSURED?

I hereby consent for Sydney Carrington & Associates, P.A. to use or disclose my health information to carry out treatment, payment, and health care operations. I authorize the use of this signature on all insurance submissions. I understand that I am financially responsible for all charges whether or not paid by the insurance. I acknowledge receipt of the practice's privacy policy.

Sarah Hughes	04/07/2003
PATIENT SIGNATURE	DATE

STEP 3   **Posting Procedures**

The patient to be treated is Mr. Hughes's wife, Sarah. Once you are at the Procedure Entry Patient Retrieval screen, key in '**200.1**' and press **ENTER** to begin the exercise. Enter the information from the encounter form shown in Figure 8-43.

Figure 8-43 Sarah Hughes's Encounter Form—Voucher 1100

Sydney Carrington & Associates P.A.
34 Sycamore Street   Suite 300
Madison, CA 95653

Date: 04/07/2003

Time: 11:00

Patient: Sarah Hughes
Guarantor: Joseph P. Hughes

Voucher No.: 1100

Patient No: 200.1
Doctor: 1 - J. Monroe

	CPT	DESCRIPTION	FEE		CPT	DESCRIPTION	FEE		CPT	DESCRIPTION	FEE
OFFICE/HOSPITAL CONSULTS				**LABORATORY/RADIOLOGY**				**PROCEDURES/TESTS**			
☐	99201	Office New:Focused Hx-Exam		☐	81000	Urinalysis		☐	00452	Anesthesia for Rad Surgery	
☐	99202	Office New:Expanded Hx-Exam		☐	81002	Urinalysis; Pregnancy Test		☐	11100	Skin Biopsy	
☐	99211	Office Estb:Min/None Hx-Exa		☐	82951	Glucose Tolerance Test		☐	15852	Dressing Change	
☐	99212	Office Estb:Focused Hx-Exam		☐	84478	Triglycerides		☐	29075	Cast Appl. - Lower Arm	
☒	99213	Office Estb:Expanded Hx-Exa	$40.00	☐	84550	Uric Acid: Blood Chemistry		☐	29530	Strapping of Knee	
☐	99214	Office Estb:Detailed Hx-Exa		☐	84830	Ovulation Test		☐	29705	Removal/Revis of Cast w/Exa	
☐	99215	Office Estb:Comprhn Hx-Exam		☐	85014	Hematocrit		☐	53670	Catheterization Incl. Suppl	
☐	99221	Hosp. Initial:Comprh Hx-		☐	85031	Hemogram, Complete Blood Wk		☐	57452	Colposcopy	
☐	99223	Hosp.Ini:Comprh Hx-Exam/Hi		☐	86403	Particle Agglutination Test		☐	57505	ECC	
☐	99231	Hosp. Subsequent: S-Fwd		☐	86485	Skin Test; Candida		☐	69420	Myringotomy	
☐	99232	Hosp. Subsequent: Comprhn Hx		☐	86580	TB Intradermal Test		☐	92081	Visual Field Examination	
☐	99233	Hosp. Subsequent: Ex/Hi		☐	86585	TB Tine Test		☐	92100	Serial Tonometry Exam	
☐	99238	Hospital Visit Discharge Ex		☐	87070	Culture		☐	92120	Tonography	
☐	99371	Telephone Consult - Simple		☐	70190	X-Ray; Optic Foramina		☐	92552	Pure Tone Audiometry	
☐	99372	Telephone Consult - Intermed		☐	70210	X-Ray Sinuses Complete		☐	92567	Tympanometry	
☐	99373	Telephone Consult - Complex		☐	71010	Radiological Exam Ent Spine		☐	93000	Electrocardiogram	
☐	90843	Counseling - 25 minutes		☐	71020	X-Ray Chest Pa & Lat		☐	93015	Exercise Stress Test (ETT)	
☐	90844	Counseling - 50 minutes		☐	72050	X-Ray Spine, Cerv (4 views)		☐	93017	ETT Tracing Only	
☐	90865	Counseling - Special Interview		☐	72090	X-Ray Spine; Scoliosis Ex		☐	93040	Electrocardiogram - Rhythm	
				☐	72110	Spine, lumbosacral; a/p & Lat		☐	96100	Psychological Testing	
IMMUNIZATIONS/INJECTIONS				☐	73030	Shoulder-Comp, min w/ 2vws		☐	99000	Specimen Handling	
☐	90585	BCG Vaccine		☐	73070	Elbow, anteropost & later vws		☐	99058	Office Emergency Care	
☐	90659	Influenza Virus Vaccine		☐	73120	X-Ray; Hand, 2 views		☐	99070	Surgical Tray - Misc.	
☒	90701	Immunization-DTP	$14.00	☐	73560	X-Ray, Knee, 1 or 2 views		☐	99080	Special Reports of Med Rec	
☐	90702	DT Vaccine		☐	74022	X-Ray; Abdomen, Complete		☐	99195	Phlebotomy	
☐	90703	Tetanus Toxoids		☐	75552	Cardiac Magnetic Res Img		☐			
☐	90732	Pneumococcal Vaccine		☐	76020	X-Ray; Bone Age Studies		☐			
☐	90746	Hepatitis B Vaccine		☐	76088	Mammary Ductogram Complete		☐			
☐	90749	Immunization; Unlisted		☐	78465	Myocardial Perfusion Img		☐			

		ICD-9 CODE DIAGNOSIS			**ICD-9 CODE DIAGNOSIS**			**ICD-9 CODE DIAGNOSIS**
☐	009.0	Ill-defined Intestinal Infect	☐	435.0	Basilar Artery Syndrome	☐	724.2	Pain: Lower Back
☐	133.2	Establish Baseline	☐	440.0	Atherosclerosis	☐	727.6	Rupture of Achilles Tendon
☐	174.9	Breast Cancer	☐	442.81	Carotid Artery	☐	780.1	Hallucinations
☐	185.0	Prostate Cancer	☒	460.0	Common Cold	☐	780.3	Convulsions
☐	250	Diabetes Mellitus	☐	461.9	Acute Sinusitis	☐	780.5	Sleep Disturbances
☐	272.4	Hyperlipidemia	☐	474.0	Tonsillitis	☐	783.0	Anorexia
☐	282.5	Anemia - Sickle Trait	☐	477.9	Hay Fever	☐	783.1	Abnormal Weight Gain
☐	282.60	Anemia - Sickle Cell	☐	487.0	Flu	☐	783.2	Abnormal Weight Loss
☐	285.9	Anemia, Unspecified	☐	496	Chronic Airway Obstruction	☐	830.6	Dislocated Hip
☐	300.4	Neurotic Depression	☐	522	Low Red Blood Count	☐	830.9	Dislocated Shoulder
☐	340	Multiple Sclerosis	☐	524.6	Temporo-Mandibular Jnt Synd	☐	841.2	Sprained Wrist
☐	342.9	Hemiplegia - Unspecified	☐	538.8	Stomach Pain	☐	842.5	Sprained Ankle
☐	346.9	Migraine Headache	☐	553.3	Hiatal Hernia	☐	891.2	Fractured Tibia
☐	352.9	Cranial Neuralgia	☐	564.1	Spastic Colon	☐	892.5	Fractured Fibula
☐	354.0	Carpal Tunnel Syndrome	☐	571.4	Chronic Hepatitis	☐	919.5	Insect Bite, Nonvenomous
☐	355.5	Sciatic Nerve Root Lesion	☐	571.5	Cirrhosis of Liver	☐	921.1	Contus Eyelid/Perioc Area
☐	366.9	Cataract	☐	573.3	Hepatitis	☐	v16.3	Fam. Hist of Breast Cancer
☐	386.0	Vertigo	☐	575.2	Obstruction of Gallbladder	☐	v17.4	Fam. Hist of Cardiovasc Dis
☐	401.1	Essential Hypertension	☐	648.2	Anemia - Compl. Pregnancy	☐	v20.2	Well Child
☐	414.9	Ischemic Hearth Disease	☐	715.90	Osteoarthritis - Unspec	☐	v22.0	Pregnancy - First Normal
☐	428.0	Congestive Heart Failure	☐	721.3	Lumbar Osteo/Spondylarthrit	☐	v22.1	Pregnancy - Normal

Previous Balance	Today's Charges	Total Due	Amount Paid	New Balance
0.00	54.00	54.00	0.00	54.00

Follow Up

PRN _____ Weeks _____   Months _____ Units _____

Next Appointment Date: _____   Time: _____

I hereby authorize release of any information acquired in the course of
examination or treatment and allow a photocopy of my signature to be used.

7. File Maintenance

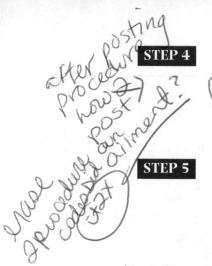

STEP 4 | ## Posting Ailment Detail

Post an ailment detail for Mrs. Hughes. Mrs. Hughes's illness, a common cold, is not at all related to her employment. The date of her first symptom is '**04/03/03**'. The date of her first consultation is '**04/07/03**'.

STEP 5 | ## Printing A Trial Daily Report

Print the Trial Daily Reports for April 7. Samples of the Trial Daily Reports are not provided for this exercise. Verify your work as you would in a medical office by comparing the amounts on the Trial Daily Report with the source documents; in this case, the encounter form.

STEP 6 | ## Performing a Final Daily Close

After you have checked the Trial Daily Report for accuracy, run a Final Daily Close for April 7.

STEP 7 | ## Advancing the Date

After you complete the Daily Close, advance the date to April 14.

STEP 8 | ## Adding a Dependent to an Existing Account

Mr. and Mrs. Hughes want to add their infant son, **Ryan**, to the account as an additional dependent. Ryan's date of birth is '**08/10/2002**'. His Social Security number is '**713-48-1365**' (Figure 8-44).

STEP 9 | ## Scheduling an Appointment

Schedule **Ryan** for a General Check-Up at **10:00** A.M. in two weeks.

Figure 8-44 Ryan Hughes—Patient Registration Form

Patient Registration Form

Sydney Carrington & Associates
34 Sycamore Street ● Madison, CA 95653

TODAY'S DATE: _04/14/2003_

PATIENT INFORMATION

Hughes	*Ryan*	
PATIENT LAST NAME	FIRST NAME	MI

Son

RELATIONSHIP TO GUARANTOR

M	*08/10/2002*	*Single*	*713-48-1365*
SEX (M/F)	DATE OF BIRTH	MARITAL STATUS	SOC. SEC. #

EMPLOYER OR SCHOOL NAME

ADDRESS OF EMPLOYER OR SCHOOL

CITY	STATE	ZIP CODE
	Leland Groves, M.D.	
EMPLOYER OR SCHOOL PHONE	REFERRED BY	

E-MAIL

GUARANTOR INFORMATION

Hughes	*Joseph*	*P.*	*M*
RESPONSIBLE PARTY LAST NAME	FIRST NAME	MI	SEX (M/F)

1916 Willow Court

MAILING ADDRESS		STREET ADDRESS (IF DIFFERENT)
Madison	*CA*	*95653*
CITY	STATE	ZIP CODE

(916)678-8205	*(916) 544-5639*
(AREA CODE) HOME PHONE	(AREA CODE) WORK PHONE

03/09/1974	*Married*	*809-32-7546*
DATE OF BIRTH	MARITAL STATUS	SOC. SEC. #

Current Manufacturing Co.

EMPLOYER NAME

9560 Albian Road

EMPLOYER ADDRESS

Madison	*CA*	*95653*
CITY	STATE	ZIP CODE

PRIMARY INSURANCE

Cross and Shield Ins. Plan

NAME OF PRIMARY INSURANCE COMPANY

435 Embarcadero

ADDRESS

Madison	*CA*	*95653*
CITY	STATE	ZIP CODE

5787653434	*Current Manufacturing Co.*
IDENTIFICATION #	GROUP NAME AND/OR #

Joseph P. Hughes

INSURED PERSON'S NAME (IF DIFFERENT FROM THE RESPONSIBLE PARTY)

1916 Willow Court

ADDRESS (IF DIFFERENT)

Madison	*CA*	*95653*
CITY	STATE	ZIP CODE

(800) 345-7689	*809-32-7546*
PRIMARY INSURANCE PHONE NUMBER	SOC. SEC. #

Self

WHAT IS THE RESPONSIBLE PARTY'S RELATIONSHIP TO THE INSURED?

SECONDARY INSURANCE

NAME OF SECONDARY INSURANCE COMPANY

ADDRESS

CITY	STATE	ZIP CODE

IDENTIFICATION #	GROUP NAME AND/OR #

INSURED PERSON'S NAME (IF DIFFERENT FROM THE RESPONSIBLE PARTY)

ADDRESS (IF DIFFERENT)

CITY	STATE	ZIP CODE

SECONDARY INSURANCE PHONE NUMBER	SOC. SEC. #

WHAT IS THE RESPONSIBLE PARTY'S RELATIONSHIP TO THE INSURED?

I hereby consent for Sydney Carrington & Associates, P.A. to use or disclose my health information to carry out treatment, payment, and health care operations. I authorize the use of this signature on all insurance submissions. I understand that I am financially responsible for all charges whether or not paid by the insurance. I acknowledge receipt of the practice's privacy policy.

Sarah Hughes (Mother)	*04/14/2003*
PATIENT SIGNATURE	DATE

STEP 10   Posting Procedures and a Patient Payment

Post the procedures listed on Mr. Hughes's encounter form (Figure 8-45), as well as a patient payment. (See Figure 8-46 for Joseph's check.) *Remember to select* '**P**' *for (P)at Due Estimate to calculate the amount of the charges Joseph Hughes is required to pay* **BEFORE** *you exit completely out of procedure entry.* Press **ENTER** at each of the amount fields to accept the default values calculated by the system. Using Figure 8-46, indicate the payment will be made by (**C**)heck, enter the voucher number on the check and other pertinent information, then **PROCESS**.

STEP 11   Posting a Return Appointment

Post a return appointment for Mr. Hughes. Refer to his encounter form for additional information.

STEP 12   Adding a Patient to Hospital Rounds

Joseph Hughes was given a Hospital Admission Physical during his visit on service (facility **4**) April 14, 2003. As a result of Mr. Hughes's back pain, Dr. Monroe would like to admit him to the hospital service (facility **4**) for further diagnostic tests. Add Mr. Hughes to Hospital Rounds. He is expected to be in the hospital for only one day. Remember to press **ENTER** to bypass any fields for which information is not provided.

STEP 13   Printing a Hospital Rounds Report

Print a Hospital Rounds Report for **Dr. James Monroe** for service facility **4**, Regional Hospital of Madison.

STEP 14   Printing a Daily List of Appointments

Create a daily list of appointments for **April 28, 2003** for **Dr. James Monroe**.

STEP 15   Printing a Daily Report

Run the Trial Daily Report for **April 14, 2003**. Do not perform a Final Daily Close at this time.

Figure 8-45 Joseph Hughes's Encounter Form—Voucher 1101

Sydney Carrington & Associates P.A.
34 Sycamore Street   Suite 300
Madison, CA 95653

Date: 04/14/2003

Time: 11:00

Patient: Joseph Hughes
Guarantor: Joseph P. Hughes

Voucher No.:   1101

Patient No: 200.0
Doctor: 1 - J. Monroe

	CPT	DESCRIPTION	FEE
	OFFICE/HOSPITAL CONSULTS		
☐	99201	Office New:Focused Hx-Exam	___
☐	99202	Office New:Expanded Hx-Exam	___
☐	99211	Office Estb:Min/None Hx-Exa	___
☐	99212	Office Estb:Focused Hx-Exam	___
☐	99213	Office Estb:Expanded Hx-Exa	___
☐	99214	Office Estb:Detailed Hx-Exa	___
☐	99215	Office Estb:Comprhn Hx-Exam	___
☐	99221	Hosp. Initial:Comprh Hx-	___
☒	99223	Hosp.Ini:Comprh Hx-Exam/Hi	$94.00
☐	99231	Hosp. Subsequent: S-Fwd	___
☐	99232	Hosp. Subsequent: Comprhn Hx	___
☐	99233	Hosp. Subsequent: Ex/Hi	___
☐	99238	Hospital Visit Discharge Ex	___
☐	99371	Telephone Consult - Simple	___
☐	99372	Telephone Consult - Intermed	___
☐	99373	Telephone Consult - Complex	___
☐	90843	Counseling - 25 minutes	___
☐	90844	Counseling - 50 minutes	___
☐	90865	Counseling - Special Interview	___
	IMMUNIZATIONS/INJECTIONS		
☐	90585	BCG Vaccine	___
☐	90659	Influenza Virus Vaccine	___
☐	90701	Immunization-DTP	___
☐	90702	DT Vaccine	___
☐	90703	Tetanus Toxoids	___
☐	90732	Pneumococcal Vaccine	___
☐	90746	Hepatitis B Vaccine	___
☐	90749	Immunization; Unlisted	___

	CPT	DESCRIPTION	FEE
	LABORATORY/RADIOLOGY		
☐	81000	Urinalysis	___
☐	81002	Urinalysis; Pregnancy Test	___
☐	82951	Glucose Tolerance Test	___
☐	84478	Triglycerides	___
☐	84550	Uric Acid: Blood Chemistry	___
☐	84830	Ovulation Test	___
☐	85014	Hematocrit	___
☐	85031	Hemogram, Complete Blood Wk	___
☐	86403	Particle Agglutination Test	___
☐	86485	Skin Test; Candida	___
☐	86580	TB Intradermal Test	___
☐	86585	TB Tine Test	___
☐	87070	Culture	___
☐	70190	X-Ray; Optic Foramina	___
☐	70210	X-Ray Sinuses Complete	___
☐	71010	Radiological Exam Ent Spine	___
☐	71020	X-Ray Chest Pa & Lat	___
☒	72050	X-Ray Spine, Cerv (4 views)	$150.00
☐	72090	X-Ray Spine; Scoliosis Ex	___
☐	72110	Spine, lumbosacral; a/p & Lat	___
☐	73030	Shoulder-Comp, min w/ 2vws	___
☐	73070	Elbow, anteropost & later vws	___
☐	73120	X-Ray; Hand, 2 views	___
☐	73560	X-Ray, Knee, 1 or 2 views	___
☐	74022	X-Ray; Abdomen, Complete	___
☐	75552	Cardiac Magnetic Res Img	___
☐	76020	X-Ray; Bone Age Studies	___
☐	76088	Mammary Ductogram Complete	___
☐	78465	Myocardial Perfusion Img	___

	CPT	DESCRIPTION	FEE
	PROCEDURES/TESTS		
☐	00452	Anesthesia for Rad Surgery	___
☐	11100	Skin Biopsy	___
☐	15852	Dressing Change	___
☐	29075	Cast Appl. - Lower Arm	___
☐	29530	Strapping of Knee	___
☐	29705	Removal/Revis of Cast w/Exa	___
☐	53670	Catheterization Incl. Suppl	___
☐	57452	Colposcopy	___
☐	57505	ECC	___
☐	69420	Myringotomy	___
☐	92081	Visual Field Examination	___
☐	92100	Serial Tonometry Exam	___
☐	92120	Tonography	___
☐	92552	Pure Tone Audiometry	___
☐	92567	Tympanometry	___
☐	93000	Electrocardiogram	___
☐	93015	Exercise Stress Test (ETT)	___
☐	93017	ETT Tracing Only	___
☐	93040	Electrocardiogram - Rhythm	___
☐	96100	Psychological Testing	___
☐	99000	Specimen Handling	___
☐	99058	Office Emergency Care	___
☐	99070	Surgical Tray - Misc.	___
☐	99080	Special Reports of Med Rec	___
☐	99195	Phlebotomy	___
☐	___	_____	___
☐	___	_____	___
☐	___	_____	___

	ICD-9 CODE DIAGNOSIS	
☐	009.0	Ill-defined Intestinal Infect
☐	133.2	Establish Baseline
☐	174.9	Breast Cancer
☐	185.0	Prostate Cancer
☐	250	Diabetes Mellitus
☐	272.4	Hyperlipidemia
☐	282.5	Anemia - Sickle Trait
☐	282.60	Anemia - Sickle Cell
☐	285.9	Anemia, Unspecified
☐	300.4	Neurotic Depression
☐	340	Multiple Sclerosis
☐	342.9	Hemiplegia - Unspecified
☐	346.9	Migraine Headache
☐	352.9	Cranial Neuralgia
☐	354.0	Carpal Tunnel Syndrome
☐	355.0	Sciatic Nerve Root Lesion
☐	366.9	Cataract
☐	386.0	Vertigo
☐	401.1	Essential Hypertension
☐	414.9	Ischemic Hearth Disease
☐	428.0	Congestive Heart Failure

	ICD-9 CODE DIAGNOSIS	
☐	435.0	Basilar Artery Syndrome
☐	440.0	Atherosclerosis
☐	442.81	Carotid Artery
☐	460.0	Common Cold
☐	461.9	Acute Sinusitis
☐	474.0	Tonsillitis
☐	477.9	Hay Fever
☐	487.0	Flu
☐	496	Chronic Airway Obstruction
☐	522	Low Red Blood Count
☐	524.6	Temporo-Mandibular Jnt Synd
☐	538.8	Stomach Pain
☐	553.3	Hiatal Hernia
☐	564.1	Spastic Colon
☐	571.4	Chronic Hepatitis
☐	571.5	Cirrhosis of Liver
☐	573.3	Hepatitis
☐	575.2	Obstruction of Gallbladder
☐	648.2	Anemia - Compl. Pregnancy
☐	715.90	Osteoarthritis - Unspec
☐	721.3	Lumbar Osteo/Spondylarthrit

	ICD-9 CODE DIAGNOSIS	
☒	724.2	Pain: Lower Back
☐	727.6	Rupture of Achilles Tendon
☐	780.1	Hallucinations
☐	780.3	Convulsions
☐	780.5	Sleep Disturbances
☐	783.0	Anorexia
☐	783.1	Abnormal Weight Gain
☐	783.2	Abnormal Weight Loss
☐	830.6	Dislocated Hip
☐	830.9	Dislocated Shoulder
☐	841.2	Sprained Wrist
☐	842.5	Sprained Ankle
☐	891.2	Fractured Tibia
☐	892.0	Fractured Fibula
☐	919.5	Insect Bite, Nonvenomous
☐	921.1	Contus Eyelid/Perioc Area
☐	v16.3	Fam. Hist of Breast Cancer
☐	v17.4	Fam. Hist of Cardiovasc Dis
☐	v20.2	Well Child
☐	v22.0	Pregnancy - First Normal
☐	v22.1	Pregnancy - Normal

Previous Balance	Today's Charges	Total Due	Amount Paid	New Balance
54.00	244.00	298.00	48.80	249.20

Follow Up

PRN _____ Weeks ___2___ Months _____ Units _____

Next Appointment Date: 04/28/03   Time: 10:00 a.m.
General check-up

I hereby authorize release of any information acquired in the course of examination or treatment and allow a photocopy of my signature to be used.

_____

Figure 8-46 Joseph Hughes's Check—Voucher 1356

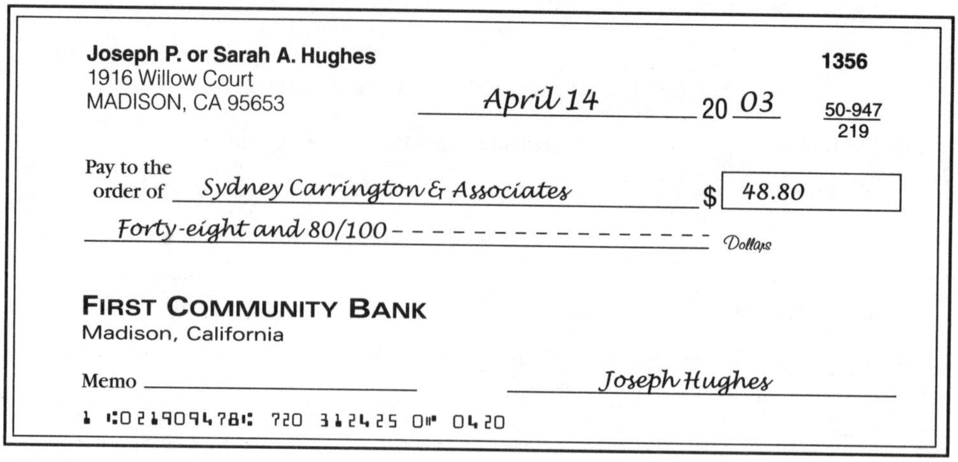

Joseph P. or Sarah A. Hughes	**1356**
1916 Willow Court	
MADISON, CA 95653	_April 14_ 20 _03_ 50-947 / 219

Pay to the order of _Sydney Carrington & Associates_ $ | 48.80 |

Forty-eight and 80/100 - - - - - - - - - - - - - - - - - Dollars

FIRST COMMUNITY BANK
Madison, California

Memo _____   _Joseph Hughes_

⑈ ⑈⑈021909478⑈ 720 312425 0⑈ 0420

STEP 16

Running a System Summary Report

Run a System Summary Report for (**A**)ll doctors.

STEP 17

Running an Account Aging Report

Run a (**D**)etailed Aging Report for Joseph Hughes's account.

STEP 18

Performing a Final Daily Close and Advancing the Date

Run a Final Daily Close for **April 14, 2003**. Advance the date to **April 15, 2003**.

Note: Remember to give your completed Final Daily Close Reports, Hospital Rounds Report, System Financial Summary Report, and Summary Aging Report by Patient to your instructor.

U N I T 9

Today's Medical Office

LEARNING OUTCOMES

After completing this unit, you should be able to:

◆ Describe the importance of information systems in a medical office.
◆ Explain how computers assist offices with changes in health care.
◆ Discuss the role of computers in communicating medical information.
◆ Discuss the clinical aspects of the medical office.
◆ Discuss Patient Privacy Regulations in the medical office.
◆ Describe the Health Insurance Portability and Accountability Act (HIPAA).
◆ Describe additional modules of **The Medical Manager** system and how they interrelate.

This course has shown how you can use **The Medical Manager** to meet the needs of a medical practice where you will be employed. As you have already learned, successful medical software must be capable of a variety of functions necessary to manage effectively a medical practice.

Today's medical offices have witnessed a steady pressure to move from the practice of medicine to the practice of office management, and now to the practice of information management. Changes in health care, billing methods, managed care, and governmental regulations require the adaptability, power, and organizational skills of a *modern* medical computer system such as the one you have just learned. However, the software must also be flexible, configurable, and adaptable to manage the ever-occurring changes in health care.

This unit explains some of the changes taking place in the health care industry and how you will be able to expand the skills you have learned with **The Medical Manager** software to help modernize the practice of medicine. Unit 9 also discusses an important federal law, the Health Insurance Portability and Accountability Act, also known as HIPAA.

ELECTRONIC DATA INTERCHANGE

Most people have used an ATM machine to withdraw money from a bank account or used a credit card and waited while their account was verified and their purchase approved. These are both examples of Electronic Data Interchange, or EDI in the banking world. In health care, EDI will become equally as important in the future.

What is Electronic Data Interchange (EDI)?

EDI provides instant, on-line connectivity to the world outside your office.

EDI is the ability to request, receive, transfer, and integrate information electronically. Electronic data interchanges connect your practice with insurance companies, hospitals, laboratories, and third-party connectivity networks. Available functions include patient referral, preauthorization and eligibility, credit card and check approval, claim status checking, electronic mail, and pharmacy and clinical data transmission. Instant online connectivity to the world outside your office ensures accurate referrals, up-to-date eligibility information, and immediate medical data.

What is an Electronic Media Claim (EMC)?

EMC allows claims to be submitted electronically, using EDI.

Electronic Media Claims (EMC), which are sometimes called *paperless claims,* allow you to submit electronic claims directly to a variety of dissimilar insurance carriers, just as you have learned to print paper claims in this class. This speeds the processing of claims, saves printing paper forms, and saves mailing fees. Electronic Media Claims are used in most offices using **The Medical Manager** and will most likely be available where you will work.

What is Electronic Remittance Advice (ERA)?

ERA eliminates the need to manually post payments.

Electronic Remittance Advice (ERA) uses information received from insurance companies about claims that have been adjudicated and paid to post payments and adjustments to patient accounts automatically. Medicare, Blue Cross/Blue Shield, and many other carriers currently can send a file to **The Medical Manager**. Offices that use this feature can save you time and make your job easier by eliminating the need for you to manually post payments from a paper Explanation of Benefits (EOB) statement, as you learned in Units 6 and 7.

Eligibility

Electronic eligibility checks patient eligibility and referral authorization in minutes.

Electronic eligibility and referral verification capabilities are particularly important to managed care practices. The ability for a primary care physician to receive his or her patient roster electronically instead of on paper is very valuable to the day-to-day operation of a practice. The capability to send the referral request electronically, check the patients' previously used plan limits, and have authorization in minutes, not days, is a tremendous asset in patient health care.

Even medical offices that are not primary care providers for managed care plans find electronic eligibility invaluable. The ability to verify a patient's insurance coverage, determine the correct visit copay amount, or the remaining deductible electronically rather than by phone saves a significant amount of time. Figure 9-1 shows a sample electronic eligibility screen.

E-Mail

Electronic mail provides the ability to send and receive messages even faster than a fax machine. This is called e-mail. When connected to an EDI network, e-mail allows you to send electronic messages to a wide variety of users in many different locations such as hospitals, insurance companies, other practices, and durable medical equipment supply companies, to name a few. This reduces paper handling and facilitates immediate communication. However, e-mail messages that contain patient information must only be transmitted using secure encryption. This differs from ordinary e-mail.

Figure 9-1 Sample Electronic Eligibility Screen

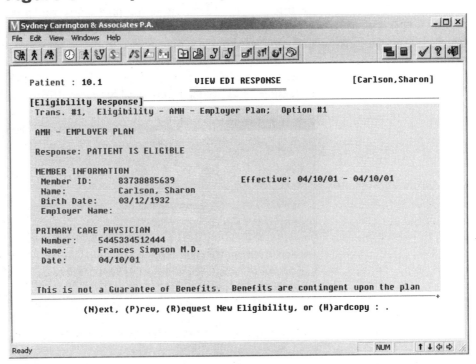

Med-Mail provides instantaneous internal communication, as well as connectivity to external e-mail networks.

Electronic mail systems give you powerful resources for performing both internal and external communications without leaving **The Medical Manager**. *Med-Mail*, the internal messaging system within **The Medical Manager** software, allows you to schedule meetings, send announcements and reminders, and share information with your staff. Incoming mail and attachments may be forwarded to either a Med-Mail user or to local e-mail networks.

Electronic Laboratory Interfaces

Electronic laboratory interfaces allow lab results to be entered automatically into the patient's medical records.

Electronic laboratory interfaces save time by allowing doctors to order tests directly from any terminal. The laboratory interface can help improve patient care by speeding the arrival of test results from the laboratory to your office. The laboratory downloads the test results directly into the patient's file within **The Medical Manager**, thus saving time and eliminating data entry errors.

The Internet

You are probably also familiar with the *Internet*, a worldwide network of computers that can be used to pass information from one computer to another until it reaches a destination determined by the sender. This allows information to be sent from a particular sender's computer to a particular recipient's computer almost any place in the world.

The Internet provides a method for unsecured communications throughout the world. Although useful for searching particular topics or transferring e-mail messages, it is not generally used for sensitive medical records. This is primarily because the number of different computers that pass messages along to their final destination makes data sent over the Internet neither private nor secure.

Intranets are private, secure EDI networks set up to work like the Internet, but within a private, closed network in which only the network participants can view the medical information. They generally offer higher reliability and better security. **The Medical Manager** and other practice management vendors have developed WebMD, a secure portal that allows physicians to view their patients' medical records from anywhere on the Internet. The advantage of this physician portal product is that it verifies the identity of the physician and scrambles data so that only the intended physician can read it. Figure 9-2 shows a sample screen from the physician portal.

Figure 9-2 Sample Patient Chart Viewed Through Physician Portal

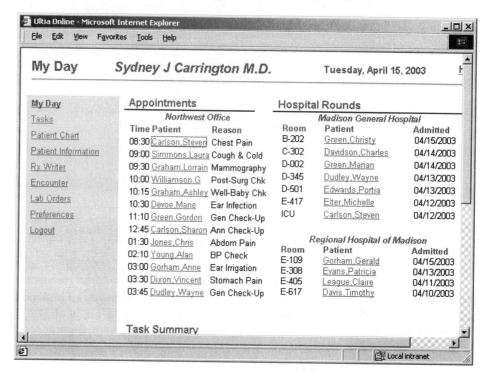

The Future of Electronic Data Interchange (EDI)

Electronic data interchange will continue to evolve in capability, and its usage will spread to other types of data. These will include connections to pharmacies, hospitals, and national medical databases. Physicians can already look up information for medical research in distant universities, or get online help from reputable clinics.

ELECTRONIC MEDICAL RECORDS

Automated records make delivering quality health care easier.

High-quality health care can be easier to deliver when a doctor has automated records and better resources with which to use them. As you learned in Unit 8, the clinical aspects of a patient's records are composed of many different types of medical information obtained from many different sources. Hospitals and universities currently have projects under development that are attempting to create and centralize electronic patient records.

Electronic Patient Charts

The Medical Manager software stores, organizes, and presents data on various aspects of a patient's medical history on demand. The ideal presentation of this data is

The Electronic Patient Chart provides the physician with a snapshot of the patient's medical record.

the *View Patient Chart* module which brings a snapshot of the patient's medical records to a single screen (Figure 9-3), and then gives the doctor instant access to almost any desired level of underlying detail. Each of 12 windows in the display access data from a particular type of medical records, such as vital signs, laboratory tests, medications, allergies, and procedure history.

Figure 9-3 Sample View Patient Chart Selection Screen

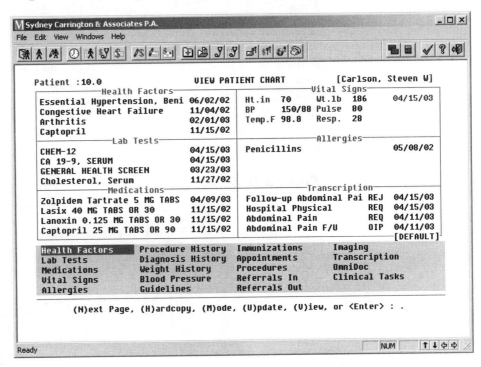

The ability to view the patient's chart elements simultaneously on a centralized display, and then bring up any needed background data with just the touch of a key, assists the physician in the examination room, the office, during dictation or chart review, and from home or hospital, as necessary.

Creating the Patient Chart

The ability to view the patient's chart must be preceded by the ability to capture the information electronically. Although electronic charts range from scanned documents to fully structured records that can be easily searched, the real question is how the information gets put into the patient's chart, by whom, and how accurately.

Electronic Laboratory Interfaces

Electronic interfaces provide the physician with patient laboratory results more quickly.

Some of the information in a patient's chart can be automatically imported, as is accomplished by the electronic laboratory interfaces discussed previously. These interfaces not only allow the doctor to order tests but to receive the results in the fastest manner possible. Results are automatically updated in the patient's record and retained for long-term comparison. The doctor, knowing the results sooner, can more quickly determine the course of the patient's treatment.

Chart History and Progress Notes

Other information can be determined from the daily posting of procedures and diagnoses, which you have learned to post in this class. Similar information will be automatically updated from the results of managed care referrals to specialists and facilities. However, much of the actual patient examination must be entered at the time the patient is seen, either as measurements taken by the nurse (weight, height, and temperature), or as transcription of the doctor's notes.

New technology is making the physician's job easier.

The examination information can be gathered in a variety of ways. New input devices are constantly being created and tested. One of the newest is the Tablet PC, which is a portable computer about the size of a notebook but with screens that are sensitive to the touch. Tapping on the screen with a special stylus selects and enters data. Similar technology in a smaller form is available in Ultia®, a *pocket PC* that fits in the palm of a doctor's hand, and uses a touch screen and a stylus, just like the larger *Tablet PC* (Figure 9-4). With this device, the doctor can order laboratory tests, write prescriptions, review the patient's chart, record the encounter electronically, dictate notes to be transcribed later, and many other tasks.

Figure 9-4 Ultia® Electronic Chart in the Physician's Hand

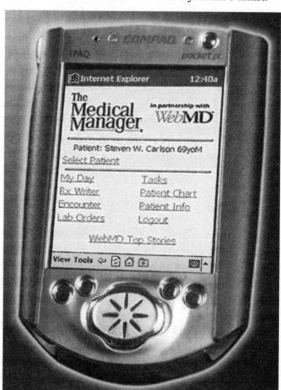

Sophisticated programs, such as *OmniDocs*, **The Medical Manager** *Electronic Medical Records System*, allow keyboard, mouse, or voice to be used; but regardless of the method of input, they store the data in a special way, not just as text you can read, but also as coded records that will someday be searched, translated, and transmitted electronically to another doctor or hospital where you are visiting. Just imagine a doctor never having to worry about locating your medical history!

Still, many offices continue to use a mouse and computer keyboard as the main method to enter information, just as you have learned to do. In these offices, the doctor may use a computer, pen pad, or Ultia to review notes, order laboratory tests, and prescriptions, but many doctors still dictate the longer examination notes. In these cases, a transcription system is used to type the information about the visit that the doctor has recorded on a small tape recorder or a pocket PC like Ultia. Once the progress note is typed, it becomes part of the patient's electronic chart, which the doctor can review online or as a printed document.

Electronic Prescriptions

The Prescription System automatically checks the patient's record for contraindications.

A patient's current medications are a major component of their medical records. Electronic prescriptions are easily written because they provide instant access to databases of pharmacy information, drugs, prescription instructions, SIG codes, standard prescriptions, and other key information. Extensive interaction checking on the drugs being prescribed, making sure they do not conflict with other medications the patient is taking, is already in place today. Electronic prescriptions can also provide checking for allergic reactions associated with specific drugs, diagnoses for which drugs are indicated and contraindicated, and potential interactions with food, alcohol, and other drugs. This checking is done automatically within **The Medical Manager** software via the *Prescription System*, which references the patient's medical history. This checking not only helps protect and educate the patient but also helps the medical practice avoid costly lawsuits and other legal actions that may arise as a result of incorrect or incomplete paper patient records.

Electronic Imaging

Electronic images can be integrated into the patient's medical record.

Of course not all medical records have words. Many would consider patient photographs, radiographs, letters, and other documents as part of the patient's record. An electronic image system can instantly retrieve images and associated image information to the screen—something that is not possible with photographic film and paper chart records today.

An image management system organizes and stores all types of images, and provides quick access to them. Each image may be associated with unlimited narrative comments such as interpretations of radiographs, commentary on photos, documents received from other practices, and remarks in response to letters from referring physicians. All of these features provide valuable additions to the patient's complete electronic medical record.

Electronic Task Management

Another important contribution of Electronic Medical Records is the improvement it makes to the workflow between the doctor and office staff. When a doctor orders a laboratory test, a medical office assistant must complete the paper work and take a specimen sample from the patient. When the results of the test are complete, the physician must be notified and the results reviewed. An Electronic Task can be used to communicate the doctor's order to the medical office assistant. A second Electronic Task then automatically notifies the physician that the test results are ready and includes a link that allows the doctor to quickly retrieve and review them.

Other examples of workflow improvements include transcription tasks, that let a transcriber know what dictation notes are ready for typing and subsequently let the physician know when the document is ready for review. Another task type might be a request from a pharmacy or patient to extend a patient's prescription.

Electronic tasks information is quickly and efficiently communicated between the doctor and staff. There is less lag time in responding to a patient's need, and overall improvements to patient care are possible.

Improving Patient Care

Unlike a paper chart, electronic medical records can be accessed by the physician from home, a hospital, or any computer terminal on the system. This feature can provide the physician with critical information whenever and wherever it is needed. Electronic medical records also allow one portion of the patient's record to be linked to another portion, which can help direct the physician's attention to important health factors for a particular patient so they are not overlooked.

Each time a procedure is performed, a laboratory result is received, or other clinical events take place, the patient's medical history is automatically updated and the appropriate quality care recommendation is considered as having been satisfied. Any new diagnoses and prescriptions for the patient are automatically added to the patient's problem list, and are then used for the next round of recall notices and guideline generation for that particular patient. This keeps patient records up to date and concisely organizes them for the patient's next visit.

An electronic patient record does not just provide a better alternative to filing charts or making them accessible. The data in the various portions of the chart can be linked to other aspects of the chart and used to improve the doctor's knowledge of the patient's total health. The records can also be analyzed to determine from many patients which treatments worked and which did not. This is called *outcome analysis*.

PROTECTING PATIENT PRIVACY

Understanding Health Insurance Portability and Accountability Act (HIPAA)

In 1996 Congress passed legislation called the Health Insurance Portability and Accountability Act (HIPAA). The law was intended to improve portability and continuity of health insurance coverage; combat waste, fraud, and abuse in health insurance and health care delivery; promote use of medical savings accounts; improve access to long-term care; and simplify administration of health insurance.

The Administrative Simplification Subsection of HIPAA (Title 2, f) covers entities such as health plans, clearinghouses, and health care providers. It has four distinct components that are being phased in over time. Each of these components is discussed briefly.

Transactions and Code Sets

Earlier in this unit EDI was discussed. When information is exchanged electronically, both sides of the transaction must agree to use the same format to make the information intelligible to the receiving system. HIPAA standardized these formats by requiring specific transaction standards be used for eight types of electronic data interchange.

In a typical EDI transaction, certain parts of the information are sent as codes. For example, in previous units, charges for patient visits were posted using procedure and diagnosis codes. These codes, instead of their long descriptions, were then sent as part of the insurance claim. Under HIPAA, any coded information within a transaction is also subject to standards. Two of the code sets you worked with in this book are required by HIPAA:

◆ Diagnoses (ICD-9) Codes
◆ Procedure (CPT-4) Codes

Uniform Identifiers

You can see how transmitting a code for a procedure or a diagnosis represents to the receiving system exactly what was done to the patient. Similarly, doctors, nurse practitioners, physician assistants, and health care businesses have ID numbers that have been assigned to them for use on insurance claims and prescriptions. This helps the receiving system ensure the proper person is reimbursed for the claim, or helps the pharmacist identify the doctor.

However, at the time HIPAA was passed, many different ID numbers were assigned by various states and companies. Although the regulations are not finalized, it is the intention of HIPAA to establish Uniform Identifier Standards, which will be used on all claims and other data transmissions. These will include:

◆ *National Provider Identifier* for doctors, nurses, and other health care providers.

◆ *Employer Identifier*, which will be the same as the Federal Employer Identification Number (FEIN) already assigned today. It will be used to identify employer-sponsored health insurance.

◆ *National Health Plan Identifier*, which will be a unique identification number assigned to each insurance plan and to the organizations that administer insurance plans, such as payers and third-party administrators.

Security

HIPAA mandates new security standards to protect an individual's health information, while permitting the appropriate access and use of that information by health care providers, clearinghouses, and health plans. The legislation is not yet final, but draft versions suggest the following ideas:

The proposed security standard does not require extraordinary measures to implement. It involves taking actions that a prudent person would agree were necessary to assure the security of the information to be protected. The standard does not dictate specific technologies, but for instance, requires that medical data transmitted over a public network be encrypted so that it could not be casually intercepted and read. The requirements of the standard may be implemented in a number of ways to meet the needs of health care entities of different size and complexity.

Privacy

The HIPAA privacy standards are designed to protect a patient's identifiable health information from unauthorized disclosure or use in any form, while permitting the practice to deliver the best health care possible. Health care providers have a strong tradition of safeguarding private health information. But in today's world, information is often held and transmitted electronically; the rule provides clear standards for all parties regarding protection of personal health information.

Medical practices of all kinds established certain basic privacy practices in their offices by April 14, 2003. For the average medical office, these practices include activities, such as:

◆ providing a copy of the office privacy policy informing patients about their privacy rights and how their information can be used.

- asking the patient to acknowledge receiving a copy of the policy and signing a consent form.
- obtaining signed authorization forms and, in some cases, tracking the disclosures of patient health information when it is to be given to a person or organization outside the practice for purposes other than treatment, billing, or payment purposes.
- adopting clear privacy procedures for its practice.
- training employees so that they understand the privacy procedures.
- designating an individual to be responsible for seeing that the privacy procedures are adopted and followed.
- securing patient records containing individually identifiable health information so that they are not readily available to those who do not need them.

As someone who will work in a medical office, it is important for you to understand two different concepts in the privacy rule. Most routine operations within the office are covered by the patient's *consent*. Most occurrences in which protected health information is sent to someone not involved in providing health care services or billing will require an *authorization* or *government request*.

Consent

Under the privacy rule, the patient gives consent to the use of his or her protected health information by the practice for purposes of treatment, payment, and operation of the health care practice. The patient does this by signing a consent form or signing an acknowledgment that they have received a copy of the office's privacy policy.

Some examples in which consent is used for treatment purposes include doctors and nurses sharing the patient's chart, and discussing what the best course of care might be. The doctor can also discuss the case with a colleague or specialist in another practice, or talk to the hospital about admitting a patient.

Consent can be used for purposes of obtaining payment. The office staff can access the patient's information to perform billing, transmit claims electronically, post payments, file the charts, type the doctor's progress notes, print, and send out patient statements.

Finally, the office can use the patient information for operation of the medical practice. For example, the office can determine how much staff it will need on a certain day, whether it should invest in a particular piece of equipment, what types of patients it sees most often, where most of the patients live, and any other uses that will help make the office operate more efficiently.

Authorization

When information is to be given to someone other than the office staff and for purposes other than treatment, payment, or office operations, an authorization form is signed by the patient or an official request is made by an authorized government agency. Unlike consent, a new authorization is signed each time there is a different purpose or need for the patient's information to be shared.

Some common examples that would require an authorization include sending the results of an employment physical to an employer or sending immunization records or the results of an athletic physical to a school. A request by the U.S. Food and Drug Administration (FDA) for information on patients who are having adverse reactions to a particular drug might be an example that would require a request from an authorized government agency instead of a patient authorization form.

Compare the differences between consent and authorization:

Patient Consent—to treat a patient, send a bill, file a claim, talk to the patient's insurance company, schedule an appointment, send the patient a reminder. A single consent covers all of these factors.

Patient Authorization—to provide records to the patient's school, the patient's attorney, the patient's employer. A new authorization must be signed by the patient or their representative for each different use of the patient's health information.

Government Requests—to fulfill legal requests from authorized government agencies. A new request must be received for each different use of the patient's health information. The request does not have to be signed by the patient; however, in most cases, the medical office must track the disclosure.

Patient Consent and Privacy Features of The Medical Manager

Many new privacy features were added to this version of **The Medical Manager**. By becoming familiar with the concepts and features of the system, you will be ready to assist your medical office in compliance with their privacy policy and these important HIPAA rules.

Although the patient privacy rule under HIPAA does not restrict the internal use of health information by the staff for treatment, payment, and office operations, you should make every effort to protect your patients' privacy and always follow the privacy policy of the practice.

Privacy Policy and Consent Forms

All medical offices have a privacy policy in effect as of April 14, 2003, and will make copies of the policy available to their patients, as required by law. Under HIPAA, the patient's acknowledgment that they have received a copy of the privacy policy is sufficient for the doctors to begin treating the patient because it supplants the requirement for a consent form. However, some practices may choose to use a patient consent form (such a form would also include an acknowledgment that the patient received a copy of the privacy policy).

In Units 2, 4, and 8, you added new patients using information supplied on the patient registration form. As is typical in many practices, the bottom of the registration form contained a statement of patient consent and an acknowledgment that the patient received a copy of the practice's privacy policy as required by law. (Refer back to Figure 8-3.)

The Medical Manager software provides a field to record for each patient when you have received the patient's signature on the proper form. As you added each patient in the exercises, you entered a '**Y**' for Yes in the patient consent field. This indicates that the practice may use the patient's identifiable information for purposes of treating the patient, including consulting with other staff and physicians, billing purposes, allowing the practice to get paid, and ordinary business of the clinic, such as managing the appointment schedule and handling paper charts.

There are other options to the consent field. These include 'No', 'Revoked', 'Unknown', and 'Restricted'. For many offices, it would not be possible to treat a patient with a consent status of No or Revoked because the doctor typically has many things that require the help of a medical office assistant, including billing. It is possible that a famous person, such as a movie star or politician, might enter into an agreement with his or her doctor to be seen on a cash basis, in which no billing was necessary. However, the more common of these special status is 'Unknown' because this is the status of every new patient who registers over the phone until they actually arrive at the medical office to sign the form. *Remember, Yes means you actually have on file a document signed by the patient or their legal guardian.*

The Medical Manager Privacy System provides a report that lets the practice monitor all or selected status of consent for patients registered in the practice. It also alerts the user whenever a patient is selected for which the consent status is other than Yes or Unknown. This is done on the Patient Retrieval screen by displaying the label "Consent" and the consent status in red.

APPLYING YOUR KNOWLEDGE

Exercise 1: Changing Consent for Ryan Hughes

In this exercise, you will learn to run the Privacy System Patient Consent Report. Before doing this, we will change the status of a recent patient.

STEP 1

From the Main Menu, choose option **7**, File Maintenance, then option **1**, Edit Patient. Key '**200.0**' and retrieve the Hughes account. Select (**D**)ependents, then position the highlight bar on Ryan Hughes and press **ENTER**. Select (**M**)odify. Use the down arrow key or your mouse to navigate to the Consent field. Change the status to '**N**'. Compare your screen with Figure 9-5, then press '**F1**' or click on the PROCESS button ('√') on the top toolbar. Press **EXIT** to return to the patient retrieval screen.

Figure 9-5 Modify Patient Consent for a Dependent

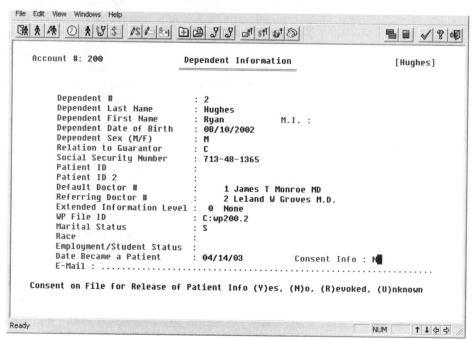

STEP 2

Key Account # '**200**' and Press **ENTER**. The Joseph Hughes family will be displayed. Using your down arrow key, move the highlight bar down to Ryan Hughes, as shown in Figure 9-6. Notice how the Consent field changes color. This alert will appear in every part of the system that has a Patient Retrieval screen. **EXIT** until you are at the Main Menu (Menu 1).

Figure 9-6 Patient Retrieval Screen for a Patient with a Special Consent Status

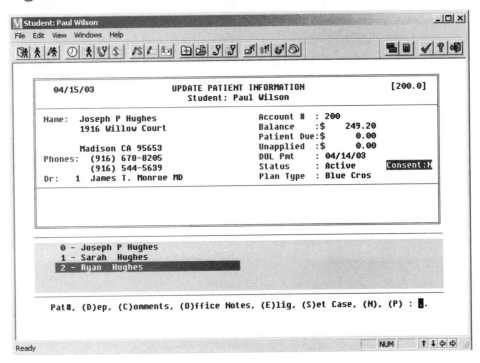

Exercise 2: Running the Patient Consent Report

STEP 1

From the Main Menu, choose option **8**, Office Management, then option **7**, Patient Privacy System, then option **3**, Patient Consent Report. The Patient Consent Report may be generated in account or name order, for all patients, or limited to those with a selected status. Because a practice might be most concerned with finding any patients who have either a No or Revoked status, a special option of the report allows you to run a report for only those two statuses. Alternatively, you may run the report selectively to find any patients with a particular status. The report may be further limited to only those patients seen since a selected date (Figure 9-7).

In this exercise, you will choose (**A**)ccount Order, and (**A**)ll status. Do not enter a date in the 'Only Patients Seen Since' field. Compare your screen with Figure 9-7, then press '**F1**' or click on the PROCESS button ('√') on the top toolbar. Compare your finished report with Figure 9-8.

Figure 9-7 Patient Consent Report Selection Screen

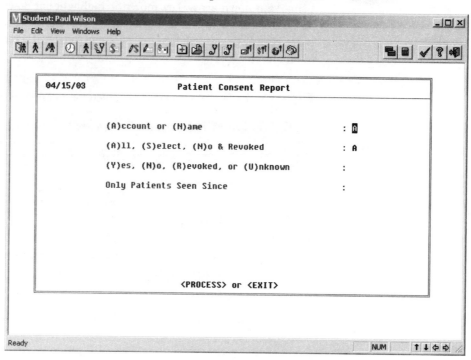

```
Student: Paul Wilson                                              _ □ ×
File  Edit  View  Windows  Help

 04/15/03                    Patient Consent Report


              (A)ccount or (N)ame                      : A

              (A)ll, (S)elect, (N)o & Revoked          : A

              (Y)es, (N)o, (R)evoked, or (U)nknown     :

              Only Patients Seen Since                 :




                         <PROCESS> or <EXIT>

Ready                                               NUM      ↑ ↓ ⇦ ⇨
```

Figure 9-8 Sample Patient Consent Report

```
04/15/03                 PATIENT CONSENT REPORT              Page 1
                          Student: Paul Wilson
                        Account Order, All Status
                               All Dates

Patient #        Name                    DOL Visit    Consent on File
--------------------------------------------------------------------
   10.0    Carlson Steven W              01/10/2003         Yes
   10.1    Carlson Sharon A              02/17/2003         Yes
   14.0    Evans Deborah A               02/17/2003         Yes
   14.1    Evans Gene S                  02/03/2003         Yes
   21.0    Edwards Portia D              02/17/2003         Yes
   21.1    Edwards Edward E                                 Yes
   21.2    Edwards Andrea L              01/10/2003         Yes
   30.0    League Claire E               02/03/2003         Yes
   34.0    Dudley Wayne R                01/10/2003         Yes
   80.0    Davis Timothy R               02/17/2003         Yes
   80.1    Davis Elizabeth S                               Yes
   80.2    Davis Mindy A                 01/10/2003         Yes
  110.0    Evans Patricia G              01/31/2003         Yes
  120.1    Simmons Laura S               01/10/2003         Yes
  120.2    Spivey Alice J                01/10/2003         Yes
  120.3    Williams Thomas C             02/03/2003         Yes
  120.4    Williams Janet L              02/03/2003         Yes
  200.0    Hughes Joseph P               04/14/2003         Yes
  200.1    Hughes Sarah                  04/07/2003         Yes
  200.2    Hughes Ryan                                      NO

                    Total Unknown :        0
                    Total No      :        1
                    Total Revoked :        0
                    Total Yes     :       19
```

Understanding Authorizations, Requests, and Disclosures

Unlike consent, authorizations are used by the patient to give permission to share a portion of his or her health care record with someone outside the office, for reasons other than treatment, billing, or operations of the medical practice. Authorizations are used for many common occurrences such as school immunization records, athletics, employment or insurance physicals, and automobile accidents.

Authorizations used in a medical office may have several different forms, but under HIPAA, all authorizations have very specific requirements to content. An authorization form must contain:

◆ the provider or practice authorized to give out the information.
◆ the authorized party (person or organization) who will receive the information.
◆ the purpose for which the patient wants the information released. (A statement, "at the request of the patient", is sufficient.)
◆ a description of the information to be released.
◆ the patient signature, date signed, and an expiration date or condition.

With a signed authorization form, the practice is not required to keep a record of when disclosures were made under the authorization, but the practice may do so.

Government agencies may request patient information from a medical office for various reasons, including verifying compliance with the HIPAA regulations, preventing the spread of disease, determining if patients are having adverse reactions to a drug or treatment, and in certain cases when ordered by a court or law enforcement agency. These requests do not require the patient to sign an authorization form but do require that the practice keeps a record of the disclosure.

A practice must record the following information about a disclosure:

◆ date of the disclosure.
◆ the person or organization (authorized party) who received the information.
◆ a description of the information released.

HIPAA also requires that the practice provide a report of disclosures to the patient upon request. **The Medical Manager** allows the practice to record authorizations or requests from a government agency and disclosure records related to either. The system includes the required Patient Disclosure Report, as well as several reports to assist the practice in managing authorizations, requests, and disclosure records.

Recording Authorizations and Requests

Each time a patient requests that you provide information on his or her behalf for a purpose other than treatment, payment, or operations, you will fill in the information on an authorization form and have the patient sign it. Each time a government agency requests information on a patient, you will make a record of the request and record all subsequent disclosures. **The Medical Manager** lets you perform all three functions from a single option, Patient Privacy Records. You can also print a copy of the completed authorization form for the patient to sign. Note that once the form is signed, it should be retained by the practice.

STEP 1

Mrs. Edwards is applying for additional life insurance, and the company requires the results of a recent physical examination. From the Main Menu (Menu 1) select option **8**, Office Management, then select option **7**, Patient Privacy System, then select option **1**, Patient Privacy Records. Enter the Patient # '**21.0**' and press **ENTER**. If she had any previous authorizations and requests on file they would be displayed in the Help window.

STEP 2

Choose (**A**)dd to add a new Authorization. Key the following Information:

Source of Authorization. Type the letter '**P**' to indicate the source of the authorization is Patient. Valid entries are as follows:

'**P**' (P)atient: Indicates that the patient requested the disclosure.

'**R**' Legal (R)epresentative: Indicates that the patient's legal guardian requested the disclosure.

'**G**' (G)overnment Agency: Indicates that a government agency requested the disclosure.

Relationship to Patient. Only when '**R**' is entered in the Source of Authorization field does the cursor move to the Relationship to Patient field. A Help window of valid entries is available by entering '**?**' in the Relationship to Patient field.

When '**P**' is entered in the Source of Authorization the field is automatically filled with '**S**' Self'.

When '**G**' is entered in the Source of Authorization field, the Relationship to Patient field (below) is automatically filled with '0' (zero) for Agency Rep

> **Tip:** Alphanumeric–(1)—Required

Date Authorization Signed. Type the date on which the authorization was signed. Press **ENTER** to default to the current date (April 15, 2003). You should complete this field only when you have received the signed form. However, if the patient is in the office and you are adding an authorization for the purpose of printing a form for the patient to sign, you may record the current date.

> **Tip:** Date–(8) When the request for disclosure is from a government agency, the field is required. When the authorization is from the patient, this field may be left blank until the actual signed document is received.

Date Authorization Expires. Type the date on which the authorization expires. Press **ENTER** and the system automatically leaves the field blank. If an authorization has an expiration date and the date has passed, disclosures should not be made for that authorization.

> **Tip:** Date–(8)–Optional

The following two fields are entered only when '**G**' for Government Agency was entered in the Source of Authorization field.

Gov. Suspend Reporting. Under certain conditions during a pending investigation, a government agency can temporarily suspend a patient's right to know of disclosures made to the agency. Key: '**Y**' for Yes if the agency requested that for a limited time the practice *not* report to the patient that a disclosure of information was requested or '**N**' for No if no suspended reporting is required. If Suspended Reporting field is '**Y**', the system will automatically omit all disclosure of information associated with the agency request from the Patient Disclosure Report until the suspension period has passed.

Tip: Alphanumeric–(1)—Required when source is '**G**'.

End Suspended Reporting. Type the date on which the suspended reporting expires. The cursor moves to this field only when '**Y**' for Yes was entered in Gov. Suspend Reporting field (above). If the Suspended Reporting field is '**Y**', press **ENTER** and the system automatically enters a date 30 days after the date entered in Date Authorization Signed field.

Tip: Date–(8)

Purpose of Disclosure. Type the purpose for which the disclosure is authorized. Key "**Insurance Physical**". The Purpose and several other text fields in the Patient Privacy Records module have an Auto Text feature that allows frequently used descriptions to be selected from a Help window and entered with a key stroke. This feature is particularly useful if the practice if frequently called upon to supply records for common requests such as insurance or pre-employment physicals. Enter '?' to access the Auto Text feature.

Tip: Alphanumeric–(2 lines–78 characters)—Required

Contact Party ID. Key '?' for help and select "Coates & Coates, Inc." from the list. This field may be used to complete quickly the contact party information if desired. Type the code that identifies the contact party and press **ENTER**, or key in '?' to view a Help window of contacts who might be frequently-used authorized parties. When a previously defined code is entered in this field or a contact party is selected from the Help window, the Authorized Party, Attention, Address, City, State, Zip Code, and Phone Number fields are automatically filled in with the appropriate information.

Tip: Alphanumeric–(6)—Optional

If you do not complete the Authorized Party information by selecting a Contact Party, the following fields must be entered:

Authorized Party: Type name of the recipient of the disclosure and press **ENTER**.

Tip: Alphanumeric–(40)—Required

Attention: Type name of the person to whom the disclosure will be sent and press **ENTER**.

Tip: Alphanumeric–(25)—Optional

Address: Type the street address of the recipient of the disclosure and press **ENTER**.

Tip: Alphanumeric–(25)—Required

City: Type the city and press **ENTER**. To display a Help window, type '?' and press **ENTER**. The Zip Code Help window from Unit 2 will be displayed.

Tip: Alphanumeric–(15)—Required

State: Type the two-letter code of the state and press **ENTER**.

Tip: Alphanumeric–(3)—Required

Zip Code: Type the zip code for the above street address and press **ENTER**. To display a Zip Code Help Window, key in '?' and press **ENTER**.

Tip: Alphanumeric–(10)—Required

Phone Number: Type the recipient's phone number and press **ENTER**. Then type the recipient's extension if necessary and press **ENTER** again.

Tip: Numeric–(10 phone, 4 extension)—Optional

Information to be Disclosed. When the cursor moves to this field, a Help window of Auto Text similar to the Purpose field appears automatically. Position the highlight bar on Free–Text and press **ENTER**. Key "**all results pertaining to insurance physical**"

Tip: Alphanumeric–HIPAA regulations require the patient to describe what information may be released, even if the description is very broad such as "all results"

STEP 3 Once you have completed the authorization information, compare your screen with Figure 9-9 and press '**F1**' or click on the PROCESS button ('√') on the top toolbar.

Figure 9-9 Authorization for Portia Edwards's Insurance Physical

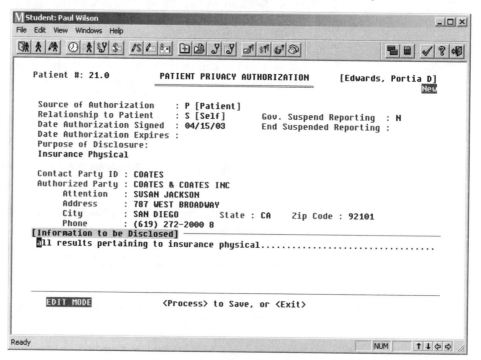

STEP 4 A medical office may print out the information on the authorization form for the patient to sign. Choose (**F**)orm, and press '**F1**' or click on the PROCESS ('√') button on the top toolbar. Compare your printout with Figure 9-10.

Figure 9-10 Authorization to Disclose Patient Records

```
AUTHORIZATION TO DISCLOSE PATIENT RECORDS


I hereby authorize [Medical Practice Name] to disclose individually identifiable
protected health information concerning the patient:

Portia D. Edwards
235 Mandolin Court

Madison CA 95653-0235

To: SUSAN JACKSON
787 WEST BROADWAY
SAN DIEGO, CA. 92101

For the purpose of:
Insurance Physical


Information to be Disclosed:
all results pertaining to insurance physical




This Authorization is to remain in effect from  04/15/2003

I understand that I have the right to revoke this authorization  by notifying
the practice in writing until such time as a disclosure has been made based on
this authorization. In addition, I understand that my signing this
authorization is not required for the practice to provide me with health care
service, except if the sole purpose of the service is for the practice to
provide health care information to the authorized party named in this document.
Finally, I understand that the information disclosed pursuant to this
authorization may be re-disclosed by the authorized party and no longer be
protected by the laws under which this authorization was created.


Signed _____   Date _____
Relation to Patient:  Self
```

APPLYING YOUR KNOWLEDGE

Exercise 3: Authorization for Andrea Edwards's Cheerleading Camp Physical

Andrea Edwards is going to a special Cheerleading Camp over spring break. The camp requires an athletic physical for each student before they can attend. Because Andrea is a minor the authorization form will be signed by her mother. Therefore choose (**R**)epresentative rather than (**P**)atient as the type.

STEP 1   If you are not already in Patient Privacy Records, from the Main Menu (Menu 1), select option **8**, Office Management, then select option **7**, Patient Privacy System, then select option **1**, Patient Privacy Records. Enter the Patient # '**21.2**' and press **ENTER** to retrieve Andrea Edwards's information.

STEP 2   Choose (**A**) and enter the following information to create a new authorization record for Andrea's camp physical.

　　　　Source of Authorization: (**R**)epresentative

　　　　Relationship to Patient: (**P**)arent

　　　　Purpose of Disclosure: **Admission to Cheerleader Camp**

　　　　Contact Party ID: (Press **ENTER** to skip this field)

Because you did not select a Contact Party, complete the following fields:

Authorized Party: **Madison High Cheerleader Camp**

Attention: **Cheerleading Coach**

Address: **111 Madison High Drive**

City: Key **Madison** and press **ENTER**

Tip: You can enter a zip code from the Help window in this field and the system will automatically complete the City, State and Zip. Remember, you must first enter '**?**' for help.

State: **CA**

Zip Code: **95653**

Phone Number:

Phone Extension:

Information to be Disclosed. Position the highlight bar on Free–Text and press **ENTER**. Key "**Results of athletic physical**".

STEP 3

Once you have completed the authorization information, compare your screen with Figure 9-11 and press '**F1**' or click on the PROCESS ('√') button on the top toolbar.

Figure 9-11 Authorization for Andrea Edwards's Athletic Physical

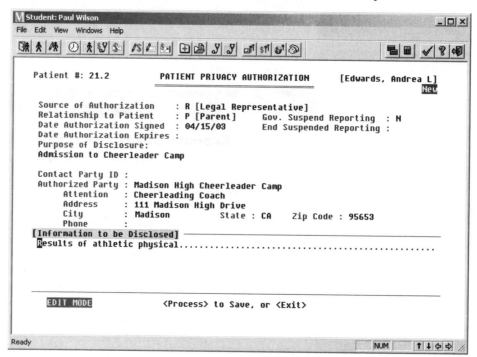

UNIT 9 Today's Medical Office

STEP 4 Choose (**F**)orm and print a form for Andrea's mother to sign. Compare your printout with Figure 9-12.

Figure 9-12 Authorization Form for Andrea Edwards

```
AUTHORIZATION TO DISCLOSE PATIENT RECORDS


I hereby authorize [Medical Practice Name] to disclose individually identifiable
protected health information concerning the patient:

Andrea L. Edwards
235 Mandolin Court

Madison CA 95653-0235

To: Cheerleading Coach
111 Madison High Drive
Madison, CA. 95653

For the purpose of:
Admission to Cheerleader Camp


Information to be Disclosed:
Results of athletic physical



This Authorization is to remain in effect from  04/15/2003

I understand that I have the right to revoke this authorization  by notifying
the practice in writing until such time as a disclosure has been made based on
this authorization. In addition, I understand that my signing this
authorization is not required for the practice to provide me with health care
service, except if the sole purpose of the service is for the practice to
provide health care information to the authorized party named in this document.
Finally, I understand that the information disclosed pursuant to this
authorization may be re-disclosed by the authorized party and no longer be
protected by the laws under which this authorization was created.


Signed _____   Date _____
Relation to Patient:  Parent
```

Recording Disclosures

Once a signed authorization or request has been entered into the system, the system may then be used to record the disclosure of authorized or requested information. A *disclosure* is a record of the actual release of a patient's health information per the authorization or request. In many cases, the disclosures will not occur on the same date that the authorization is signed. In some cases, such as an accident, a patient being treated over a period of time may have numerous disclosures.

However in this case, Mrs. Edwards and her daughter have their physicals on April 15 and the doctor is able to send the records out the same date.

STEP 1 If you are not already in the Patient Privacy Records module, enter the module by following the instructions in the previous exercise. At the Patient Retrieval screen key '**21.0**' and press **ENTER** to retrieve Portia Edwards's authorization records. The Help window should display the authorization for her "Insurance Physical" as shown in Figure 9-13.

Figure 9-13 Authorization for Portia Edwards

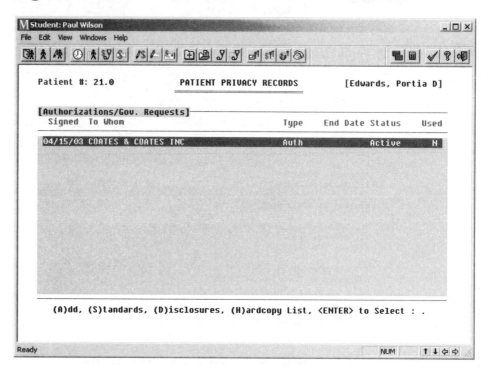

STEP 2   Choose (**D**)isclosures. A Help window of Disclosure Records related to the authorization "Insurance Physical" will be displayed. Because there have not been any previous disclosures, the window will display the message "Record of Disclosures Not Found" (Figure 9-14).

Figure 9-14 Add Disclosure Screen

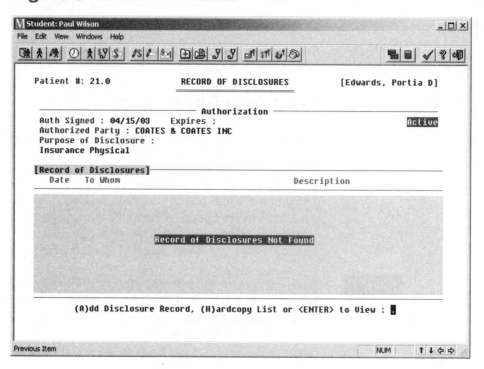

Choose (**A**)dd to add a new Disclosure Record. Enter the following information:

Date of Disclosure: Key the date on which the disclosure of information was made. Press **ENTER** to default to 04152003.

Tip: Date–(8)—Required.

Disclosed To: Press **ENTER** to default to the Authorized Party "Coates & Coates."

Type name of the recipient of the disclosure or press **ENTER** to default to the Authorized Party information on the authorization form. Note that the information entered in this field does not modify any information entered when the authorization was created, thus allowing the practice to be very specific about who received the actual disclosure.

Tip: Alphanumeric–(40)—Required

Information Disclosed: When the cursor moves to this field, a Help window of Auto Text automatically appears, similar to Figure 9-15. Position the highlight bar on the first entry in the Help window '*AUTH*', and press **ENTER** to default the Information Disclosed from the text that was entered in the authorization.

This field is used to describe the information that was disclosed. The Auto Text feature allows the user to automatically enter whatever text was entered in the Information to be Disclosed field when the authorization was created (making it much quicker to complete disclosure records).

Tip: Alphanumeric—Required

Figure 9-15 Information Disclosed Help Window

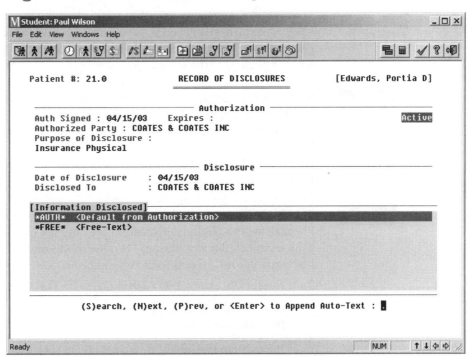

STEP 4

Once you have completed the disclosure information, compare your screen with Figure 9-16 and press '**F1**' or click on the PROCESS ('√') button on the top toolbar.

Figure 9-16 Completed Disclosure Record for Portia Edwards

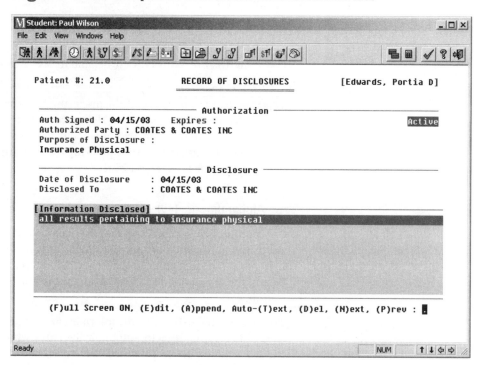

APPLYING YOUR KNOWLEDGE

Exercise 4: Recording a Disclosure for Andrea Edwards

The results of Andrea's camp physical are ready to be mailed to the school. Using the knowledge you have learned in this exercise, retrieve the patient Andrea Edwards in the Patient Privacy Records module. Add a record of disclosure, indicating that you have sent her physical to the school cheerleading coach (Figure 9-17).

STEP 1

If you are not already in the Patient Privacy Records module, enter the module by following the instructions in the previous exercise. At the Patient Retrieval screen, key '**21.2**' and press **ENTER** to retrieve Andrea Edwards's authorization records.

STEP 2

Position the highlight bar in the Authorization Help window on the "Cheerleading Physical" authorization as shown in Figure 9-17. Choose (**D**)isclosures.

STEP 3

A Help window of Disclosure Records related to the Authorization "Insurance Physical" will be displayed. Because there have not been any previous disclosures, the window will display the message "No Disclosures on File". Choose (**A**)dd to add a new Disclosure Record. Enter the following information:

Date of Disclosure: **04152003** (Press **ENTER** to default)

Disclosed To: "Madison High Cheerleader Camp" (Press **ENTER** to default to the Authorized Party)

Information Disclosed: "Results of athletic physical" (Press **ENTER** to default)

Figure 9-17 Authorizations for Andrea Edwards

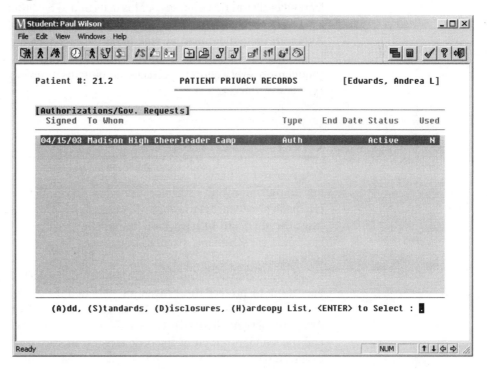

STEP 4

Once you have completed the disclosure information, compare your screen with Figure 9-18 and press '**F1**' or click on the PROCESS ('√') button on the top toolbar.

In these exercises, you have learned how to use **The Medical Manager** to keep records of patient authorization forms, requests by government agencies, and records of disclosures made under them. These are generally cases in which the information is not being disclosed for treatment, payment, or health care operations (Figure 9-18).

Figure 9-18 Andrea Edwards's Completed Disclosure Record

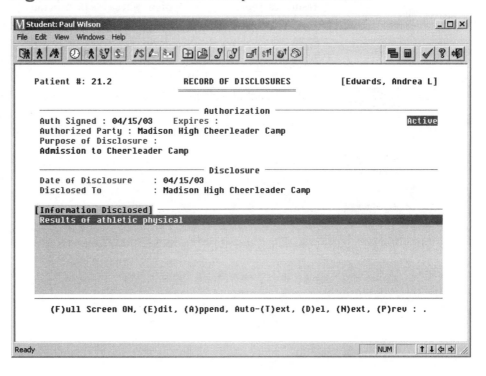

Information is used internally in the practice based on the patient's consent. As you learned earlier in this unit, consent is determined by either a signed consent form or a signed acknowledgment that the patient received a copy of the practice privacy policy. Although the patient privacy rule under HIPAA does not restrict the internal use of health information by the staff for treatment, payment, and office operations, you should make every effort to protect your patients' privacy and always follow the privacy policy of the practice.

UNIT 9 SUMMARY

This course has focused primarily on the financial billing and scheduling aspects of managing a physician's practice. However, an equally important component in modern medical software is the ability to computerize the patient's medical information to assist the physician with tracking the care and treatment of the patient. This includes electronic prescriptions, examination notes, laboratory results and other medical information.

In addition to computerizing the clinical aspects of the physician's office, it is also important to protect the privacy of patient information in the physician's office. Standards were established under a federal law called Health Insurance Portability and Accountability Act (HIPAA). HIPAA also includes regulations on security transactions and the standardization of the code sets. A practice establishes a privacy policy and assigns a person in the practice to act as a privacy officer to ensure that the policy is enforced. Copies of the practice's privacy policy must be made available to each patient and a good faith attempt made to get the patients to acknowledge receiving a copy of the policy. By acknowledging receipt of the privacy policy or signing a consent form, the patient agrees that the practice can use the patient's personally identifiable information for the purposes of treating the patient, operating the clinic, and billing to receive payment for services the physician performed.

When information needs to be released to outside organizations for purposes other than treatment, payment, or operation, an authorization form needs to be signed by the patient. Authorizations might be used when the practice is asked to report the results of sports or employment physicals or provide accident records to an attorney. Disclosures made for purposes other than treatment, payment, or operation also need to be recorded and tracked. Under the HIPAA regulations, patients have certain rights, including the right to review or amend their medical records and to receive a report or list of any disclosures that were made for purposes other than treatment, payment, or health care operations of the practice.

TESTING YOUR KNOWLEDGE

1. Define EDI and provide examples of how it may be used. What benefits does it offer for the medical office?

2. Explain the benefits of using the Intranet, rather than the Internet, to transmit electronic medical records.

3. Discuss how the patient's electronic medical record may be used to improve the overall quality of his or her health care.

4. Discuss ways in which computers are being used to communicate medical information.

5. What does the acronym HIPAA stand for?

(continues)

6. Name three EDI transactions that are regulated by HIPAA.

7. Name three reasons you can use patient's health information under HIPAA Consent.

8. Under what circumstances will you need the patient to sign an authorization Form?

9. Why should you protect the privacy of the patient's medical information?

UNITS 5-9 CONCEPTS EVALUATION

I. Office Management—Match the terms from Column 1 with a related phrase from Column 2

Column 1

1. _____ Appointment worklist
2. _____ Double book
3. _____ Multiple slots
4. _____ Secondary insurance plan
5. _____ Jump
6. _____ Follow-up appointment
7. _____ General check-up
8. _____ Hospital round

Column 2

a. the plan billed for remaining charges
b. general appointment using one slot
c. may be used for more in-depth patient visits
d. appointment for patient's condition to be re-evaluated
e. appointment schedule for the day
f. visits the physician makes to patients
g. a command used to schedule appointments
h. scheduling two patients for the same time

II. Financial Management—Match the terms from Column 1 with a related phrase from Column 2

Column 1

1. _____ Unique payments
2. _____ Billing routine
3. _____ Insurance Billing worksheet
4. _____ Split check
5. _____ Negative adjustment
6. _____ Batch billing
7. _____ Current period
8. _____ Copayment

Column 2

a. used to generate bills
b. this billing cycle
c. patient portion of bill
d. payment is to be divided among patients
e. prints bills according to a formula
f. may require several steps to complete
g. increases the patient's balance
h. used to help verify billing

III. Give a one- or two-sentence explanation of the following concepts:

1. Posting zero adjustments
2. Dual insurance coverage
3. Transfer responsibility to patient
4. Account aging

IV. Explain the difference between Auto Pay and individual allocation of payments.

(continues)

V. Name two types of reports and describe the purpose of each.

VI. Medical Records

1. List three types of information in a paper chart that could be kept electronically.

2. How could an Electronic Medical Record improve patient care?

VII. Privacy

1. What are HIPAA Privacy Standards designed to protect?

2. Explain the difference between patient consent and patient authorization.

Glossary

A

Account Adjustment: This refers to the posting of a payment (either positive or negative) to keep the doctor's books and the patient's account in balance. Any change in the original charge must be clearly documented and justified. A finished entry is called an adjustment and is used to increase or decrease the initial charge amount. For example, if a patient's check is returned due to insufficient funds, the amount originally credited to his or her account for the payment must be adjusted to account for the non-payment. Similarly, the doctor's account must be adjusted to reflect the fact that payment was actually not made on the account (i.e., the doctor did not yet receive any payment for these services).

Account Aging: This refers to a function performed to determine the financial status of patient accounts. The options chosen when an Account Aging Report is performed print a report based on how long patient account balances have been due (this is sometimes called the accounts 'age'). Frequently, accounts are aged by category: for example, 30 to 60 days overdue, 60 to 90 days overdue, 90 to 120 days overdue, 121 to 150 or over 151 days overdue. Aging Accounts Receivable allows the practice to determine which accounts need the most attention for collections purposes.

Accounts Receivable: The unpaid accounts in a medical office. This is also sometimes referred to as the practice's 'AR'.

Adjustment for Zero Dollars: This is an account adjustment made by crediting a payment amount of $0.00 to a patient's account. An adjustment for zero dollars is usually done when it is necessary to rebill a lost insurance claim but may also be used in place of the (T)ransfer option to transfer responsibility for a charge.

Adjustments: To keep the doctor's books and the patient's ledger in balance, any change in the original charge must be accounted for. A finished entry called an adjustment is used to increase or decrease the initial charge amount.

Aged Accounts Receivable: This refers to how long an account has been due, sometimes called its age. Frequently, accounts are aged by category: for example, 30 to 60 days overdue, 60 to 90 days overdue, 90 to 120 days overdue, 121 to 150 or over 151 days overdue. Aging Accounts Receivable allows the practice to determine which accounts need the most attention for collections purposes.

Aging Report: This refers to a report generated for the purposes of determining how long patient account balances have been due. *Also see* Account Aging.

Ailment Detail: In-depth information about an illness or injury that is always required for Worker's Compensation claims and sometimes needed for other claims. This is also the name of a screen found in the Procedure Entry phase of **The Medical Manager** software. Ailment Detail can be thought of as the "other information" needed on the CMS-1500 form.

391

Allocate Payment: This refers to assigning a payment amount to an outstanding charge or charges. For example, a payment of $100.00 may be allocated to two line items charges for $50.00 each. This may also be referred to as 'Posting Payment.'

Appointment Schedule: This is a list of all the patients to be seen in the practice for a particular time period (e.g., a day, a week). Appointments may be scheduled manually in a daily appointment book or by computer using **The Medical Manager** software. All practice activities are based on the Appointment Schedule.

Appointment Slot: This is a single space or hole in the appointment schedule. Although practices may have different methods of determining the slot length used on their appointment schedules, a typical slot is 15 minutes long; generally the time necessary for the physician to see the patient for a general check-up.

Approved Profile: The schedule used to estimate the amount of reimbursement to expect from the insurance company. The profile determines how much the practice will be paid for a particular procedure performed for the patient.

Approved Provider: A physician or health care facility contracted with an insurance plan to provide services to the plan members. Under the rules of the plan contract, referrals must be issued to an approved provider; generally, an approved provider is a member of the same plan as the referring provider.

Assignment of Claim: This (Y)es/(N)o option within the software designates who will receive payment from the insurance company. If you answer (Y)es to the 'Accept Assignment' for the doctor field, the doctor agrees to wait to collect payment for the services provided to the patient until he or she is reimbursed by the insurance company. If you answer (N)o at this field, this indicates that the physician will not wait to collect payment from the insurance company and requires that the patient pay in full for all charges at the time of the visit. In this case, the insurance company would reimburse the patient for the out of pocket expenses he or she incurred as a result of the visit. For the purposes of the Student Edition course, you will always answer (Y)es at this field.

Audit Trail: The ability to trace information from the time it is entered into the computer until it is purged. For example, if a payment is removed from an account because a check was returned by the bank, it will be important to note the reason for the check being returned, and to document that the payment was removed from the patient's account and the doctor's accounts receivable.

Authorization: An authorization form signed by the patient or an official request from an authorized government agency to provide patient health information for purposes other than treatment, payment, or office operations. Unlike consent, a new authorization is signed each time there is a different purpose or nee for the patient's information to be shared.

Auto Pay: A method in the Payment Entry phase of **The Medical Manager** system that allows the computer to allocate automatically payments to several open items, rather than requiring the operator to allocate individually payment. An example of this is when an insurance company sends full payment for several insurance billed charges on an account. In this case, the (A)uto Pay option can be used to allocated the full amount of the check to the full balance of all outstanding insurance billed charges. This is sometimes referred to as 'autopay.'

B

Batch: A group of charges or payments posted in one session, or a group of insurance claims transmitted together electronically.

Batch Total: This is a running total, calculated by the system, which is shown throughout the duration of a posting session. This total amount reflects all payments made on a group of charges or payments posted in one session. The batch total is helpful during a charge posting session because when posting is complete, the batch total should equal the total of the amounts shown on the patient's encounter form. The batch total is especially useful when payments are being posted for a claim (e.g., from an insurance company) because it allows the poster to easily keep track of how much of the check has been posted and how much still remains to be allocated.

Basic Insurance Coverage: This insurance generally covers the physician's fee, hospital expenses up to a maximum amount, and surgical fees (as defined in each contract). With basic insurance coverage, the patient is typically responsible for the first hundred dollars or more charged for medical services (this amount is called a deductible), in addition to a copayment amount for each service or treatment provided.

Billing Routine: This refers to the function of generating bills and month-end statements and sending them to guarantors and their insurance companies. This process usually starts with running the Insurance Billing Worksheet and ends with the practice filing paper or electronic claims with the insurance companies and sending paper billing statements to guarantors.

Bill Type: Two numeric characters that tell the computer the type of bill a patient receives and the type of statement the patient receives. For the purposes of the Student Edition course, this will usually be Bill Type '11.'

Bill-Thru Date: A stopping point for billing. Items posted through the bill-thru date will be billed, and those posted after that date will not be billed.

Budget Payment: A smaller, regular payment made toward the patient due amount. Some practices will allow patients to pay small installments (i.e., monthly or weekly) toward their total account balance. This is often called a budget payment because the total amount due is broken down, or budgeted, for the patient.

C

Cancel Reason Code: This is a code, often defined by the practice, to indicate why an appointment is cancelled. For example, if a patient's appointment is cancelled because the physician has an emergency and is not available, a Cancel Reason Code of 'NODOC' will be chosen, because the physician was not available to meet with the patient.

Capitation Payment: This refers to a monthly payment offered by insurance companies to doctors for each patient who has chosen him or her as their primary care physician (PCP). This amount is based on a flat rate of reimbursement (i.e., a specific amount of money for every patient), rather than a fee-for-service (i.e., a specific amount for every service performed) basis. This situation is typical in a managed care program, such as a Health Maintenance Organization (HMO).

CHAMPVA: A government insurance program for veterans and their dependents. *Also see* TRICARE.

Charting: When a patient is seen, the doctor writes or dictates notes on everything significantly relating to the patient's illness. These medical notes are called patient charts and are unrelated to billing. Because charting is usually done manually by the physician, there is limited practical value to putting the entire chart on a computer, especially considering the time needed to enter the data into the computer. However, entering key points into the computer, such as medication, allergies, or surgery, is practical for many offices.

Check Register: This is part of the Daily Close function that lists all checks posted during 1 day. For example, a practice check register would contain a list of all checks posted for each doctor in the practice for that day of business. The check register would include the check number, amount, and for whom the payment was posted into the system. This allows the practice to easily reconcile the bank deposit made at the end of the day.

Claim Form: This is the document sent to the insurance company to request payment for services that were performed for the patient. In cases in which the doctor accepts assignment, the doctor will submit the claim for the patient and wait to receive payment. In cases in which the doctor does not accept assignment, the patient may be required to pay the doctor and then submit the completed claim form himself or herself (sometimes the practice will still file the claim for the patient) and wait to be reimbursed. Note that the claim form may also be submitted electronically to the plan.

Clinic Without Walls: This term is used to describe physicians who have formed a group as a financial entity for negotiating managed care contracts but do not practice in the same building. In this situation, physicians keep their individual offices but work together as a single unit to provide services by referring patients to other physicians within their own network.

CMS-1500 Form: This is a standardized form created by the American Medical Association for insurance billing purposes. This health insurance claims form contains spaces for information that is most typically requested by insurance companies and is accepted by most government and private insurance companies (Formerly designated as HCFA-1500).

Comment Field: This is a field on the Ailment Detail screen that allows the user to enter a specific comment about why the Ailment Detail is being created for the patient. For example, if a patient is being treated for a work-related injury (such as a back injury) that will be billed to the patient's employer's Worker's Compensation Policy, it will be necessary for the physician to enter a complete Ailment Detail for the patient. In the Comment field on the Ailment Detail screen, the physician may enter "WC Back" to indicate that this is a back injury that will be billed to Worker's Compensation.

Comprehensive Insurance Coverage: This insurance combines the benefits of both basic insurance coverage and major medical insurance (explained below). With comprehensive insurance coverage, a small deductible usually covers broad medical treatment under one policy.

Consent: Under the HIPAA Privacy rule, the patient gives consent to the use of his or her protected health information by practice for purposes of treatment, payment, and operation of the health care practice. The patient does this by signing a consent form or signing an acknowledgment that thay have received a copy of the office's privacy policy.

Console: The console is the computer screen. When used in **The Medical Manager** system, choosing "console" means that you want to generate the report to the computer screen instead of to the printer.

Contractual Rate: In a managed care system, this term refers to a pre-defined price the insurance company pays for services the physician performs. The physician's contract with the managed care plan specifies how much he or she will be reimbursed for each, specific service or type of service he or she provides to each of the plan's patients.

Copayment (Copay): This is an amount each patient is required to pay for a particular service he or she receives from the physician or other managed care provider. Copay amounts are determined by the managed care plan and each patient's type of coverage. For example, most plans require a Visit Copay which is a flat amount (usually between $10.00 and $20.00) the patient pays each time he or she visits the doctor. Many plans also require Procedure Copays, which are copayments required for specific procedures (e.g., surgery, radiographs).

Coverage: The treatment or services the insurance plan will agree to allow for a patient. These services are what the insurance plan will, at least in part, pay for. *Also see* Service Limitations.

CPT-4: CPT stands for Current Procedural Terminology, a standard medical coding system developed by the American Medical Association. The "4" stands for the fourth edition of the coding system, currently in use. CPT-4 codes are standardized codes used to identify the treatment performed for a patient. This coding system is used by insurance carriers and medical offices to identify the services, procedures, and treatments performed for patients by the medical staff.

Credit: An accounting term that means to lower an amount. For example, to credit an account for a payment of $50.00 means that the account balance will be lowered by $50.00.

Current Period Report: This is a report of all payments, charges, and adjustments that were performed within the current period. The purpose of the Current Period Report is to show the changes in the guarantor's financial status during the present period. The report begins with this period's beginning balance, itemizes all charges, adjustments, payments, write-offs, and refunds for the period, and shows the ending balance. It differs from other financial activity reports for the patient because it details financial information only for the current period.

D

Daily Close: An end-of-day report detailing all of the transactions that were posted during the day. The daily close is similar to a daysheet or daily log. You may run a Trial Daily Close to check that the information you entered was correctly posted, and then run the Final Daily Close to actually close the day's business. This is also called the Daily Report.

Daily Files Backup: This refers to a floppy diskette (used in the Student Edition course) or tape (often used in a practice) that contains all the data that has been entered about patients, insurance companies, procedures and treatments, appointments, and other related information. In the event of system difficulties, the daily files backup permits the practice to recover data needed to maintain updated patient records and other important practice-related information.

Daily Log: A listing of all charges and payments made by patients during one day. Usually one line is used for each patient treated.

Daily Report: An end-of-day report detailing all of the transactions that were posted during the day. This is also called the Daily Close. You may run a Trial Daily Close to check that the information you entered was correctly posted, and then run the Final Daily Close to actually close the day's business.

Database: The information stored on the computer disk. In a database, information from different files is connected to each other; that is, a record in one file may require information from two or three other files.

Date of Post: This is the date a transaction was posted into the system. In the Student Edition course, you will generally press ENTER at this field to accept the default system date as the date of post.

Daysheet: A journal listing the charge and payment transactions incurred during the day. It is listed in chronological order; each patient seen during the day will have one or more entries on the daysheet. Usually one line is used for each patient treated. This daysheet is balanced at the end of the day to ensure accuracy of addition and is totaled for bookkeeping purposes. The sheet is used to determine how much was billed and collected on a daily basis for each doctor and the entire practice.

Debit: A debit is an accounting term that means to increase an amount. For example, posting an account for a debit of $50.00 (i.e., a charge of $50.00) will increase the account balance by $50.00.

Deductible: This is the amount the patient is expected to pay before the insurance plan will begin paying. The deductible is used when a patient is expected to pay a portion of their medical expenses. For example, the charges for a patient's visit may total $120.00. However, because the patient's deductible for this plan is $100.00 annually, the insurance company will only be billed for the remaining $20.00, whereas the patient will have to pay the $100.00 deductible amount.

Default Response: The information that appears automatically when ENTER is pressed. Default responses speed up data entry and report selections. A default response is generally the most common response for a given entry. In general, during the Student Edition course, you may press ENTER to accept the default response for any field for which information is not provided.

Dependent: This is a person who may receive services on someone else's account. A dependent is not the guarantor of the account but the guarantor does agree to be financially responsible for the care the dependent receives. A dependent may be a spouse, significant other, a child, a parent, or other similarly defined relationship (as permitted by the insurance laws in each state).

Diagnosis Code: The physician's determination of what is wrong with each patient is called the diagnosis. Insurance companies normally require that each service performed by the physician be related to a specific diagnosis. A uniform description and numbering system of diagnosis codes called ICD, or International Classification of Diseases, has been adopted for use by physicians and insurance carriers.

Diagnosis Code Group: A group of diagnosis codes used in defining a plan limit. For example, all diagnosis codes associated with substance abuse can be defined as a group.

Direct Chaining: This is a way to move from place to place within **The Medical Manager** system without going through all the other screens that would normally be required to do so. Direct chaining may also be used to move quickly between menus.

Disability: A condition that prevents the patient from being able to perform certain activities. A disability may be temporary (e.g., a broken leg) or permanent (e.g., a severed spinal cord).

Display Patient Data: This is a function in the system that allows the user to look at every computerized record about a given patient. Through Display Patient Data, the user has immediate access to every piece of account data found in the Guarantor reports, the Financial Activity reports, the Ailment File report, and the Office Management reports. Display Patient Data provides the user with an immediate, full screen look at an account's activities without printing a long report. Every screen also provides a hard copy option.

Double Book: This is the practice scheduling more patients than the physician can see during a reasonable period of time. Double booking may also be called double scheduling or overbooking.

Dual Insurance Coverage: This refers to the case in which a patient is insured by more than one insurance plan. For example, a Medicare patient is generally covered for 80 percent of charges for a physician visit. In this case, he or she would usually be responsible for the remaining 20 percent of charges. However, if he or she has dual insurance coverage and is also covered by a supplemental plan, Medicare Plus, this secondary plan would generally pay the amount not covered by the patient's primary insurance plan, Medicare.

E

Edit Activity Records: A procedure that is used to modify or delete charges that were posted through Procedure Entry. Deletion can only occur on charges before they are daily closed. After daily close, the activity may be edited, but neither the doctor number nor the amount of the charge can be changed.

Edit Ailment Detail Screen: This is a screen used to modify the Ailment Detail (explained above) that was entered for a patient. For example, when the patient's Ailment Detail was originally created, the physician may have entered a beginning date for partial disability for the patient. As the patient's condition improves, the physician will use the Edit Ailment Detail screen to enter an end date for partial disability (i.e., this is the generally the date the patient's condition has improved to such a degree as he or she is able to resume normal activity).

Edit Patient Screen: This is a screen used to modify patient information already in the system. For example, you would use the Edit Patient screen to change the name of a patient's employer, add additional insurance plans for the patient, or create additional dependents on the patient's account.

Elective Surgery: Any surgery the patient decides, or chooses to have that is not absolutely necessary. Two examples of elective surgery are tubal ligation (the cutting and tying off of the fallopian tubes to prevent future pregnancy) and breast augmentation (the surgical enlargement of the breasts).

Electronic Data Interchange (EDI): The ability to request, retrieve, transfer, and integrate information electronically. For example, physicians often use EDI to submit claims to insurance carriers.

Eligibility Roster: This is a list of all the members of an insurance plan that selected a particular primary care physician. Each physician in the plan is provided with access to the eligibility roster so that he or she is aware of the specific patients that he or she must provide health care services for. During a typical visit to the PCP's office, the patient's eligibility for treatment (i.e., proof the plan will pay for services provided to the patient) is verified against the eligibility roster. Then, the patient is seen by the PCP and treated or referred to a specialist or facility for further care.

Electronic Media Claims (EMC): This refers to electronic claims that are sent over the telephone, using a modem. Filing insurance claims electronically saves time the practice would normally spend waiting on mailed claims to be received, processed, and returned. EMC allows for accurate, well-documented claims to be created and sent to the insurance company electronically, reducing the time it takes for the physician to be paid, as well as fully documenting all associated actions within the system.

Electronic Remittance Advice (ERA): This feature uses the information received electronically from insurance companies (specific information about claims which have been adjudicated and paid) to post payments and adjustments to patient accounts automatically. This eliminates the need to post payments manually.

EMC Billing: Producing insurance claims electronically. *Also see* Electronic Data Interchange (EDI).

Encounter Form: This is a printed list of the most common procedures and treatment performed by the doctor. The doctor uses this paper form to indicate the procedure(s) or treatment performed for the patient, as well as the diagnosis for the patient's condition.

EPSTD: This term stands for Early Periodic Screen and Testing Diagnostics. This is a program sponsored by Medicaid that focuses on the early diagnosis of conditions in children (e.g., mental retardation, autism, etc.).

Existing Appointment: This is an option from a prompt line on the patient's Appointment screen that allows you to view all existing appointments for a particular patient. Note that this is in addition to the red flag ('Exists') that appears on a patient's Appointment screen to indicate that there is an existing appointment for that patient in the system.

Explanation of Benefits (EOB): This is an insurance company document that accompanies payment (or explains the lack of payment) for a particular patient's charges. For example, an EOB from Medicare might advise that for the three line items billed to Medicare for that patient, items one and two have been approved, but payment is being applied to the patient's deductible; therefore, no money is included in the check for these items. To ensure accurate records for this patient, the items listed on the EOB should be reduced to the amount approved by Medicare and then transferred to patient responsibility.

Extended Information Level: A screen of 18 fields for recording information unique to a single practice and not normally kept by other medical practices.

F

Facility: A provider of services such as a laboratory or hospital. *Also see* Place of Service (POS).

Family Accounts: When several members of a family receive care from the same group of physicians, only the head of the family normally receives the bill. All patients designated as members of the same family appear in the family's ledger. This is called family account billing.

Fatal Error Message: A fatal error message indicates something is wrong with the data you are using with your program. The most common cause of these errors is shutting off the computer or removing your student data diskette before you have properly exited **The Medical Manager** system. In either case, this can cause data to be only partially written, or copied, to the diskette. If you see a message on your screen that begins with the word "fatal," do not continue working. Notify your instructor immediately.

Fee Schedule: A schedule of defined charges that a provider can use when billing.

Field: The location for specific pieces of information typed in the computer by the user (e.g., a field for "Last Name" would require that the patient's last name be entered at this point).

File Maintenance: When information is stored in a computer, it is said to be filed. File maintenance is a series of programs that allows previously stored information to be modified or deleted.

File Rebuild Routine: This is a powerful program by which **The Medical Manager** system attempts to recover from a fatal error.

Financial Activity Reports: A menu of reports about the finances of the practice and the patients.

Form #, Format #: These identify the type of insurance form to be used for a patient and the method in which the information is to be filled out for a specific insurance plan.

Form Alignment Pass: This is an option presented to you by the system when you are printing information onto a form. The form alignment pass allows you to make sure that the form you will be printing on is properly aligned so that the information you are printing will print in the correct form spaces. The layout (i.e., the way the information will be printed on the form) of the information is determined by the use of Format Files.

Format File: This refers to specially coded files that specify the layout of printed insurance claim information. These files determine what prints where on the insurance form and are necessary since each insurance company could require that the CMS-1500 claim be filled out a different way. Format Files are maintained in the system's Support Files.

Format File Maintenance: A program for customizing or changing format files.

G

General Ledger (GL): The overall financial accounting for the entire practice. This includes the accounts receivable, the accounts payable, the payroll, and other accounting stages, **The Medical Manager** software is the accounts receivable portion of a general ledger.

General Ledger Transfer/Distribution Report: This is a component of the Daily Close Report that describes how the current day's transactions affect the general ledger. The General Ledger is the overall financial accounting for the entire practice (this includes the accounts receivable, the accounts payable, the payroll, and other accounting stages). This is also referred to as the GL Daily Distribution Report.

Group Name: This is a field on the Insurance Policy screen that allows you to specify who the group policy belongs to. For example, if a patient is insured through his employer, the employer name would be entered at the 'Group Name' field.

Guarantor: This is the person who agrees to be financially responsible for the account. In other words, this is the person who will have to pay for any services provided to him or her and his or her dependents. This will most likely also be the person to whom all account notices or billing statements will be sent.

Guarantor Report: This is a report that provides patient personal information, extended information, and insurance information from the guarantor's file. This report may be printed for all or specific guarantors of all accounts in the system.

H

Health Insurance Portability and Accountability Act (HIPPA): Federal legislation intended to improve portability and continuity of health insurance coverage; combat waste, fraud, and abuse in health insurance and health care delivery; promote use of medical savings accounts; improve access to long-term care; and simplify administration of health insurance. The Administrative Simplification Subsection covers entities such as health plans, clearinghouses, and health care providers.

Health Maintenance Organization (HMO): A group of physicians usually operating within one facility. In an HMO, the patient will initially be seen by his or her PCP. If the PCP believes the patient needs further testing or specialized treatment, the PCP will refer the patient to the appropriate specialist.

Help File: A file of messages that give the user more information about each field. These messages change automatically on the screen as you pass through the fields.

Help Window: A list of information that appears when '?' and ENTER are pressed at a field, or when the user clicks on the Help button ('?') on the top toolbar. The user may choose from the information in the list to complete the field in question. Examples of the help window are the Zip Code Help Window, the Procedure Code Help Window, and the Referring Doctor Help Window.

HMO Write-Offs: These are adjustments that are calculated automatically by the software and are based on the Profile/Fee information set up for each insurance policy. These adjustments will appear on Daily Close statements as a per line 'HMO Write-Off' and do not represent student entries.

Hospital Rounds: These are the visits a physician makes to patients who are in the hospital. The Hospital Rounds Report is a list of the patients in the hospital, their room numbers, their estimated length of stay, the referring doctor's name and phone number, the diagnosis, and any other remarks or comments the physicians need to remember for each patient. Physicians refer to this report as they visit each of their hospitalized patients, add comments, and return this report to the front desk. In this way, the Hospital Rounds Report may be used instead of an encounter form.

Hospital Rounds Report: A list of the patients in the hospital, their room numbers, their estimated length of stay, the referring doctor's name and phone number, the diagnosis, and any other records or comments the physicians need to remember for each patient. Physicians refer to this report as they visit each of their patients, add comments, and return this report to the front desk. In this way, the Hospital Rounds Report may be used instead of an encounter form.

IBNR: This refers to approved services that are Incurred But Not yet Realized or Incurred But Not Yet Reported. Services are incurred when a referral is created. The value of the referral is deducted from the remaining dollars and visits of the plan limit. When results are posted against the referral or the referral is closed, the unused dollar and visit amounts can be transferred from IBNR back into remaining dollars and visits in the plan limits.

ICD-9: This stands for "International Classification of Diseases, 9th Edition," which is a book that is published by the American Medical Association. ICD-9 codes are standardized codes used to identify a patient's medical condition. The first three digits of an ICD-9 code identify the primary diagnosis, and any additional digits define the diagnosis area further. Many insurance companies require diagnosis codes, which make processing claims easier and faster, on their claim forms.

Independent Physicians Association (IPA): This refers to a group of physicians who have formed a financial group to contract with the insurance plan for managed care contracts and provide gatekeeper services for these plans. Physicians in these associations retain control and ownership of their own practices but agree to be bound by the rules and stipulations set by the plans.

Inpatient: A person who is required to stay at a facility overnight for in-depth medical treatment, such as a surgical procedure, is referred to as an inpatient.

Insurance Billing Worksheet: The insurance billing worksheet allows you to verify that previous information was entered correctly before you print claim forms and send them to the insurance company for payment. Information that may be reviewed on an insurance billing worksheet include procedure, diagnosis, and assignment information for each patient.

Insurance Carrier: The name and address to which insurance claims are sent. This is sometimes called insurance plan, insurance company or claim center.

Insurance Claim: Most people have health insurance that pays all or a portion of expenses incurred when they have an illness or injury. An insurance claim form must be completed and filed with the insurance company before reimbursement will be made.

Insurance Coverage Priority: This is information set in the Insurance Coverage Priority screen in the system that establishes the insurance policy or policies a patient is covered by. This determines which plan is to be billed first for the patient's charges and, if applicable, which plan is to be billed for the remaining charges. Dependent's insurance coverage priority may often be different from the coverage the guarantor of the account has.

Insurance ID #: An identification number is assigned by the insurance company to identify a particular insurance policy. It is sometimes called a subscriber number or a policy number.

Insurance Policy Information: The name and location of the insurance company to which claims are to be sent for each patient. Each patient's insurance plan information must be entered completely so that the practice will know what insurance the patient is covered by and what medical procedures are covered by the insurance plan for that patient. It is common for a patient to have more than one insurance plan. This is sometimes called Insurance Plan Information.

Insured Party: This is the person in whose name the insurance coverage is held. This person is sometimes also referred to as the subscriber. The guarantor and the insured party may be the same person.

Intelligent Insurance Billing Process: This process allows **The Medical Manager** system to determine which items, out of a number of open items, should be assembled on the same claim.

Interface, Laboratory: An electronic connection that allows communication between a practice and a laboratory, using **The Medical Manager** software. For example, the practice orders a test (e.g., urinalysis) for a patient via **The Medical Manager**. The laboratory electronically notifies the practice when the results are ready and automatically downloads the patient's laboratory results into his or her medical record within **The Medical Manager** system.

J

Jump: Also seen as (J)ump, this is a command in the Appointment Schedule that allows you to move to any date in this century and schedule an appointment. This is a field on the Appointments screen.

L

Last Period Close: The date on which the last financial period ended is called the last period close.

M

Main Menu (Menu 1): The screen that appears after the date is entered. This is the starting place for accomplishing any function in the system.

Major Medical Insurance: This is sometimes called catastrophe insurance because it is designed to help offset huge medical expenses that result from a lengthy illness of serious accident. With major medical insurance, the patient is typically responsible for a deductible amount, as well as a copayment amount for each service or treatment provided. However, this amount is typically less than the deductible amount required with basic insurance coverage.

Malpractice: This is a term used to indicate that the treatment a physician provided to a patient was incorrect or improper. Most physicians are required to maintain malpractice insurance, which helps protect them and their practice from costly settlements that may arise out of legal action taken against them by a patient.

Managed Care: This is insurance coverage that attempts to keep medical costs under control by providing incentives for the physician to keep the patient healthy. Costs are also controlled by predefining a price, a contractual rate, for services the physician performs and negotiating with the managed care plan to determine which medical services will or will not be covered, the service limitations, under the plan. Managed care insurance coverage is also sometimes referred to as 'Pay-In-Advance' healthcare.

Managed Services: This term describes the limits set at the carrier level. Carrier limits are defined by three factors: the place of service (inpatient or outpatient), procedure codes, and diagnosis codes. Each limit can have annual, lifetime, and two user-defined dollar and visit limits associated with it.

Management Service Organization (MSO): This is a financial organization that consists of business people, rather than physicians. These organizations are formed to assist physicians in managed care plan contract negotiations and management functions (including billing and reporting). MSOs generally represent a large number of individual medical practices or groups of physicians. In many cases, the MSO actually purchases the physician group practices and the physicians become employees of the MSO.

Master Patient Index (MPI): This refers to an electronic patient index that contains every patient in the enterprise. In an MSO, each individual practice within the network can automatically register patients with the MSO. Any practice in the MSO network will have access to this MPI, which enables any changes to patient data made at the master or practice location to be automatically updated throughout the MSO network of medical providers.

Medicaid: This is a financial assistance program sponsored jointly by the federal government and the states to provide healthcare for the poor. Medicaid generally pays the deductible amount charged under Medicare (explained below), as well as the 20 percent of charges not covered by Medicare medical insurance for eligible patients. In general, Medicaid patients do not have to pay for health care services.

Medicare: This is an insurance program sponsored by the federal government to protect the elderly and disabled population. Medicare medical insurance pays 80 percent of reasonable physician's fees and related medical charges, minus a deductible amount. Medicare hospital insurance pays for most but not all of a patient's hospital treatment and related expenses.

Medicare Adjustment: A Medicare adjustment lowers the physician's charge to the amount that Medicare approves. This adjustment must be made if the physician is a "participating provider" in Medicare.

Medicare-Approved Amount: The maximum amount that a Medicare participating provider may collect for performing a procedure.

Medicare Pay Level: **The Medical Manager** software stores different percentages that Medicare will pay in a file called Medicare Pay Level.

Medicare Plus: This is a supplemental Medicare insurance policy that generally pays the 20 percent not covered by Medicare, plus the patient copayment required by Medicare. Note that Medicare plus insurance also requires a patient deductible amount and may also require certain procedural copayment amounts.

Medicare Profile: A list of the amounts Medicare will approve for specific medical procedures.

Medicare Profile %: Even though Medicare approves a certain amount for a procedure, the full amount is not paid. The Medicare Profile % is the percentage of the approved amount that Medicare will pay. The patient must pay the difference between the amount Medicare paid and the amount Medicare approved.

Modifier: This is a two-digit code added to a procedure code including why the procedure is not being charged at its normal fee.

Multiple Slots: Multiple slots are needed when a patient requires more than one time slot for a visit. For example, an appointment for a General Check-Up requires one slot, whereas an appointment for a Personal Consult requires multiple slots (i.e.: two slots). A patient's appointment is scheduled in terms of slots, to indicate the amount of time required for the proper examination to be given or proper treatment to be administered.

N

Narrative: Text written by the physician about the patient that includes items such as patient history, subjective and objective findings, and recommendations.

Negative Adjustment: This type of adjustment allows money that has been allocated to individual open items (explained below) on a patient's account to be removed from that item. Negative adjustments do not cause the money to leave the patient's account but simply move it from an open item into unapplied credit.

New Patient Entry: This is a **Medical Manager** routine for entering the patient's personal and insurance information.

O

Open Items: This refers to charges that were posted previously but have not yet been paid in full or adjusted off the account. During a Period Close performed in a medical office, open items with a balance of $0.00 are purged from the system, unless they are pending because of insurance billing.

Operating System: This is the set of internal programs that runs the computer. Two examples of this include DOS and Windows.

Outcome Analysis: This refers to a process in which records of many patients are analyzed to determine which treatments for particular medical conditions are successful and which are not. The goal of this process is to determine if a particular condition responds to a particular treatment performed. This determination is only made after a large number of patient records have been analyzed. Of course, this is a function more easily accomplished with concise, well-organized electronic medical records.

Outpatient: A person who receives in-depth medical treatment, such as a surgical procedure, from a facility such as a hospital, but is not required to stay at that facility overnight.

Overbooking: This is the practice scheduling more patients than the physician can see during a reasonable period of time. Overbooking may also be called double scheduling or double booking.

P

Password: This is a private word, phrase, or numeric combination used as a safety device for entering the software. In the Student Edition, the student password is 'ICAN.' In a practice, however, the password will be set to some meaningful phrase that allows only authorized personnel (i.e., people who know the password) to enter the system.

Patient Billing: This is an option that produces bills to the patient for charges that have been posted into the system. Patients often receive their first bill at the time of the visit. This statement may be as simple as a copy of the encounter form marked by the physician, or it may be a computerized listing of services performed. When a bill is printed after posting a patient payment, it is sometimes used as a payment receipt.

Patient Checkout Payments: This option on the Payment Posting Menu (Menu 31) allows payments to be made for all of the charges posted on the current day for the current patient. Patient Checkout Payments also includes an estimate of the patient due portion of the day's charges, and allows pre-collected copay and other unapplied credit to be easily applied to the day's charges. This option is normally accessed automatically by the system from within Procedure Entry at the end of a posting session, and includes only charges posted during that session.

Patient Extended Information: This is information about the patient's employer or school and is, generally, unrelated to the patient's other file information. Extended information provides another way for the practice to get in touch with the patient for billing or other communications.

Patient Due: The amount the patient is responsible for paying for medical services rendered. The patient due amount may represent the patient's deductible, copay, or balance due, after the insurance plan pays the covered amount.

Patient Ledger: A file card (or a computer version of a file card) for each patient that lists charges, payments, and adjustments and usually includes responsible party and insurance information. The patient ledger is used by the office to keep track of all financial activity on the patient's account.

Patient Notification: This is a form sent to notify the patient when the referred services have been authorized, denied, or are still pending approval by the insurance plan. These forms are easily formatted to fit the desired text, then generated when the referral is issued.

Patient Number: This is the unique number assigned to every patient at the time he or she is entered into the system during New Patient Entry. Each dependent on the patient's account will be assigned automatically by **The Medical Manager**. In the Student Edition course, each patient will be assigned a specific number, as indicated on his or her Patient Registration Form. In an actual medical practice, the system is generally set up to assign patient numbers automatically and sequentially as patients are entered into the system. A patient's number may never be changed.

Patient % of Profile: The amount a Medicare patient will owe.

Patient Registration Form: This is the form the patient completes when he or she first sets up his or her account at the medical practice. The Patient Registration Form typically contains the patient's full name, complete address and telephone number, social security number, date of birth, employment information, insurance plan information, and similar information for each of his or her dependents.

Patient Statement: The patient statement feature produces a list of outstanding charges in a patient's account. The patient statement is generally sent to the guarantor at the end of the month prior to Period Close, but it may be sent as many times as desired, until the account has been paid in full.

Payment Allocation: The amount of a payment made that is applied toward the fee for each procedure performed.

Payment Entry: A program that posts payments, adjustments, and refunds to patients' accounts.

PCP: *See* Primary Care Physician

PCP Bills Plan: The PCP may have an arrangement with the insurance plan whereby he or she can bill the insurance plan for the services rendered by the specialist. In this case, the insurance plan would reimburse the PCP for the specialist's services. Normally, the PCP would bill the insurance plan at a higher rate than what he or she is paying the specialist in order to cover administrative expenses.

PCP Pays Referring Doctor: Under some capitated plans, the PCP will pay the referring specialist for services rendered. This is typically referred to as a "global cap." The PCP negotiates with the specialist for an approved amount to be reimbursed to the specialist each time he sees one of the PCP's patients. In other words, the PCP acts like an insurance carrier and pays the specialist for referral services.

Percentage ##%: A numeric entry field used in Procedure Entry Payment to calculate the patient-due portion of charges just posted.

Period Close: The period close is performed at the end of each financial month to purge paid-off items from the system. This function will not be performed in the Student Edition course.

Period Purge: The Period Purge removes all paid-off items from outstanding accounts. This allows the practice to start the new billing period with all accounts up to date. This function will not be performed in the Student Edition course.

Period-To-Date: Period-to-date covers the time from the last period close to the current system date.

Physical Form: The CMS-1500 claim form is a standard form. However, some insurance companies still require a different form. The Student Edition course uses physical form 1. A working medical office may also have a physical form 2 for a given insurance company. When printing the insurance claim for, the software asks the student to line up the form in the printer. As part of the form alignment question, it asks which form to line up. Always answer form 1.

Physical Form Number: This number indicates the type of form on which insurance information is to be printed.

Plan Limits: Plan limits are carrier limits (managed services) defined at a plan level. The carrier level may be set up with general procedures or diagnoses, but the plan limit may have more specific procedures and diagnoses associated with it.

Point and Select: This is a way to make selections on menus within **The Medical Manager** system. To use the Point and Select feature, the user points by using the arrow keys or the mouse to move the cursor to a desired location (this highlights the selection) and then selects by pressing ENTER or double-clicking the mouse. This is sometimes referred to as Point and Shoot.

Policyholder: This is the individual who owns the insurance policy. In other words, the policyholder is the person who brings the insurance policy to the family account. This person must be the guarantor or one of the dependents on the account. In general, this is also usually the guarantor.

POS (Place of Service): This is a series of standardized codes that indicate the place where the doctor saw the patient or performed the procedure (e.g., the physician's office, the hospital). These codes are stored in the support files of the system and may be quickly ascertained using a help window.

Posted Window: This is a completed screen. For example, a completed Insurance Policy Information or Guarantor Information screen may each be referred to as a posted window.

Posting a Procedure without Insurance: This is keying information, including procedure and diagnosis codes, into a patient's account when the patient is not covered by insurance. In this case, during Procedure Entry the software will automatically skip the insurance fields, because no insurance plans are listed for the patient. Additionally, all charges will be automatically listed as patient ('PT') responsibility.

Posting an Account: Keying payments, credits, and adjustments to accounts. For example, if you enter information into the system in order to credit a patient's account for a check the patient gives you, you are posting an account.

Posting Partial Payments: This refers to entering payments for charges for part of an item on a guarantor's account. For example, an insurance company may pay only 80 percent of an original charge of $100.00. When you post the insurance company's partial payment, only $80.00, you will need to transfer responsibility for the remaining 20 percent of the charge (i.e., $20.00) to patient responsibility. Posting a partial payment usually means that the remaining amount must be transferred either to secondary insurance ('2nd') responsibility or patient ('PT') responsibility.

Posting Payment: Entering payments made on a guarantor's account into **The Medical Manager** system. This is normally done through the payment entry screen but, if payment is made at the time of the patient's visit, may also be done through the procedure entry screen.

Preferred Provider Organization (PPO): An organization of physicians participating in a plan. Generally, PPO plans allow the patient to see a participating physician or a nonparticipating physician of his or her choice. However, the patient tends to pay less if he or she is treated by a participating doctor.

Preventing Billing: This refers to an activity performed to prevent a specific item or items from being billed to an insurance company. An example of this is when a patient is incorrectly charged for two procedures (e.g., an examination and a cast removal) when he or she should have only been charged for one procedure (e.g., the examination that includes the cast removal). In this case, it is necessary to prevent the patient's insurance company from being billed for both procedures. This is done through Edit Activity Records and involves editing the insurance plan listed for the procedure to '00,' as well as voiding the incorrect charge from the patient's record.

Primary Care Physician (PCP): This is a doctor who has contracted with a managed care plan and has agreed to be responsible for providing the healthcare for specific patients participating in the plan. Each patient with a managed care plan must choose a PCP from a list, or directory, of physicians who are providing services for the plan. Under the terms of most managed care plans, the patient must contact his or her PCP before he or she receives care from any other healthcare provider (except in the case of an emergency). Because the PCP is required to monitor and administer the healthcare of the plan's patients, the PCP is often referred to as the 'Gatekeeper' of managed care.

Primary Insurance: This is the insurance company that is mainly responsible for paying a claim. Therefore, this is the company that is billed first.

Prior Authorization: A number issued by the insurance company to indicate that the procedures have been pre-approved.

Procedure: The service performed by the doctor. A treatment or other medical service provided by the doctor, or at the direction of the doctor by his or her staff, is also be considered a procedure.

Procedure Code: The services the doctor provides to a patient are called procedures and are identified by a procedure code number. Typical procedures include office visits, injections, radiographs, appendectomy sutures, and other services. Current Procedure Terminology, fourth edition (CPT-4) is used in **The Medical Manager** system for coding.

Procedure Code Group: A group of procedure codes used to define a plan limit. For example, physical therapy services may be grouped together as a procedure code group with a limit of $2,000 per year. Any procedure that is associated with physical therapy would fall into this group.

Procedure Entry: The procedure entry routine allows charges to be posted in **The Medical Manager** system.

Procedure History: A chronological listing of all procedures and associated diagnoses for the account.

Prompt: This is the cursor on the computer screen. When it is blinking, it is waiting for the user to do something. In other words, it is prompting the user to take action.

Provider: Any health care specialist rendering service. Providers are physicians, hospitals, laboratories, physical therapists, chiropractors, and others. For billing purposes, each provider is assigned one or more provider numbers by government agencies.

Purge: Remove items from computer records. *Also see* Period Close with Purge.

Q

Quality Care Guidelines: These are guidelines that reflect recommended intervals of tests and other medical care events specific to the patient. Care guidelines are usually generated based on the patient's age, sex, diagnosis, and other health factors. Quality Care Guidelines are established by the U.S. Preventative Services Task Force and other groups.

R

Recall Notices: Reminders, sent to patients to advise them of upcoming appointments, to request they call for future appointments, to remind them of overdue accounts and for a wide variety of other uses (including the recall of selected groups of patients).

Recall Report: A listing of all patients in the system who have been set up for a recall appointment.

Receipts: This refers to all payments received during a particular time period. For example, the practice's day's receipts may be verified against the Cash Analysis Report produced during a Trial Daily Close. This includes all forms of payment from patients and insurance companies.

Referral Template: Each referral in **The Medical Manager** system will have the same base information. In addition, a second screen can be created, called the referral template. Referral Templates can be unique to each plan and gather different information for facility and specialist referrals.

Referring Doctor: This is a physician who refers his or her patients to another physician, often a specialist, for more in-depth care. For example, a family physician would probably refer a patient with a broken arm to an Orthopedic specialist.

Refund Reason Code: This is a code, often defined by the practice, to indicate why a refund needs to be made to the patient or insurance plan. For example, if an overpayment refund must be made because the medical office made a mistake, a Refund Reason Code of '01' (for 'Incorrect Data Entry') will be chosen, because the overpayment refund is required due to a data entry error by the practice's staff.

Refunding an Overpayment: This refers to a procedure done to perform a refund when a patient or insurance carrier overpays an account. An overpayment may be the result of the patient's or carrier's mistake when preparing a check, a mistake by the medical office during the posting procedure, or an incorrect treatment indicated by the physician. An overpayment is any amount of payment that exceeds the total amount due.

Reimbursement: Payment of a medical claim.

Reschedule Reason Code: This is a code, often defined by the practice, to indicate why an appointment needs to be rescheduled. For example, if a patient's appointment must be rescheduled because the physician is waiting on the results of some lab work he or she requested for the patient, a Reschedule Reason Code of 'LABS' will be chosen, because the physician is awaiting the patient's laboratory results.

Responsible Party: The person or, in some cases, the organization responsible for paying part or all of the patient's bills.

Results: Results are the information supplied by the physician or facility in response to a referral. Referral results may consist of actual procedure codes performed or narrative text concerning the visit.

S

Scheduling Formula: This refers to a particular way each practice has of determining how long it takes to provide each service to a patient. For example, a practice may establish that a General Check-Up requires 15 minutes (i.e., one slot) whereas a Personal Consult requires 30 minutes (i.e., two slots).

Secondary Insurance: This is the insurance company that is billed for any remaining charges (minus copayments and deductibles) after the primary insurance company has been billed. It is not uncommon for patients to have secondary and sometimes even tertiary insurance coverage.

Self-formatting Field: This is a field in which hyphens, slashes, and other formatting text are automatically entered by the system. For example, date fields, telephone number fields, and the social security number field are all self-formatting.

Service Limitations: This refers to specific details in each managed care contract that determine which services will or will not be covered. For example, a physician's contract with the managed care plan may specify that plastic surgery to correct birth defects or injury caused by an accident is covered (i.e., this is within the service limitations of the plan and the doctor will be paid for the charges for this procedure). However, the contract may also specify that plastic surgery for any other reason, such as for cosmetic purposes, would not be covered (i.e., this is outside of the service limitations of the plan and the doctor will not be paid for the charges for this procedure).

Simultaneous Billing: The capability of **The Medical Manager** system to print both the primary and secondary insurance claim forms at the same time.

Specialist: This refers to a provider who has specialized training in a particular area of medicine. The managed care plan will contract with this physician to provide services within his or her area of specialty to patients who are covered by the plan.

Split Check: This refers to a check that includes payment for more than one guarantor's account. Checks like this, which include payment toward multiple account balances, are often from insurance plans. For example, an insurance plan might send payment for three of a practice's guarantor accounts. With split checks, careful attention must be paid to post only the amount designated for each patient.

Standard Referral: The most commonly used referrals can be set up as standard referrals. Standard referrals can be modified for patient-specific information when they are being entered.

Statement: The bill sent by the doctor to each patient or family detailing the services rendered. Most offices send statements on a monthly basis, and only to patients with outstanding balances.

Stop Loss Limit: The maximum value of services rendered if they were fee-for-service. Once a provider's services have reached the stop loss limit, the patient is usually transferred to a discounted, fee-for-service contract, allowing the doctor to obtain additional funds for his or her services.

Support Files: These are files of information stored within **The Medical Manager** system for later (and generally repeated) use by the practice. Examples of information contained within support files are procedure codes, diagnosis codes, insurance plans, service facilities, referring doctors, etc. They provide a way to enter a short code instead of typing a long description.

Support Reports: These reports show information that was entered through Support File Maintenance, including procedure codes, diagnosis codes, claim centers, service facilities, and referring doctors.

System Date: This is the date set within **The Medical Manager** system. In the Student Edition course, this date is set to start off as January 10, 2003 (i.e., 01/10/2003). This date is set at the beginning of the course, and advanced several times during the progression of the course, so it will match the sample screens, reports, and other information provided. In an actual practice, the system date should normally equal the current calendar date.

System Financial Summary Report: This is a financial report that shows period-to-date and year-to-date totals for each doctor or for the practice. The System Financial

Summary Report provides a quick look at the practice's accounts receivable and practice totals for the period-to-date and year-to-date. The summary can be printed for the practice as a whole or for all or selective doctors. This report shows total charges, receipts, adjustments, accounts receivable, net accounts receivable, total number of procedures performed, and the percentage of net charges that have been collected. This report is sometimes called the System Summary Report.

T

Transfer Responsibility: This refers to the ability in Payment Entry to change responsibility for the charges on an open item from one insurance company to another, or from insurance responsibility to patient responsibility. This may be accomplished by using the (T)ransfer option on the Payment Entry screen.

Treatment Plan: A specific itemization of services to be performed on the patient by the specialist or facility. These can be defined as specific, procedure codes, a group of procedure codes, or write-in codes. If a treatment plan is attached to a referral, the allowed dollar and visit limits will override the plan's limits.

Trial Insurance Billing: Trial insurance billing is used only for creating new insurance formats. It produces a claim form but does not mark the item as insurance billed.

TRICARE: A government insurance program for military personnel and their dependents. This program was formerly referred to as CHAMPUS.

Type of Service (TOS): This is a series of standardized codes that indicate the type service performed for the patient (e.g., Medical Care, Surgery). These codes are maintained in the support files of the system for ease of use and access.

U

Unapplied Credit: Payments for a patient's account that have not been allocated to individual open items are called unapplied credit. Unintentional overpayment of items may also be credited to the patient's unapplied credit balance. For example, if a patient sends in a payment for $55.00 when he or she was only billed for $45.00, the additional $10.00 will be posted to the patient's unapplied credit. This unapplied credit may be refunded to the patient or left in the patient's unapplied credit to be allocated to a future charge.

Units: This refers to the number of times the procedure was repeated during the date or dates of service. The procedure must have been performed by the same doctor on the same patient. This field is found on the Procedure Entry screen.

User Note: The User Note is a field in the insurance plan screen that is typically used to designate which insurance company should be billed for the services provided to the patient (e.g., primary, secondary, Worker's Compensation, Medicare, or self-pay).

Utilization: The analysis of referrals and patient visits by carrier, insurance plan, PCP, and specialty. A monthly report provides a comparison between the actual usage and the projected dollar and visit amounts defined in the plan contract.

V

View Patient Chart (VPC): This module within **The Medical Manager** system generates a virtual snapshot of the patient's medical records to a single screen and then gives the doctor instant access to almost any desired level of underlying detail. Each of 12 windows in the display access data from a particular type of medical records (e.g., vital signs, laboratory tests, medications, allergies, and procedure history).

Voiding Transactions: This refers to marking out an item in a patient's file in the system. Voiding transactions does not remove the item from the patient's file, but rather marks it as having been voided and removes either the amount posted for charges or the amount of payments made to the patient's account. Voiding an item will correct the patient's balance and ensure correct productivity reports.

Voucher: The check or other type of payment that is used to pay an account. For example, the number on the upper right corner of a patient's Encounter Form is called the voucher number. A check number, such as the number on a check sent to the practice from the insurance company or patient, is also referred to as a voucher number.

W

Worker's Compensation: This is insurance that covers medical expenses incurred as a result of a work-related injury or disability. This insurance, paid for by employers, also pays the salary of an employee who is unable to work, due to the injury or disability. Worker's Compensation laws vary, somewhat, by state.

Work-In: This refers to a patient who is accommodated, or "worked-in" to the practice's appointment schedule, rather than having a scheduled appointment. For example, if a patient brings her child with her to the doctor's during her normally scheduled appointment because her child is ill, an encounter form will need to be created for that child. However, because the voucher numbers on encounter forms are generally pre-assigned to the patients scheduled to see the physician that day, an encounter form with a sequentially assigned voucher number will not be available. Therefore, it will be necessary to create an encounter form using 'Work-In' as the voucher number.

Write-In: This refers to the ability to write somebody's name in the appointment schedule without adding the name to the computer list of appointments.

Index

Messages, fatal error, 48
Mouse, 18

N

O

P

The Medical Manager®
Quick Reference Guide

EXITING THE MEDICAL MANAGER SOFTWARE

ESCAPE Key

Used to return to previous screen without saving; used repeatedly, this key will eventually invoke the prompt: 'Do You Wish to Exit **The Medical Manager**? (Y/N).'

Exit Button

Used to return user to previous screen without saving; used repeatedly, this key will eventually invoke the prompt: 'Do You Wish to Exit **The Medical Manager**? (Y/N).'

Close Button

Used in Windows programs to exit the current application; to exit **The Medical Manager** software use at any menu or patient retrieval screen.

File-Exit

Drop-down Menu options selected, in order, to exit **The Medical Manager** software use at any menu or patient retrieval screen.

/quit

Direct chaining command keyed at any menu or patient retrieval screen; used to exit **The Medical Manager** software session.

CONTROL BUTTONS ON THE MAIN TOOLBAR

FUNCTION	BUTTON	KEY
New Window Opens a new window of **The Medical Manger**		
Calculator Invokes a math calculator. If invoked in a numeric field, results are automatically entered in the field upon exit of the calculator		
Process/Save Saves information or starts a report		F1
Help Invokes help window in most fields Invokes calendar in date fields		? or Home
Exit Escapes without storing information		ESC

CONTROL BUTTONS ON THE STATUS TOOLBAR

	BUTTON	KEY
Up Arrow Moves the cursor to the previous field and moves the light bar up in a help window	↑	↑
Down Arrow Moves the cursor to the next field and moves the light bar down in a help window	↓	↓
Page Up Scrolls a help window to the previous page	⇐	PgUp
Page Down Scrolls a help window to the next page	⇨	PgDn

SPECIAL KEYS

		KEY
Left Arrow Moves the cursor left within a field or a help window		←
Right Arrow Moves the cursor right within a field or a help window		→
Insert Toggles the type over mode off/on. The normal mode is type over		Ins
Delete Deletes the character currently under the cursor		Del
END Moves Cursor beyond the last character in a field		End

Detach at perforation

Key	Function
F12	CLINICAL FORMS
F11	CLINICAL ITEMS
F10	CLEAR FIELD
F9	DISPLAY PATIENT
F8	APPTS
F7	EDIT PAYMENT
F6	EDIT ACTIVITY (PROC.)
F5	EDIT PATIENT
F4	PAYMENT ENTRY
F3	PROCEDURE ENTRY
F2	NEW PATIENT ENTRY
F1	SAVE/ PROCESS
ESC	EXIT

The Medical Manager

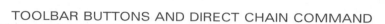

TOOLBAR BUTTONS AND DIRECT CHAIN COMMAND

Direct chain commands allow you to go quickly from one module to another. Direct Chain commands may be used from any menu or patient retrieval screen. Buttons on **The Medical Manager** Toolbar allow you to change modules quickly and will automatically open a second window if you are not on a menu or patient retrieval screen

DESCRIPTION	DIRECT CHAIN	BUTTON
New Patient Entry Add new accounts, set up guarantors, dependents and insurance policies	/pat	
Display Patient Data View almost any information about an account or patient	/dis	
Edit Patient Records Modify guarantor and patient demographic information; add dependents or insurance policies	/epat	
Appointment Entry View schedule for the day; make, reschedule, and cancel appointments	/app	
Encounter Forms Print Encounter forms	/enc	
Procedure Entry Post charges for procedures performed also collect patient payments at the time charge is posted	/pro	
Payment Entry Post insurance or patient payments; post adjustments and refunds	/pay	
Edit Activity Records Edit charges that were posted through Procedure Entry; delete charges that have not been daily closed or billed	/epro	
Edit Payment Records Delete payments, adjustments and refunds that were posted in error and have not been daily closed	/epay	
Collections System Monitor accounts and insurance plans that have items due longer than a designated number of days	/col	
Electronic Chart Menu Maintain all aspects of a patient's computerized medical record	/m28	
View Patient Chart View and update all aspects of a patient's computerized medical record	/vpc	
Clinical History Enter Allergy and other clinical information about a patient	/m10	
Managed Care System Manage and issue referrals for patients who have managed care insurance plans	/mcs	
Electronic Media Claims Create and transmit insurance claims electronically	/emc	
Electronic Remittance Receive and automatically post electronic payments	/ers	
Medical Manager Network Services Verify patient's insurance eligibility and status of claims electronically	/mmns	
Phone System Record and track incoming phone messages for doctors and medical office staff	/phone	